KAPLAN ALLIED HEALTH
Allied Health Careers and Communications

KAPLAN ALLIED HEALTH

Allied Health Careers and Communications

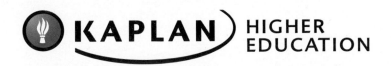

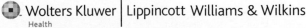

Wolters Kluwer | Lippincott Williams & Wilkins
Health
Philadelphia · Baltimore · New York · London
Buenos Aires · Hong Kong · Sydney · Tokyo

Chapters 1–3, and 12–14 from Molle EA, et al. *Comprehensive Medical Assisting*, 2nd ed.
Copyright 2005, Lippincott Williams & Wilkins, Philadelphia, Pa.
Study guides and worksheets for chapters 1, 3, and 12–14 from West-Stack C and Howe BB.
Study Guide: Comprehensive Medical Assisting, 2nd ed.
Copyright 2005, Lippincott Williams & Wilkins, Philadelphia, Pa.

Excerpts in chapters 1 and 2
Copyright 2007, Lippincott Williams & Wilkins, Philadelphia, Pa.

Chapter 4 and appendices from Willis MC. *Medical Terminology: The Language of Health Care.* 2nd ed.
Copyright 2006, Marjorie Canfield Willis. Lippincott Williams & Wilkins, Philadelphia, Pa.

Chapters 5–9 from Cohen BJ, Taylor J. *Memmler's Structure and Function of the Human Body.* 8th ed.
Copyright 2005, Lippincott Williams & Wilkins, Philadelphia, Pa.
Study guides and worksheets for chapters 5–9 from Cohen BJ, Hull KL, and Taylor J.
Study Guide for Memmler's Structure and Function of the Human Body. 8th ed.
Copyright 2005, Lippincott Williams & Wilkins, Philadelphia, Pa.

Chapters 10–11 and study guides and worksheets for chapters 10–11 from Womble DM.
Introductory Mental Health Nursing.
Copyright 2005, Lippincott Williams & Wilkins, Philadelphia, Pa.

Publisher: Julie K. Stegman
Acquisitions Editor: John Goucher
Project Manager: Matt Hauber
Production Manager: Eric Branger
Art Coordinator: Jennifer Clements
Cover Design: Armen Kojoyian
Compositor: Aptara, Inc.

KAPLAN MISSION STATEMENT

Kaplan helps individuals achieve their educational and career goals.
We build futures one success story at a time.

ABOUT KAPLAN HIGHER EDUCATION

Kaplan Higher Education offers certificate and degree programs, on campus and online, that prepare students for employment in fields including health care, business, criminal justice, fashion, design and graphic arts, information technology, and paralegal studies. At campuses in the United States and abroad, as well as via online programs through Kaplan University and Concord Law School, we offer educational opportunities that help people advance their careers and improve their lives. Each of our schools is separately accredited by one of several national or regional accrediting agencies approved by the U.S. Department of Education.

Kaplan is responsive to the needs of adult learners, many of whom juggle work, family, and other responsibilities. Our comprehensive support system provides financial aid counseling, academic advising, study skills workshops, time management guidance, and more. Our faculty is committed to ensuring that our students get the maximum value from their experience.

Kaplan, Inc., entered the postsecondary education industry in 2000, with the acquisition of Quest Education Corp., a network of 30 schools. Today, Kaplan Higher Education has become Kaplan's largest business, serving 68,000 students through more than 70 schools in 21 states and online programs in the United States and abroad. The company is market-driven, adding locations and programs in areas that will best serve local employment needs. The company's curricula include programs designed to lead to entry-level employment in many of the country's fastest growing occupations, as projected by the U.S. Department of Labor.

ACKNOWLEDGMENTS

We are pleased to present to you the *Kaplan Allied Health* module series, a compilation of materials focusing on fundamental principles that help develop proficient and sensitive medical professionals.

Designed to serve a broad audience of medical, therapeutic, pharmacy, and dental students, this guide offers interdisciplinary readings and activities for English fundamentals, computer applications, anatomy and physiology, and behavior and communications.

Primary acknowledgment must go to the many dedicated instructors who continually take on challenges of all shapes and sizes aimed at improving education. The professional literature and journals acknowledge individual contributions, but textbooks cannot adequately pay such tribute. Albert Einstein identified this problem, commenting that although "there are plenty of well-endowed (professionals) . . . it strikes me as unfair to select a few of them for recognition." We are indebted to all these unnamed people.

On a more immediate level, we would first like to thank our consulting editor and publisher, Lippincott Williams & Wilkins, for their expert and exhaustive work. We are especially grateful to Susan Katz, John Goucher, Matt Hauber, Eric Branger, Julie Stegman, Dale Gray, Dana Knighten, Leigh Wells, and Michael Marino for their enthusiasm and cooperation in making these books a reality. They have processed a formidable number of materials with dedication, attention to detail, knowledge, and editorial skill.

In addition, we thank the Kaplan Higher Education Faculty Advisory Board for providing educational guidance. They deserve grateful recognition for their indispensable help.

We gratefully acknowledge the following Faculty Advisory Board members:

Anthony Devore, Texas Careers
Denise Gemmel, Technology Education College
Bruce Gilden, Maric College, North County Campus
Mary Hitchens, Maric College
Tereas O'Mara, Professional Careers Institute
Thomas Reynolds, Texas Careers
Lisa Stephens, Professional Careers Institute

CAAHEP COMPETENCIES

Upon completion of this unit, students will be able to demonstrate mastery of the following CAAHEP competencies:

C   GENERAL COMPETENCIES
   1   Professional Communications
      b   Recognize and respond to verbal communications
      c   Recognize and respond to nonverbal communications
   3   Patient Instruction
      d   Identify community resources

CONTENTS

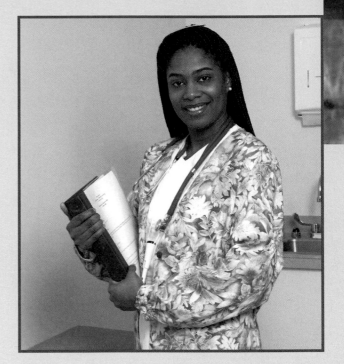

English Fundamentals

English Fundamentals and Written Communications

I

CHAPTER OBJECTIVES

In this chapter, you'll learn:
1. To spell and define the key terms.
2. To discuss the basic guidelines for grammar, punctuation, and spelling.
3. To describe six key guidelines for medical writing.
4. To discuss the eleven key components of a business letter.
5. To describe the three steps to writing a business letter.
6. To describe the process of writing a memorandum.

PERFORMANCE OBJECTIVES
In this chapter, you'll learn:
1. To write a business letter.
2. To write a memorandum.

KEY TERMS

BiCaps	font	margin	salutation
block	full block	memorandum	semiblock
enclosure	intercaps	proofread	template

THE ABILITY TO WRITE WELL IS an important skill for allied health professionals. Your written communication must be clear, concise, and correct. Poorly written documents reflect negatively both on the physician's practice and on you. You will be responsible for creating and handling many types of written communication. Examples of written communication include letters, consultation reports, agendas, and minutes from meetings. Written communication may be sent or received through the postal service, facsimile machines, or electronic mail. This chapter discusses guidelines for professional writing, letter development, memorandum writing, sending written communication, handling incoming mail, and composing agendas and minutes.

PROFESSIONAL WRITING

Professional writing is different from writing letters to your friends or family members. The goal of professional writing is to communicate information in a concise, accurate, and comprehensible manner. Slang or idiomatic terms that are commonly used in writing letters to friends are not appropriate for business letters. For example, "Drop by and say hi" is not suitable for a professional letter, even if you know the recipient personally.

Basic Grammar and Punctuation Guidelines

Grammatical rules seem to be an endless maze of twists and turns! And each rule comes with numerous exceptions. You must be familiar with these rules and be able to apply them to your writing. Key rules of punctuation and grammar are listed in Box 1-1.

Basic Spelling Guidelines

Good spelling skills take time to acquire. Box 1-2 gives you basic tips for spelling. Many words sound exactly alike but are spelled differently and have different meanings. Be very careful with these words. Which of the following sentences has a spelling error?

- Wound cultures were taken from the left lower leg site.
- Wound cultures were taken from the left lower leg cite.

The first sentence is correct. Site and cite sound alike, and both are spelled correctly, but in the second sentence, the wrong word was used. These types of errors occur as a result of poor word usage and poor spelling. Box 1-3 lists words that are most likely to be misused or misspelled.

FORMING A SENTENCE

A sentence will always consist of two parts and express a complete idea. These two parts are the subject and the predicate. The subject is *what* or *whom* the sentence is about. The predicate tells us something about the subject; for example, what they are doing or where they are.

Box 1-1

BASIC GRAMMAR AND PUNCTUATION TIPS

Punctuation
- Period (.)—Used at end of sentences and following abbreviations.
- Comma (,)—Used to separate words or phrases that are part of a series of three or more. The final comma before the "and" may be omitted. A comma can also be used after a long introductory clause or to separate independent clauses joined by and, but, yet, or, and nor.
- Semicolon (;)—Used to separate a long list of items in a series and to separate independent clauses not joined by a conjunction (e.g., and, but, or).
- Colon (:)—Used to introduce a series of items, to follow formal salutations, and to separate the hours from minutes indicating time.
- Apostrophe (')—Used to denote omissions of letters and to denote the possessive case of nouns.
- Quotation marks (" ")—Used to set off spoken dialogue, some titles (e.g., journal articles, newspaper articles, television and radio program episodes), and words used in a special way.
- Parentheses [( )]—Used to indicate a part of a sentence that is not part of the main sentence but is essential for the meaning of the sentence. Also used to enclose a number, for confirmation, that is spelled out in a sentence.
- Ellipsis (. . .)—Used in place of a period to indicate a prolonged continuation of a conversation or list. Also used to display individual items or to connect phrases that are loosely connected.
- Diagonal (/)—Used in abbreviations (c/o), dates (2003/2004), fractions (3/4), and to indicate two or more options (AM/FM).

Sentence Structure
- Avoid long, run-on sentences.
- A verb must always agree with its subject in number and person.
- Ensure that the proper pronoun (he or she) is used.
- Adjectives should be used when they add an important message. Don't overuse adjectives or adverbs. Remember, double negatives used in one sentence make the sentence positive.

Capitalization
- Capitalize the first word in a sentence, proper nouns, the pronoun "I," book titles, and known geographical names.
- Names of persons, holidays, and trademark items should be capitalized.
- Expressions of time (a.m. and p.m.) should not be capitalized.

BASIC SPELLING TIPS

When in doubt about the spelling of a word, always use a dictionary or a spell check. Keep in mind that a computer spell check will check for spelling but will not alert you to inappropriate word usage.

- Remember this rhyme: I comes before e, except after c, or when sounded like a as in neighbor and weigh. Examples: achieve, receive. (The exceptions are either, neither, weird, leisure, and conscience.)
- Words ending in -ie drop the e and change the i to y before adding -ing. Examples: die, dying; lie, lying.
- Words ending in -o that are preceded by a vowel are made plural by adding s. Example: studio, studios; trio, trios. Words ending in o that are preceded by a consonant form the plural by adding es. Examples: potato, potatoes; hero, heroes.
- Words ending in -y preceded by a vowel form the plural by adding s. Examples: attorney, attorneys; day, days. Words ending in -y that are preceded by a consonant change the y to i and add es. Examples: berry, berries; lady, ladies.
- The final consonant of a one-syllable word is doubled before adding a suffix beginning with a vowel. Examples: run, running; pin, pinning. If the final consonant is preceded by another consonant or by two vowels, do not double the consonant. Examples: look, looked; act, acting.
- Words ending in a silent -e generally drop the e before adding a suffix beginning with a vowel. Examples: ice, icing; judge, judging. The exceptions are dye, eye, shoe, and toe. The e is not dropped, however, in suffixes beginning with a consonant unless another vowel precedes the final e. Examples: pale, paleness; argue, argument.
- For all words ending in -c, insert a k before adding a suffix beginning with e, i, or y. Examples: picnic, picnicking; traffic, trafficker.

To find the subject of a sentence, look for the verb, or action in a sentence. Ask yourself who or what is undertaking the action. The answer to this question is your subject.

For example, in the sentence, "The patient left his coat on the chair," the verb is "left," from the past tense of "to leave." The patient is the person who left his coat, so the patient must be the subject of the sentence. If you are still not sure, another way of identifying the subject is to see if you can replace that part of the sentence with a pronoun (we, they, he, she, I, it, you). If it can be replaced by a pronoun, you have found your subject. So, using the above example, "the patient" could be replaced by "he."

Once you have established the subject of the sentence, finding the predicate is easy. It is simply everything else remaining in the sentence. Take a look at these examples:

1. Dr. Phillips wanted to leave early.
2. The canteen was very noisy.

Here are the same sentences divided into subject and predicate:

	Subject	Predicate
(1)	Dr. Phillips	wanted to leave early.
(2)	The canteen	was very noisy.

Note that "Dr. Phillips" can be replaced with either "he" or "she," depending on whether the doctor is male or female. "The canteen" can be replaced by "it." This means that they must all be the subject in the sentence.

You will notice that not all sentences appear to have a subject. For example, imperative sentences, or sentences that give a command, have subjects that are implied, rather than stated. For example, "Don't do that!"

You can still find the subjects using the techniques mentioned above. For example, if someone is saying "don't do that," which pronoun would make sense? If one person is talking to someone else, she is effectively saying, "You! Don't do that!" So, the subject is you (or whomever the person is talking to). In imperative sentences, the listener is always the subject.

To give you a more in-depth idea of what forms subjects and predicates, we will discuss each topic separately.

What Is a subject?

We have already established that a subject is *who* or *what* the sentence is about. But we can get a bit more specific than that. Take a look at these sentences; their subjects are in bold type:

1. **The elderly lady** said she was sore.
2. **John** told the doctor he felt sick.

As you can see, a subject can contain a number of words or just consist of one word. What these subjects have in common is that they all contain either a noun (lady, John) or a pronoun (she).

Nouns

A noun is a word used to name a person, animal, place, or object. It can also be used to describe an abstract idea. For example, "justice" is a noun, even though we cannot see, hear, or touch it.

There many types of nouns, but the two most important to consider when structuring sentences are *proper nouns* and *common nouns*. A proper noun is the exact name of a person (Dr. Rogers), place (Northwestern Memorial Hospital), or thing (Eiffel Tower). Take a look at this sentence:

The nurse asked doctor jones if she had seen her patient yet.

Because "Doctor Jones" is the name and title of a person, it is a proper noun and should be capitalized. All proper nouns require capital letters.

The nurse asked Doctor Jones if she had seen her patient yet.

A common noun is a general name for a person (patient), place (ward), or object (prescription). It only needs to be capitalized if it is at the beginning of a sentence or if it is part of a more specific title, where it becomes a proper noun. For example, the "Northwestern Memorial Hospital cafeteria" does not require the word "cafeteria" to be capitalized. It is used as a general term. But if the hospital has a cafeteria that is specifically named "Chicago Cafeteria," it becomes a proper noun and should therefore be capitalized.

Person	Place	Object	Abstract Idea
patient	ward	stethoscope	pain
doctor	corridor	needle	discomfort

When you write sentences, you will notice that nouns have several things in common:

- Nouns can be made plural to show that there is more than one ("doctor" becomes "doctors").
- Nouns can be made possessive to show ownership ("doctor" becomes "doctor's").
- Nouns can be made more specific by adding the words "the," "hers," and "my" (called "determiners" because they specify which noun you are talking about; for example, "his wound" instead of "your wound").

Pronouns

A pronoun is a word that takes the place of a noun in a sentence. Examples of pronouns include: "he," "it," "we," "I," and "you." Look at the sentence:

Dr. Roberts and Dr. Flanders requested a larger budget for the following year.

"They" could replace "Dr. Roberts" and "Dr. Flanders," and the sentence would still make sense.

They requested a larger budget for the following year.

Pronouns are used so that we don't have to repeat ourselves too frequently when we write. We can replace the name of the person or object we are talking about with a pronoun. Usually, writers alternate between the two in a paragraph.

What Is a Predicate?

We now know that a predicate is the part of the sentence that does not contain the subject. Returning to our original examples, we have:

	Subject	Predicate
(1)	Dr. Phillips	wanted to leave early.
(2)	The canteen	was very noisy.

If you take a look at the examples above, you will see that the predicates contain verbs, or action words: "wanted" and "was." Both predicates contain a verb. The verb is the action that is undertaken by the subject in the sentence.

One of the most important functions of a verb is to give a sense of time:

- By adding "ed" to most verbs, you can show that something happened in the past ("perform" becomes "performed").
- By adding "will" in front of the verb, you can show that something will happen in the future ("perform" becomes "will perform").
- By adding a form of the verb "to be" before the verb, and "ing" at the end of it, you can show that something is happening in the present ("she is performing").

Some sentences have more than one verb in them. For example, "She is performing" contains two verbs—"is" and "performing." The verb "is" is called a *helping verb*. It is not the main verb in the predicate, but it helps give us a sense of what the main verb means. There are many helping verbs that we use frequently when we are speaking and writing. Here are some more examples, with the helping verb in bold type and the main verb underlined:

WHAT IF

You are writing a letter and can't find out how to spell a word. What should you do?

Begin with your computer's spell check software. Spell check is generally under the heading Tools at the top of the screen. Most programs offer suggestions for the misspelled word. Be very careful that you do not select the wrong word on the suggestion list. You may also either look up the word in a dictionary or use an online dictionary. Two Web addresses that offer online dictionaries are given in this chapter. You may ask a colleague for spelling assistance. An option is to exchange the word for another word from a thesaurus. Be sure that the meaning of the sentence does not change if you use a different word. If these steps do not work, print the letter, mark the word with a question mark, and leave it for the physician. Never mail a letter with a spelling error.

To do: do, does, did
Dr. Flatley **did not** <u>like</u> figs.
To be: were, be, been, being, am, are, is
She **was** <u>operating</u> on the patient.
Can: can, could
Doctors **can** <u>help</u> many people.

Let's reassess what we have learned so far. Sentences are composed of two parts: the subject and the predicate. The subject is what or whom the sentence is about, and it always contains a noun or pronoun. The predicate is the action performed in the sentence, and it always contains a verb.

COMPOSING PARAGRAPHS

Once you have an outline for your paper, you will need to structure the information by organizing it into paragraphs. Here are the things you need to ask yourself when you are composing a paragraph:

- What type of paragraph are you writing?
- Does the paragraph contain the required information?
- Is the paragraph structured correctly?

Structuring Paragraphs

A well-written paragraph should contain three things: an introductory sentence, supporting details, and a conclusion. The **introductory sentence** informs the reader about the paragraph by introducing an idea. The **supporting details** give additional information about the idea. They make up the main part of the paragraph. The **conclusion** is written at the end of the paragraph, to reiterate the information you have just given. It is a summary of the main idea.

Here is an example of a paragraph, divided into its three parts:

Introductory sentence:
Practicing basic hygiene is a fundamental aspect of working in a hospital.

Supporting details:
It is vital for doctors and nurses to pay attention to personal hygiene while they are at work, as it directly affects the welfare of their patients. Simple techniques, such as washing hands thoroughly with antibacterial soap after all physical contact with patients, can help prevent infection. Other good habits include tying back long hair, ensuring uniforms are clean, and wearing face masks when dealing with vulnerable patients.

Conclusion:
It is difficult to stress how important it is that doctors and nurses maintain good personal hygiene on the wards to help prevent infection.

Purpose of Writing

The type of paragraph that you compose will depend on the purpose of your paper. The main types of writing are narrative, descriptive, expository, and persuasive.

Narrative Writing is sequential. It expresses something that takes place in time order. Stories and diaries are examples of narrative writing. When you write a narrative paragraph, you should use words that show the order in which events take place. Examples of these include *next*, *then*, *first*, *finally*, and *afterward*. This is an example of a narrative paragraph:

Sister Peters began her rounds by making sure that all the information on the chart was up to date. She then visited her patients to ask them how they were feeling. Finally, she consulted the white board to ensure that all her nurses got to work on time. She was so busy that she would not be able to take a break until much later that day.

Descriptive writing tries to create a picture in the reader's mind by describing something in as much detail as possible. You should use the five senses to describe how the subject looks, smells, feels, tastes, or sounds. This is an example of a descriptive paragraph:

John had none of his usual sparkle about him. His eyes were dull and lifeless. His cheeks were sunken, as if the very essence of his face had been sucked away. As he tried to speak, his hands trembled violently; the effort of raising them to gesticulate was almost too much for his twig-like arms.

Expository writing is informational. The purpose of an expository paragraph is to explain something to the reader. It should be based on facts, rather than opinions, and written from an unbiased viewpoint. Textbooks and newspapers are examples of expository writing. This is an example of an expository paragraph:

Man has been studying medicine for many centuries. We have records of medicinal practices used by the ancient Greeks as early as 460 BCE, when they believed that the body was made up of four humors. The Greeks believed that each of these humors had to be in balance for a person to stay healthy.

Persuasive writing is biased. As a writer, you will compose a persuasive paragraph if you want the reader to agree with your viewpoint, or if you want to encourage them to carry out a particular action. Advertisements and newspaper editorials are examples of persuasive writing. They will often use words such as *you should*, *you will*, *only*, and *just*. Other persuasive techniques include asking the reader rhetorical questions, repeating information to make sure the reader remembers it, and using a catchy slogan that will stick in people's minds. This is an example of a persuasive paragraph:

Save time and money by lunching at your friendly hospital cafeteria. Not only will you avoid having to make the same old sandwich every morning, but you will also have a wide selection of hot and cold meals that are ready to eat. With prices starting at only $2.00, what are you waiting for?

Guidelines for Medical Writing

Writing letters to medical professionals follows many of the standard guidelines. There are, however, some specific guidelines of which you need to be aware. They are discussed next.

Accuracy

Many of the medical documents or letters that you will write contain information that requires precision, accuracy, and careful attention to details. Inaccurate information in some letters can lead to injury of a patient and lawsuits and can harm the physician's practice. Some of your letters will be placed in the patient's permanent medical record. Most letters will start with the physician asking you to draft a letter. He may or may not give you some notes to follow. Either way, your responsibility in typing the letter is to be as accurate as possible and to question anything about which you are unsure. Here are some examples of inaccuracy:

- You wrote, "The patient was started on the MVP chemotherapy regimen." The physician, however, had written "MVPP." These are two completely different regimens. MVP is used for treating lung cancer, and MVPP is used for Hodgkin's lymphoma.
- The physician wrote, "Patient was told to take Dristan Cold tablets." You rearranged the sentence, however, and wrote "The patient had a cold and was told to take Dristan tablets." Dristan Cold contains an antihistamine medication that plain Dristan does not. Never edit a physician's sentence unless you are sure that it will not affect the meaning.
- The physician wrote, "There is no reason for him to start radiation therapy at this time." You wrote, however, "There is reason for him to start radiation therapy at this time." The simple elimination of the word "no" completely changes the meaning of the sentence and can lead to errors in patient care.
- The physician wrote, "Hospitalization is needed because the patient continues to be violent." You typed, however, "Hospitalization is needed because the patient continues to be violet." The meaning of the sentence has been changed by the elimination of one "n" in violent.

? Checkpoint Question

1. What are three consequences that could arise from inaccurate information in a business letter?

Spelling

Spell check in word processing programs can be a great asset, but it has limitations. Medical terminology spell check software should be added to your computer and be updated frequently.

You can add medical terms into your computer's spell check dictionary, but make sure that any word you add is spelled correctly! Spell checks can never be 100 percent stocked with all the needed terms, especially in the medical profession, as new technologies, medications, and treatments arise daily. Remember, spell check will not recognize words that are spelled correctly but misused. Which of the following sentences has a spelling error?

- The patient's mucus was yellow.
- The patient's mucous was yellow.

Mucus (noun) refers to a sticky secretion. Mucous is a type of membrane that secretes mucus. The second sentence is wrong. Here is another example:

- The physician received a plague.
- The physician received a plaque.

There is a big difference between plaque (commemorative item) and plague (bacterial disease)! Box 1-3 lists some commonly used medical words that can easily be misspelled or misused.

Capitalization

Pay particular attention to how words, names, and abbreviations are capitalized. Words or phrases with unusual capitalization are called **intercaps** or **BiCaps**. Never change how a word is capitalized unless directed to do so. Ask for clarification and mark the proof letter with a question mark for the physician to answer. For example m-BACOD is a very different medication regimen from M-BACOD. Here are some other common medical intercaps: pH, RhoGam, rPA, ReoPro, aVR.

Box 1-3

COMMONLY MISUSED OR MISSPELLED MEDICAL TERMS

- anoxia and anorexia
- aphagia and aphasia
- bowl and bowel
- emphysema and empyema
- fundus and fungus
- lactose and lactase
- metatarsals and metacarpals
- mucus and mucous
- parental and parenteral
- postnatal and postnasal
- pubic and pubis
- rubella and rubeola
- serum and sebum
- uvula and vulva

Abbreviations and Symbols

Abbreviations and symbols can save time in long handwriting and with typing. Use abbreviations sparingly. When typing professional letters, you should spell out all abbreviations that are not universally accepted (e.g., p.m.). Become familiar with the abbreviations and symbols that are used where you work. Most offices have a policy listing their approved ones. Following are some ways abbreviations can be misinterpreted:

- The physician wrote, "The patient had good BS." You assumed that BS meant bowel sounds, so you typed "The patient had good bowel sounds," but the physician meant the abbreviation BS to mean breath sounds.
- Do not change < or > signs to *less than* or *greater than* unless you are sure of what the statement is saying. For example, "The patient will not be admitted to the hospital until her hemoglobin is less than 13." If you made a mistake and typed "greater than 13," confusion could occur.
- The symbols for male (♂) and female (♀) are commonly used in handwritten notes, but you should replace these symbols with words when writing a business or professional letter.

Plural and Possessive

Converting words to plural or possessive form can be tricky in English. Refer to your medical terminology book or a dictionary when you are unsure. Which of the following sentences is correct?

- The patient had multiple bullas.
- The patient had multiple bullae.

The second sentence is correct. *Bullae* means multiple blisters; *bulla* is one blister.

Numbers

In general, numbers one to ten should be spelled out, except when used with units of measurement (e.g., 5 mg), and those over 10 may be expressed as a numeral. Here are some important tips you will need to remember about numbers:

- Numbers referring to an obstetrical patient's medical history are not written out: "The patient is a gravida 3, para 2." Do not convert these numbers.
- Watch decimal point placement. There is a huge difference in medication between 12.5 mg and 1.25 mg.
- Double-check that you have not transposed numbers. For example, you typed, "The patient's red blood cell count was 1.5," but it was actually 5.1. A red blood cell count of 1.5 is incompatible with life.
- Roman numerals should never be changed to words. For example, "lead II of the patient's electrocardiogram" should never be changed to "lead two of the patient's electrocardiogram."

- Many health care professionals use military time. Time that is written in military style does not have to be changed if the recipient of the letter is familiar with it (doctors, nurses). If the letter is going to a patient or other person who may not be able to interpret it, however, either convert the time or express the standard time in parentheses; for example, "The patient's next appointment is at 1430 hours (2:30 P.M.)." No colons are used in military time.
- Temperatures must always have the correct symbol for Celsius or Fahrenheit included (98.6°F or 37°C).
- Telephone numbers should include the area code in parentheses or followed by a hyphen, then the number with a hyphen. Add extensions to the number by placing a comma after the last digit of the number, then type Ext. and the number: (800) 555-0000, Ext. 6480. Periods may replace hyphens and parentheses: 800.555.0000.

LETTER DEVELOPMENT

Writing effective business letters is a skill that requires practice and careful attention to detail. To write a professional business letter, you must:

- Understand the components of a letter
- Use the correct letter format
- Ensure that the message is clear, concise, and accurate

These skills are described in the following sections.

Components of a Letter

A typical business letter has 11 components. We will explore each one, beginning at the top of the page. For easy reference, Figure 1-1 displays a sample business letter with these components marked.

1. *Letterhead.* The letterhead consists of the name of the practice or physician, address, telephone number, fax number, and sometimes the company logo. The letterhead is often embossed in color and centered on the top of the page. The letterhead may also be preset into a **template**. (Templates are discussed later in the chapter.)
2. *Date.* The date includes the month, day, and year. It should be positioned two to four spaces below the letterhead. The date must be typed on only one line and abbreviations should not be used.
3. *Inside address.* The inside address refers to the name and address of the person to whom the letter is being sent. A nine-digit zip code should be used if available. The inside address is placed four spaces down from the date unless the letter is being mailed with a window envelope and it will not be aligned correctly. Never abbreviate city or town names. States can be abbreviated. Never abbreviate busi-

Benjamin Matthews, MD
999 Oak Road, Suite 313
Middletown, CT 06457
860-344-6000

①

February 2, 2003 ②

Adam Meza, MD
Medical Director   ③
Family Practice Associates
134 N. Tater Drive
West Hartford, CT 06157

Re: Ms. Beatrice Suess ④

Dear Dr. Meza: ⑤

Thank you for asking me to evaluate Ms. Suess. I agree with your diagnosis of rheumatoid arthritis.
Her prodromal symptoms include vague articular pain and stiffness, weight loss and general malaise.
Ms. Suess states that the joint discomfort is most prominent in the mornings, gradually improving
throughout the day.

My physical examination shows a 40-year-old female patient in good health. Heart sounds normal,
no murmurs or gallops noted. Lung sounds clear. Enlarged lymph nodes were noted. Abdomen
soft, bowel sounds present, and the spleen was not enlarged. Extremities showed subcutaneous
nodules and flexion contractures on both hands.

⑥

Laboratory findings were indicative of rheumatoid arthritis. See attached laboratory data. I do
not feel x-rays are warranted at this time.

My recommendations are to continue Ms. Suess on salicylate therapy, rest and physical therapy.
I suggest that you have Ms. Suess attend physical therapy at the American Rehabilitation Center
on Main Street.

Thank you for this interesting consultation.

Yours truly,   ⑦

Benjamin Matthews, MD
                            ⑧
Benjamin Matthews, MD

BM/es ⑨

Enc. (2) ⑩

cc: Dr. Samuel Adams ⑪

F I G U R E   I - I.   Components of a business letter. This letter is done in full block format and contains these elements: (1) letter-head, (2) date, (3) inside address, (4) subject line, (5) salutation, (6) body, (7) closing, (8) signature and typed name, (9) identification line, (10) enclosure, (11) copy.

ness titles (e.g., President, Chief Executive Officer). Here are some other points to remember:

- If the letter is going to a business, type the name of the addressee, followed by his or her title, then the name of the business on the next line, then the address.
- If the letter is being addressed to two or more people at different addresses, type the individual address block one line space under the other or place the addresses side by side.
- If the letter is going to two people at the same address but with different last names, type the woman's name on the first line, man's name on the second line, then the address. If the sexes are the same, do them in alphabetical order, followed by the address.

4. *Subject line.* The subject line, an optional component, is used to state the intent of a letter or to indicate what the letter is regarding. It is placed on the third line below the inside address and is written as Re: (an abbreviation for regarding) followed by the subject. For example, Re: Blood tests.

5. *Salutation.* The **salutation** is the greeting of the letter. It is placed two spaces down from the inside address or the subject line. Capitalize the first letter of each word in the phrase and end the phrase with a colon. It is permissible to eliminate the salutation if the letter is informal or if a subject line has been used. When writing to a physician, write out the word doctor. Here are some recommendations when writing salutations:

- If the letter is going to one person and the gender is known write, Dear Mr. Rogers.
- If the letter is going to one person and the gender is *not* known, write, Dear Pat Smith (use the person's first name).
- If the letter is going to a woman and a man with different last names, always address the woman first: Dear Ms. Ray and Mr. Oscar.
- If the letter is going to several people, place them in alphabetical order: Dear Mr. Andersen, Mr. Cats, Ms. Dart, and Mr. Raymond.
- To Whom It May Concern, Dear Sir, or Dear Madam should not be used.

6. *Body of the letter.* The body of the letter contains the message. It should be single-spaced with double spacing between the paragraphs. Here are some guidelines for writing the body of the letter:

- If the letter is more than one page long, try to avoid dividing a paragraph at the end of a page. If you must, leave at least two sentences at the bottom of the first page. Use the widow and orphan control feature of your word processor program to prevent orphan lines from appearing.
- Tables and graphs should not be broken. They should appear on one page only.

- Web addresses and e-mail addresses should fit on one line and never be continued to another page.
- If the letter is more than one page long, page numbers should be used.
- Use a bulleted format to highlight key points for the reader. For example, "The possible side effects of this medication are:" (then list them vertically with a bullet symbol).
- Letterhead is used only on the first page of the letter. The second page should be the same quality paper as the letterhead. Start the second page with a continuation line (name of person the letter is going to and the date of the letter). Continue the letter two lines down from the continuation line. Your margins must be the same as those on page 1. Most templates type the continuation line for you.

7. *Closing.* The closing concludes the letter. Some common closings are: Sincerely, Yours truly, Regards, Respectfully, and Cordially yours. Only the first word is capitalized and a comma follows the phrase. Closings are placed two spaces down from the end of the letter. Never put the closing alone on a page.

8. *Signature and typed name.* The name of the person sending the document is typed four spaces below the closing, with the person's title typed directly below. The physician will read and sign the letter above the typed name. If you are instructed to sign the letter, sign the physician's name followed by a slash mark and your name, e.g., Susan James, MD/Raymond Smith, RMA.

9. *Identification line.* The identification line, an optional component, indicates who dictated the letter and who wrote it. It consists of abbreviations only. The initials of the person who dictated the letter are capitalized (generally the physician); the initials of the writer of the letter are in lower case (generally these will be yours). The identification line can also be called the reference line.

10. *Enclosure.* An **enclosure** is something that is included with a letter. It is abbreviated Enc. and is placed two spaces down from the identification line. The number of documents included is placed in parentheses; if only one document is included, just the abbreviation Enc. is used.

11. *Copy.* The abbreviation c is used to indicate that a duplicate letter has been sent. It is typed two spaces below the enclosure line. Usually, letters are copied to managers, supervisors, or to the physician who requested that the given information be dispersed.

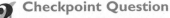

Checkpoint Question

2. Whose address is typed as the inside address? What is the purpose of the salutation? What is the purpose of the identification line?

Letter Formats

There are three basic types of letter formats: *full block*, *semiblock*, and *block*. Office policy or the physician's preference will dictate which format you use.

Full Block

In **full block** format, each line is flush left. Full block is the most formal format and is most commonly used for professional letters. Figure 1-1 shows a letter in full block format.

Block

In **block** format, the date, subject line, closing, and signatures are flush right. All other lines are flush left (Fig. 1-2).

Semiblock

In **semiblock** format, the first sentence of each paragraph is indented five spaces, if done on a typewriter, or is tabbed, if done on a computer (Fig. 1-3). Semiblock is also referred to as modified block.

Writing a Business Letter

To create a professional business letter, follow these three steps: preparation, composition, and editing. Box 1-4 gives you some guidelines for starting to write a letter.

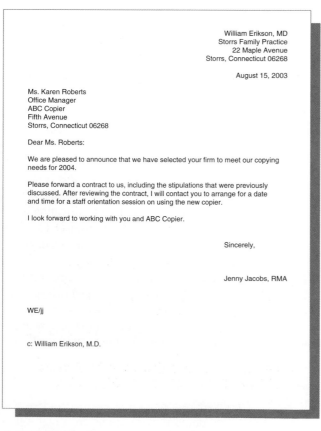

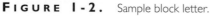

FIGURE 1-2.   Sample block letter.

BOX 1-4

HOW TO START WRITING A LETTER

By determining the answers to these four questions, you can better prepare the message of your letter.

1. Who is my reader?

   It is very important that you use proper gender identification. Be especially careful with names that can be used for males or females (e.g., Sam, Kelly, Ronnie, Alex, Tracy). Determine the reader's comprehension level. Letters to physicians will be more technical and will use medical terminology. Letters to patients will be less technical and use medical terminology sparingly.

2. What do I want my reader to do?

   This is your call to action; make it clear and specific. For example, you might write, "Please complete the enclosed insurance form (2 pages). Be sure to include all necessary information and sign your name. Place the form in the enclosed envelope and return it to our office by June 15, 2003." Avoid using "at your earliest convenience"; include a date for the required action. If possible, include a response mechanism, such as a self-addressed, stamped envelope.

3. What do I want to say?

   Briefly list the necessary information. To help you remember all of the necessary information, ask yourself who, what, where, when, why, and how.

4. How will I organize my message?

   Here are three basic ways that you can organize your message:

   - *Chronological:* Discuss items in a sequential manner, beginning with the earliest date and proceeding to the most recent date. For example, when discussing the physician's career, list his or her earlier experiences before the most recent career achievements.
   - *Problem oriented:* Let the reader know about a specific problem and provide instructions for correcting the problem. For example, if a patient's blood work came back with abnormal findings, a letter would be sent, identifying the problem (e.g., low hematocrit) and advising the patient on the possible causes, treatments, and follow-up procedures.
   - *Comparison:* Evaluate the effectiveness of two or more items. For example, as an office manager, you may have to write to the physician comparing two service contracts or two sample computer software packages.

Elizabeth Jones, M.D.
750 East Street, Suite 205
Hialeah, Florida 33013
305-311-2666

June 12, 2003

Margaret Trent
18 Cambridge Street
Hialeah, Florida 33013

Dear Ms. Trent:

As per our phone conversation, your blood glucose level remains elevated. It is essential that we stabilize your blood sugar level.

In order to achieve normal blood sugar levels, you must follow the enclosed diet. A meeting with a Registered Dietitian can be arranged for you to discuss any dietary concerns you may have.

I am also enclosing patient education instructions for the use of a glucometer. You must test your blood sugar every morning and keep a diary of your results. Glucometers can be purchased from any pharmacy. If you need assistance in using the glucometer, please contact Raymond Smith, CMA, at 555-6423.

Presently, I do not wish to prescribe any medications. If we are unable to get your blood sugar under control, I will prescribe an oral diabetic medication.

Please call my office and schedule an appointment for the week of June 20 for a blood draw and a follow-up visit.

Sincerely,

Elizabeth Jones, M.D.

EJ/rs

enc. (2)

F IGURE 1 - 3. Sample semiblock letter.

Preparation

Good preparation is a key element in writing professional business letters. Preparation consists of planning the content and the mechanics of the letter.

Mental Preparation. Before you begin to compose a letter, mentally prepare your message. You might start formulating the message by envisioning yourself talking to the person to whom you are sending the letter. Preparation offers three benefits:

1. It helps eliminate writer's block.
2. It gets you to focus on the message, not the mechanics (e.g., spelling, grammar, punctuation).
3. It enhances your organization.

Using cue cards or note cards will help ensure all the necessary information is covered in the letter.

Mechanics of the Letter. Before you begin to type the letter, select the appropriate *template*, *margin*, and *font*. A template provides you with the skeleton of the letter. The key elements are already set and spaced correctly, so you just type in the pertinent information. Most computers have numerous letter templates or a letter wizard. These programs will make the process of letter writing easy, fast, and professional. You may

use macros in your template to make repetitive tasks faster.

The **margin** is the blank space around the letter. A 1-inch margin is used for both left and right sides of the letter and the bottom. Margins are used to center the components of the letter in a standarized manner. If you select a template, your margins will be set for you.

Next, select the font. A **font** is the typeface; it affects the way words look and how easy it will be to read the letter. **Choose a font that is easy to read and that is appropriate in size.** Avoid cute or elegant fonts that can be difficult to read or see. The most common fonts used in business letters are Times New Roman, Garamond, and Arial. Box 1-5 gives you some examples of fonts and their sizes.

 Checkpoint Question

3. Before you begin to type a letter, name three mechanics that you need to select.

Composition

The goal of composition is to ensure that your message is transmitted clearly, concisely, and accurately to your reader. As you did during preparation, focus on the message, not on the mechanics.

A clear message ensures that your reader knows precisely what is expected; an unclear message leaves room for doubt.

Unclear: Please contact me.
Clear: Please contact me by Thursday, October 1.
Unclear: You need to make an appointment for blood work.
Clear: Call Temple Hospital laboratories (555-4010) and make an appointment for a blood glucose test on March 13.

B ox 1 - 5

FONTS

Here are fonts that would be suitable for a business letter:

- This is 12-point Times New Roman.
- This is 10-point Times New Roman.
- This is 12-point Garamond.
- **This is 12-point Arial.**

Here are fonts and sizes that would not be appropriate:

- This is 8-point Times New Roman.
- **This is 12-point Colossalis Black.**
- THIS IS 12-POINT COTTONWOOD.
- This is 12-point Tekton.
- **This is 12-point impact.**

A concise message is short and to the point. Wordy phrases with many adjectives should not be used.

Not concise: Please enclose a check in an envelope for exactly $50.
Concise: Please enclose a $50 check.

An accurate message includes the correct date, time, figures, and information. Inaccurate messages cause delays and confusion and can lead to poor public relations.

Editing

After you have composed the letter, edit it for both grammatical errors and factual information. Editing is a key step in making your letter a success. Editing entails two steps: proofreading and corrections.

Proofreading. Whenever possible, have a colleague **proofread** (read text and check for accuracy) your letter and provide constructive criticism. Be sure to maintain confidentiality. If you are using a computer, consider printing out a hard copy of your document for proofreading; some individuals find it difficult to proofread a document on the computer screen. Check for the following items:

- Accuracy of all information
- Clarity and conciseness
- Grammar
- Spelling
- Punctuation
- Paragraphs appropriate in length and limited to one subject
- Capitalization
- Logical organization and flow

Use proofreader's marks (Box 1-6) to speed up the editing process. These are standard marks used to indicate corrections. You should become familiar with the basic marks.

Checkpoint Question

4. What is the purpose of proofreading?

Corrections. After making corrections, print a final copy of the letter. As discussed earlier in the chapter, a computer spell check should be used with caution, as it highlights misspelled words but not incorrectly used words.

Types of Business Letters

You will be asked to create and type various letters. Letters that you write will be sent to patients, insurance companies, other health care providers, pharmaceutical companies, and various businesses. Here are some common types of letters that you may write:

Box 1-6

STANDARD PROOFREADER MARKS

- ℐ or ℽ or ⁊ delete; take it out
- ⌒ close up; print as one word
- ℈ delete and close up
- ∧ or ˃ or ⋀ caret; insert here —(something
- # insert a space
- eq # space evenly where indicated
- stet let marked text stand as set
- tr transpose; change order the
- / used to separate two or more marks and often as a concluding stroke at the end of an insertion
- [set farther to the left
-] set farther to the right
- ⌒ set ae or fl as ligatures æ or fl
- = straighten alignment
- ‖ straighten or align
- X imperfect or broken character
- □ indent or insert em quad space
- ⁋ begin a new paragraph
- ⓈⱣ spell out (set 5 lbs as five pounds)
- cap set in capitals (CAPITALS)
- sm cap or s.c. set in small capitals (SMALL CAPITALS)
- ℓc set in lowercase (lowercase)
- *ital* set in italic (*italic*)
- rom set in roman (roman)
- bf set in boldface (**boldface**)
- = or – or ≐ or ⊢ hyphen
- $\frac{1}{N}$ or en or /N/ en dash (1965–72)
- $\frac{1}{M}$ or em or /M/ em—or long—dash
- ⋁ superscript or superior ($\overset{2}{\vee}$ as in πr^2)
- ⋀ subscript or inferior ($\overset{2}{\wedge}$ as in H_2O)
- ◇ or ╳ centered (◇ for a centered dot in $p \cdot q$)
- ⋀ comma
- ⋁ apostrophe
- ⊙ period
- ; or ;/ semicolon
- : or ⊙ colon
- ⋁⋁ or ⋁⋁ quotation marks
- (/) parentheses
- [/] brackets
- OK/? query to author: has this been set as intended
- ⊥ or ⋀¹ push down a work-up
- ℘¹ turn over an inverted letter
- *wf*¹ wrong font; a character of the wrong size or esp. style

¹ The last three symbols are unlikely to be needed in making proofs of photocomposed matter.

- Letters welcoming new patients to the practice
- Letters to patients regarding their test results
- Consultation reports to other health care professionals
- Workers' compensation letters verifying the patient's injury or treatment
- Justification or explanation of treatments to insurance companies
- Cover letters for transferring patients' records to another practice
- Clarification or explanation to patients regarding fees or billing concerns
- Thank you letters to sales representatives
- Physician changes for on-call schedules (generally sent to the hospital and covering physicians)
- Announcements of new services, hours, or office location changes.

MEMORANDUM DEVELOPMENT

A **memorandum** (often called a memo) is for communication within the office or with another department only; it is never sent to patients. It is less formal than a letter and is generally used for brief announcements.

Components of a Memorandum

A memorandum contains the standard elements in the following list. Use these guidelines to complete each element. Figure 1-4 shows a sample memorandum.

1. *Heading.* The word Memorandum is typed across the top of the page.
2. *Date.* Use the same rules for letters when typing the date for memorandums.
3. *To.* List the names of all recipients in either alphabetic or hierarchic order. If the memorandum is going to a particular group (e.g., all department managers, all employees), it can be addressed to the group.
4. *From.* List the name and title of the person sending the memorandum.
5. *Subject.* Insert a brief phrase describing the purpose of the memorandum.
6. *Body.* Write the message of the memorandum here.
7. *Copy (c).* Use the same rules as for letters when sending duplicate copies of memorandums.

Salutations and closings are not used in memorandums. All lines in a memorandum are justified left, and 1-inch margins are used. Writing a memorandum entails the same steps (preparation, composition, editing) as writing a business letter. The memorandum should be read and initialed by the physician before it is distributed. Your computer software will have a memorandum template.

Checkpoint Question

5. What are memorandums used for?

Summary

As an allied health professional, you need excellent written communication skills. Careful attention to detail is essential. Good grammar, punctuation, and spelling are key skills. Be careful when you use your computer spell check. It will not recognize words that are misused. You will use these skills to write letters, memorandums, and other correspondence. These letters will be sent to patients, physicians, and businesses. After writing these documents, you must be able to select the appropriate service for mailing your letters. Your primary goal with all written communication is to get your message across in a clear, concise, and accurate manner.

Critical Thinking Challenges

1. Create a business letter. Include all the components and use the full block format. Print your unedited copy and, using proofreader's marks, indicate your corrections. Make the corrections and reprint a final copy. Ask your instructor to review both copies.
2. Write 10 sentences using terms from Box 1-3. Use some terms correctly and others incorrectly. Exchange your sentences with another student. Correct your peer's sentences.

Answers to Checkpoint Questions

1. Inaccurate information in a business letter can lead to injuries to the patient and lawsuits and can harm the physician's practice.
2. The inside address is the address of the person to whom the letter is going. The salutation is the

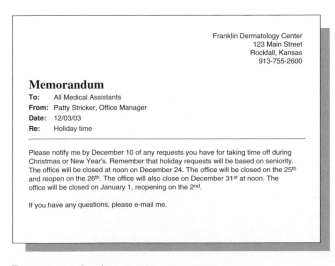

Franklin Dermatology Center
123 Main Street
Rockfall, Kansas
913-755-2600

Memorandum

To: All Medical Assistants
From: Patty Stricker, Office Manager
Date: 12/03/03
Re: Holiday time

Please notify me by December 10 of any requests you have for taking time off during Christmas or New Year's. Remember that holiday requests will be based on seniority. The office will be closed at noon on December 24. The office will be closed on the 25th and reopen on the 26th. The office will also close on December 31st at noon. The office will be closed on January 1, reopening on the 2nd.

If you have any questions, please e-mail me.

FIGURE 1-4. Sample memorandum.

greeting. The identification line shows the initials of the person who dictated the letters and the initials of the person who typed the letter.

3. Before you begin to type a letter, select the template, font, and margins that you will use.

4. Proofreading allows you to check the accuracy and content of the letter.

5. Memorandums are used for communication within the office and with other departments.

 Websites

Here are some Web addresses that may help you:

Airborne Express
www.airborne.com

Medical dictionary
www.medical-dictionary.com

Merriam-Webster's Dictionary
www.m-w.com

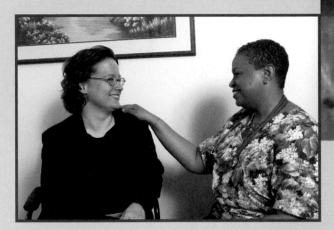

Computer Applications and the Internet

Introduction to the Computer

CHAPTER OBJECTIVES

In this chapter, you'll learn:

1. To identify the basic computer components.
2. To understand the basics of a computer operating system and how to set your preferences.
3. To understand how to create and manage files and folders.
4. To identify the appropriate office software to use for specific tasks.
5. To understand how to create, format, save, and print Word documents.
6. To understand how to create, format, save, and print PowerPoint presentations.
7. To understand how to create, format, save, and print Excel spreadsheets.

COMPUTERS PLAY A MAJOR ROLE in the health care facility. Computers promote communication among health care professionals and provide access to new treatment options. You will need excellent computer skills to work as an allied health professional. This chapter will help you to improve your existing skills. It provides a basic review of computer components. You will learn how the Internet is used in health care settings and some precautions. Various software applications will also be discussed.

THE COMPUTER

A computer system is roughly divided into two areas, hardware and peripherals.

Hardware

Computer hardware consists of seven key elements. Here is a review of their parts:

- *Central processing unit.* The central processing unit (CPU), or microprocessor, is the circuitry imprinted on a silicon chip that processes information. The CPU consists of a variety of electronic and magnetic cells. These cells read, analyze, and process data and instruct the computer on how to operate a given program. All CPUs function basically the same way, but chips differ dramatically in capabilities and speeds. Your CPU has many ports to connect the printer, mouse, and speakers. At minimum, it has two serial ports, one parallel port, and two universal serial bus (USB) ports. Serial ports are used for items like modems; parallel ports are used for connecting printers and backup drives to the CPU; and USB ports allow the computer to connect with various instruments.
- *Keyboard.* The keyboard is the primary means by which information is entered into the computer. Besides the typical letter and number keys, you will find special function keys that provide increased capabilities. Examples of special function keys are Alt, Ctrl, Insert, and Esc. Each of these keys has a specific function that is determined by the software program. These functions may include searching for and replacing words, moving blocks of text, indenting or centering text, and spell checking.
- *Monitor.* Monitors, also called the visual display terminals, come in various sizes and qualities. The quality of the image is based on the DPIs (dots per inch). The more DPIs, the clearer the picture. There are adjustment dials for brightness and contrast.
- *Hard drive.* The hard drive provides storage for programs, data, and files. The capacity of a hard drive (i.e., the quantity of programs and data it can hold) is measured in megabytes or gigabytes. Originally, hard drives could hold 5 MB (equivalent to about 2,000 typed pages), but today they have much more capacity.

- *Printer.* The printer transfers information to paper (hard copy). Printers use various technologies, operate at various speeds, and print in either black or color. The printer allows you to generate bills, print letters, and produce a daily schedule.
- *Scanner.* A scanner allows you to take a picture or report and read it into the computer. You may scan laboratory reports, radiology reports, and discharge summaries into a patient's file. Patient education materials can also be scanned into the computer and then adjusted to meet the needs of your office. Keep in mind that you need to adhere to copyright laws.
- *Secondary storage systems.* All computers have multiple methods for saving data. Examples include floppy diskettes, compact discs (CDs), digital video discs (DVDs), zip drives, and jump drives. Cartridges are used by hospitals for large storage systems. When saving any type of data, remember that good organization skills are essential. Name your files appropriately and place files in properly identified folders. Most computers have preset timing systems that automatically save data. Check your default setting and readjust as needed.

 Checkpoint Question

1. What do the CPU cells do?

Peripherals

Computers can have many peripheral connections. Three key computer peripherals that you need to know are:

- *Mouse.* The mouse can be used to control the cursor on the display screen. Although you cannot type in characters using the mouse, you can move or delete individual characters, words, or entire blocks of text with it. The track ball is an alternative to a mouse. Your finger rotates the ball to move the pointer. It takes less space than a mouse and is used based on personal preference.
- *Battery backup.* A battery backup allows the computer system to function in the event of a power failure. Batteries come in various sizes depending on the size of your computer and the amount of work to be done during a power failure.
- *Modem.* A modem is a communication device that connects your computer with other computers, including the Internet, online services such as bulletin boards, and electronic mail systems. The faster the modem, the faster the transmission. Modems may be connected through cable systems or through the telephone. Digital subscriber line (DSL) is the preferred method. To use a cable or DSL connection, your computer must have an **Ethernet** port or an Ethernet interface card.

Box 2-1

BASIC CARE OF DISKS

Whether you are using a diskette, CD, or DVD, follow these guidelines:

- Always handle the disk by the label or jacket.
- Do not touch the inside of the disk.
- Store in a safe, cool dry place. Avoid high-moisture areas.
- Keep all food and liquids away.
- Never store near a magnetic field, such as a television screen or cellular telephone.
- Store in a vertical container designed for that purpose.
- Always label before storing. Write on the label sticker before sticking the label to the disk.

Checkpoint Question

2. Why should your computer have an Ethernet port or Ethernet interface card?

Care and Maintenance of the System and Equipment

As with any piece of equipment in the health care facility, it is necessary to maintain your computer on a regular basis. Some general care guidelines follow:

- Place the monitor, keyboard, and printer in a cool dry area out of direct sunlight.
- Static electricity can cause memory loss, inaccurate data collection, and other adverse reactions. To control this problem, place the computer desk on an antistatic floor mat or carpet, or purchase a specific antistatic device.
- Use available accessories to care for your system. For example, use dust covers for the keyboard and the monitor when they are not in use. Antistatic wipes are available to use on the screen, and they should be used as an alternative to glass cleaners.
- When moving the computer, lock the hard drive to protect the CPU and disk drives.
- Keep keyboards free of debris and liquids, which can be hazardous to the keyboard, as it is directly plugged into the computer. Vacuum the keyboard periodically to eliminate dust particles under the key pads. Do not eat or drink while working on the computer.
- Be aware of any maintenance and warranty contracts for the computer system and do not hesitate to contact the service representative when needed. Some maintenance agreements require that a service representative clean and inspect the system on a regular basis.
- Handle data storage disks with special care. Box 2-1 provides some general guidelines.

THE COMPUTER OPERATING SYSTEM

The computer operating system controls your computer and allows you to use all the programs and software that are loaded on it. Your computer at work might be a desktop or a laptop computer — either way, it has an operating system. If you are working on a PC, you will likely be using the Microsoft Windows operating system. If your computer is a Mac, the operating system is a bit different. Either way, the operating system helps you navigate the computer and get your work done.

Setting Your Preferences

When you turn your computer on, the first thing you'll notice is the desktop. The desktop is the screen that is the gateway to the software that's available on your computer.

Just as you organize the items on top of your desk, you can set up your computer's "desktop" according to your preferences. You can have easy access to the files and folders that you use the most. You also can create shortcuts to get to certain programs.

When you set your preferences, you can create a screensaver, or an image that pops up on the screen when you're away from your computer. However, it's important to keep in mind that your work computer is just that — a computer that is used for work. It belongs to the health care facility and is not your own personal computer. That means you shouldn't set your preferences to create screensavers that include personal pictures or images that are not related to work.

Managing Files and Folders

For a computer to be useful, the information needs to be organized. Just as we use manila folders and file cabinets to sort and file information, Windows uses this familiar concept to organize electronic files. A disk is like a filing cabinet that holds many folders. A file is like a piece of paper or several pages stapled together.

Files

A computer file can be a document or spreadsheet that you create. Originally, file names could only be eight characters long, but Windows no longer has these restrictions. Here are some hints to keep in mind when creating file names:

- Spaces are okay in file names.
- You cannot use the following symbols and punctuation marks in a file name: * ? " < > |:\ /:
- The file name should always end with a period followed by a three-character identifier called an extension. The three characters identify the type of file and the applications that created it: ".doc" for a document created in Word, ".xls" for a spreadsheet created in Excel, ".txt" for a plain text file that can be opened in many applications.

Folders

A computer folder works just like a manila folder to hold related files together. Folders also may be called *directories*. Within a folder, you can have files and/or more folders. These are called *subfolders*.

Windows locates and identifies each file or folder by its unique address, called a *path* (or path name). The path lists the disk, folders, and subfolders that contain the file. Each folder in the path is separated by a backslash (\). For example, a typical path might look like this:

C:\Documents and Settings\Laura\My Documents\ Referrals.doc

Windows creates certain folders called *system folders* to locate the information it needs to run your computer. System folders and their files must remain in their exact location with folder names intact for Windows to operate, but otherwise you are free to create as many folders as you like. Windows gives you unlimited options for creating folders and sorting information.

USING OFFICE SOFTWARE

As an allied health professional, you should be familiar with the basic computer software you might use at work. You might be asked to type a letter or to create a list or chart for your supervisor. In some cases, you might be called on to assist with creating computer presentations with numerous slides. Thankfully, the computer can help you achieve all these goals easily.

Discovering Word

One of the most common computer programs is Microsoft Word, a word processing program. You can use Word to create documents ranging from business letters to patient education materials.

Creating and Formatting Word Documents

One of the easiest ways to learn about Word is to search the toolbar at the top of the page. If you move the cursor over the toolbar, the computer will explain what each icon does. You can click on the "blank page" icon to open a new document.

Word allows you to customize your document to fit your needs. Once you've begun to create your document, you can use the toolbar to adjust the formatting. The toolbar gives you many simple formatting options, including:

- copy and paste
- change font style and size
- align text
- check your spelling
- add bulleted or numbered lists

Saving and Printing Word Documents

You can use the toolbar to save or print your document. A good rule of thumb is to save your document as soon as you create it. Then you should save the file multiple times again while you're working on it. This will ensure that your work has been saved, even if other systems on your computer go down.

To save a document, you can either click on the "disk" icon, or click on "File." "Save As" will allow you to name your document and save it in a particular folder on the network.

To print your document, you can either click on the "print" icon, or click on "File" and scroll down to "Print." The latter option often allows you to choose which printer you'd like to use, as well as the number of copies you'd like to print.

Discovering PowerPoint

As an allied health professional, you might be asked to create a presentation. The most popular program used to write presentations is Microsoft PowerPoint.

Creating and Formatting Presentations

Once you open PowerPoint, you can choose to open the AutoContent Wizard, a Design Template, or a blank presentation. Click on "blank presentation" and select the layout of your first slide. You can format and add new slides to your slide show using the toolbar. Add clip art or pictures by clicking on "Insert."

You can view your slide show by doing one of the following:

- Click "Slide Show" at the lower left of the PowerPoint window.
- On the Slide Show menu, click "View Show."
- On the View menu, click "Slide Show."
- Press F5 on the keyboard.

Saving and Printing Presentations

You can use the toolbar to save your presentation the same way you would save a Word document. "Save As" will allow you to name your presentation and save it in a specific folder on the network. Clicking on "File" and "Print" will allow you to choose from more options, such as which printer you'd like to use and how many copies you'd like to print. Printing copies is often encouraged so that your audience can view the presentation at their own pace.

Discovering Excel

As an allied health professional, you might be asked to organize information. Excel can create spreadsheets to record and keep track of data ranging from patients' records to office supplies.

Creating and Formatting Spreadsheets

To create a new spreadsheet, you can click on the "new document" icon. The rows and columns can be organized much like a chart. To add text to an individual cell, simply click on it. Cells can be expanded or retracted using the toolbar. The toolbar also allows you to format your spreadsheet with many different options, such as copy and paste and highlighting. You can even write formulas that will add or subtract numbers in the rows and columns and perform the math for you. To find out more about these features, you can use the "Help" feature.

Saving and Printing Spreadsheets

To save your spreadsheet, you can click on the "disk" icon or on "File." "Save As" allows you to name the spreadsheet and save it in a particular file on the network. To print your document, you can either click on the icon or "File." The latter option allows you to choose which printer you'd like use, as well as the number of copies you'd like to print.

3

Computer Applications in the Health Care Setting

CHAPTER OBJECTIVES

In this chapter, you'll learn:

1. To spell and define the key words.
2. To explain the basics of connecting to the Internet.
3. To discuss the safety concerns for online searching.
4. To describe how to use a search engine.
5. To list sites that can be used by professionals and sites geared for patients.
6. To describe the benefits of an intranet and explain how it differs from the Internet.
7. To describe the various types of clinical software that might be used in a health care facility.
8. To describe the various types of administrative software that might be used in a health care facility.
9. To describe the benefits of a handheld computer.
10. To describe various training options.
11. To discuss the ethics related to computer access.

PERFORMANCE OBJECTIVES

In this chapter, you'll learn:

1. To search a given topic on the Internet.
2. To conduct a basic literary search.

KEY TERMS

cookies
downloading
encryption

Ethernet
Internet
intranet

literary search
search engine
surfing

virtual
virus

INTERNET BASICS

Most health care facilities can connect to the **Internet.** The first thing you need to know is how to get your computer connected to the internet.

Getting Started and Connected

The Internet is used for access to the World Wide Web (www) and for electronic mail. To get connected, you will need an Internet connection company and appropriate Internet software.

There are three ways that your computer can connect to the Internet. One is an Internet service provider (ISP). The ISP is a company that connects your computer's modem to the Internet through the phone line. It is often called a dial-up service. This method provides the slowest service but is the cheapest. The second option is your cable television company. This system provides a faster connection. The third option is a digital subscriber line (DSL). This is the fastest connection but is not available in all areas. DSL is the most expensive connection system. If you need to download large files through the Internet, you should use either a DSL or cable connection. If you are having trouble accessing the Internet because of either slow service or connection troubles, speak to your supervisor or office manager to determine whether a different connection or ISP is needed.

Second, your computer will need a Web browser. A Web browser is software that communicates with your computer and the Internet. Two common examples are Internet Explorer and Netscape Navigator. Most computers are preloaded with a Web browser.

Clicking on the Web browser icon makes the actual connection to the Internet. Depending on how your system is set up, you may have to use a password. Box 3-1 gives you some guidelines on password use.

Box 3-1

PASSWORD USE

Here are some guidelines for passwords:

- make unique passwords (combine letters and numbers).
- do not use your initials, birth date, or phone number
- systemwide passwords that allow access to the computer should be changed after an employee has been fired
- do not share your password with your colleagues
- do not tape your password on the computer monitor or leave it on your desk
- it is a good idea to have additional password verifications for certain secure sites.

Checkpoint Question

1. Which two types of Internet connection are recommended for downloading large files?

Security

If you choose correct sites and follow some general safety tips, the Internet is a safe way to obtain and transfer patient information. Here are a few key points:

- never send *any* patient information over the Internet to a site that does not have a secure sockets layer (SSL). This scrambles your information as it leaves your computer and unscrambles it when it arrives at its designated address
- look for a lock icon on the status bar
- set limits on your Web browser for **cookies.** A cookie is a tiny file left on your computer's hard drive from a website without your permission. By examining your cookies, a website can learn what sites you have visited, products that you have been searching, and files that you have downloaded. You may control your computer's cookies by setting limits on your Web browser software. Limit setters can generally be found on your toolbar under Internet options, then under either privacy or security.

Viruses

Virus protection is an important security issue. A virus is a dangerous invader that enters your computer through some source and can destroy your files, software programs, and possibly even the hard drive. A worm is a specific type of virus that affects e-mail. Most computers come with virus protection software. This software will identify and stop harmful transmission. No virus protection is, however, 100% guaranteed. Some ways that you can protect your computer are:

- do not open any attachments that are from unknown or suspicious sites
- update your virus protection software regularly. Most virus protection programs offer an updating service Virus protection updates address new worms, as well
- remember, new viruses are detected daily.

Downloading Information

The Internet is filled with great patient teaching resources and other information. You may decide to copy some of this material into your computer. This is **downloading.** Downloading transfers information from an outside location to your computer's hard drive. Download only files that pertain to work. Do not download screen savers, news releases, recipes, or other personal information. Do not assume that you can photocopy any material that you have downloaded and distribute it. Always ask for permission from the author. Some government and professional medical websites state that their material can be freely copied and used. A good example of this is the United States Department of Agriculture (USDA) website that allows the food pyramid to be copied and used for teaching.

Working Offline

It is possible to access Web pages without connecting your computer to the Internet. To do this, save your commonly accessed sites on your Web browser. (If you are unsure how to do this, search your help topics for working offline). Then, to view the pages off line, click on the connection icon, select work off line, and locate your file. Remember, Web pages are regularly updated, and a page that you have saved to view off line may not be the latest version. Periodically view the online site and resave the site.

ELECTRONIC MAIL

Electronic mail (e-mail) provides many benefits to the health care system. It is estimated that about 6.6 trillion e-mail messages are sent every year. E-mail promotes good patient care, enhances communication, promotes teamwork, eliminates phone tag, and provides written documentation of messages. E-mail messages can't be guaranteed to provide confidentiality. Some general tips for using e-mail follow:

- use the office e-mail address only to send work-related messages. Do not send personal messages
- do not participate in chain letters
- download your e-mail and read it off line unless you are using a DSL or cable connection
- all e-mail messages should be professional
- read your e-mail's **encryption** feature and activate it. Encryption is a process of scrambling messages so that they cannot be read until they reach the recipient
- always leave a message on your e-mail system when you will be away for a vacation or other reason. This message is automatically sent to the incoming e-mail senders. This alerts the sender that you will not be reading their message. Include the date when you will be returning to the office and instructions on whom they should contact in case of emergencies. This feature is often called "out-of-office assistant." An example of a good message: "I will be out from 1/20 through 1/28. If your message requires immediate attention, please forward it to Barbara Smith. I will respond to your e-mail when I return."

Checkpoint Question

2. What does the encryption feature do?

Access

Access to your e-mail account is through either Internet or intranet. The intranet is discussed later in the chapter. To access your e-mail, locate the mail icon, double-click it, and enter appropriate information. A password is generally required.

Composing Messages

Here are a few tips for composing e-mail messages:

- check your spelling, grammar, and punctuation before sending any messages
- keep messages short, concise, and to the point
- flag messages of high importance. This will alert the recipient that the message is important and should be read first. Do not overuse this feature. Flag only messages that warrant immediate response or attention.
- use appropriate fonts and an appropriate font size
- generic or plain stationery should be used. Do not use stationery that has cute figures or looks busy
- always complete the subject line. Keep the subject line short and use only a few key words, for example, Staff meeting tomorrow
- it is a good idea to restrict e-mail messages to only one topic
- paragraphs are not indented on e-mail messages. Skip a line between paragraphs
- you can add a permanent signature to all outgoing e-mails. Your signature should include your name and phone number.

Address Books

Your e-mail software will allow you to create address books. An address book is a collection of e-mail addresses. Additional information, such as phone numbers, fax numbers, and street addresses, can be added. A few tips regarding address books are:

- keep your addresses up to date
- organize your addresses in folders or categories. For example, one folder may contain all the cardiologists in the area, and another may contain just insurance-related addresses.

Attachments

An attachment is a file that is sent along with an e-mail. You can attach a single file (letter) or several documents at one time. Remember these guidelines:

- when you receive an e-mail with an attachment, open the attached file or letter. File it in an appropriate place on your computer. If appropriate, print the attachment and distribute it as needed
- if you are sending an e-mail and need to attach a file, compose your message first. Then attach the file by going into the tool bar and locating the menu for file attachments. Find the file on your computer and click to attach it. It is a good idea before sending the attachment to open it to be sure that you have selected the correct file or version of the document.

Opening Electronic Mail

Some general guidelines regarding opening an e-mail message follow:

- open only your own e-mail messages unless otherwise instructed
- after reading the e-mail, either delete it or place it in a folder. Do not allow multiple e-mails to clog your inbox
- always open flagged messages first and respond to them immediately
- if you receive a message that you cannot address or resolve, forward the message to your supervisor and alert the sender that the message has been forwarded
- if you start receiving bulk mail, either block the sender or ask to be deleted from that mailing list. This can be accomplished by clicking on "unsubscribe," usually at the end of the message.

Checkpoint Question

3. Can you be 100% guaranteed that your e-mail transmissions are safe?

MEDICAL APPLICATIONS OF THE INTERNET

Besides e-mail, the Internet offers the World Wide Web, which provides health care professionals with great resources and information. Navigating through the Web quickly and efficiently takes skill and practice. The process of searching the Internet is called **surfing**. Surfing that is unorganized and not focused can be time consuming and unproductive.

Before surfing for information, you need to remember one important rule: Not all of the information on the Web is accurate or truthful. Anyone can post anything or make any claim. Since the information that you obtain from the Web will affect patient care, all steps must be taken to ensure that only accurate information is found and used. First, look for the HON (Health on the Net) seal. The HON seal is a voluntary seal that indicates that the site has met certain standards for reliability and credibility. It does not certify that the information is correct or truthful, but it is a good starting point. Keep in mind that many good sites, for example governmental sites, do not have this seal. Box 3-2 provides you with some guidelines for selecting safe sites.

Search Engines

A **search engine** allows you to find sites that have the information that you need. There are numerous search engines (Google, Yahoo, Lycos, Excite, Dogpile). These sites are best used for searching out general information. Once you arrive at the search engine page, you must enter some key words. Your key words should be focused to limit the

---

Box 3-2

SAFE SITE SELECTION GUIDELINES

Remember these key points when reading information on a website:

- beware of phrases like breakthrough, medical miracle, secret formula
- avoid sites that advertise that they have cured a disease
- use caution when you see the phrase "ancient remedy"
- use caution when you find a site that will treat a whole list of diseases with the same treatment
- do not believe every testimonial that you read
- if the site claims that the government is hiding information to cure a disease, use extreme caution
- use caution when the treatment can "only be bought here"
- If the site suggests that you not tell your doctor about it, stay away
- do not try to learn lifesaving skills, such as cardiopulmonary resuscitation, on the Internet. No matter how good the information or site is, you need to take a professional class.

---

number of responses that you will get. For example, if you type in the key word "heart," you will get thousands of sites that pertain to the heart. Some of these sites will be referring to the heart as an organ and other sites will address how to mend a broken heart. If you had selected your key words to be "heart attack," however, you would narrow your search tremendously. To further narrow your search use the advanced search feature. Click on advanced search and use the key words "heart and attack and prevention." By doing this, you will obtain the information you want faster and more efficiently. Unless you are using a medical search engine, avoid using medical terms. For example, use the word lung instead of pulmonary. When you need to find medical information, use a medical search or a megamedical site with links. See the listing of websites at the end of this chapter for some good places to start searching for medical information.

Checkpoint Question

4. What is a search engine?

Professional Medical Sites

At the end of the chapters in this book you will see various Web addresses listed that provide you with more information on that chapter's content. These are good starting points for professional topics. But keep in mind that Web addresses

Box 3-3

SITES HEALTH CARE PROFESSIONALS USE

Health care professionals are likely to use these sites:

Journal of the American Medical Association	*www.jama.com*
New England Journal of Medicine	*www.nejm.org*
Annals of Internal Medicine	*www.annals.org*
AMA	*www.ama-assn.org*
JCAHO	*www.jointcommission.org*
CDC	*www.cdc.gov*
Clinical trials	*www.clinicaltrials.gov*

change frequently. If you are unable to access a site, try eliminating the letters and symbols after a slash (/). Use the primary site address. For example, suppose you want to enter this site: *www.fda.gov/cder/drug/consumer/buyonline/guide.htm*. If you cannot access that site, try *www.fda.gov* and advance from there. Most sites will link you automatically to a new home page. Also, depending on your Web browser, you may not have to type in www. In this case, you would just type in fda.gov.

The Internet can help you communicate with patients who speak a foreign language. Some websites translate phrases and words. Box 3-3 lists sites that physicians are most likely to use. All medical specialties have their own special site. Hospitals have their own sites also.

Literary Searches

Most research information is found through a **literary search**. A literary search involves finding journal articles that present new facts or data about a given topic. Physicians who specialize in a given area and have conducted a controlled research study write these articles. Various databases can be used to do a literary search:

- OVID will search for articles as far back as 1966. It contains access to more than 4,000 professional journals
- PubMed will search for journal articles back to 1966 from the National Library of Medicine
- CINAHL contains journal articles published since 1982. It has primarily journals for nurses and other allied health care professionals.

Most literary search databases require an annual subscription fee. Once you arrive at the site, you can start to search for the information. First, enter your key words. To narrow the search, you can request journal articles from all countries or limit it to the United States. You can also limit the search by selecting a time line, such as the past 6 months. Once you have done your search, a list of articles will be displayed, and you can highlight the ones you wish to see. You will be asked whether you want to see the whole article or only the abstract. An abstract is a summary of the article. It is always a good idea to print only the abstracts and then decide which full articles you want to see. Fees for downloading the complete journal article vary. Abstracts can generally be downloaded free. Your local hospital librarian is often available to assist you with literary searches and may be able to get the article for free.

Checkpoint Question

5. How is a literary search different from a search on an internet website?

Insurance-Related Sites

The insurance world can seem like an endless maze of papers and regulations. The Internet can help you sort through and clarify some information. Your first stop should be the patient's insurance company. Its Web address is usually listed on the back of the patient's insurance card. Bookmark these sites. A few sites that can also help you and your patients follow:

- for information on buying health insurance online: *www.ehealthinsurance.com*
- the Medicare site (*www.medicare.gov*) discusses the basics of Medicare programs, eligibility, enrollment, drug assistance programs, and many frequently asked questions. This site will link you to various other options. You will also find links to report Medicare fraud and abuse.

Patient Teaching Issues Regarding the Internet

Some of your patients will be very skilled at using the Internet. They can find enormous amounts of information regarding their disease, treatment options, medications. The guidelines discussed in Box 3-2 pertain to patients who surf the Internet. You cannot stop or limit the information that patients will search and find. Keep in mind that patients often turn to the Internet when they feel confused or hopeless about their disease or anger about the medical profession.

Teach patients to acquire reliable medical information and advise them of the dangers on the Web. Some facilities print brochures with recommended Web addresses. This is a very good education tool for patients. Box 3-4 gives you some good patient education sites. Some areas you should be aware of are discussed below.

Buying Medications Online

As the cost of prescription medications soars, patients look for options. It is possible to buy prescription medications over the Internet. A good Internet pharmacy will provide information on what the medication is used for, possible side effects, dosage recommendation, and safety concerns.

Box 3-4

GOOD PATIENT EDUCATION SITES

These sites provide good patient information:
American Dental Association
  www.ada.org/public/index.asp
American Sleep Apnea Association
  www.sleepapnea.org
Consumer Health Publications
  www.health.nih.gov
Merck Manual Home Edition
  www.merckhomeedition.com
National Attention Deficit Disorder Association
  www.add.org
American Association of Poison Control Centers
  www.aapcc.org
Smoking cessation
  www.QuitNet.org
Sources for people with cancer
  www.cancersource.com
Travel health
  www.cdc.gov/travel

If patients want to purchase prescriptions online, advise them to use only sites that are certified by the Verified Internet Pharmacy Practice Site (VIPPS). This certification comes from the National Association of Boards of Pharmacy and indicates that the site has been checked and is monitored for safety and quality care. Advise patients to purchase only medications that have been prescribed by their physician. Warn patients never to purchase medications from sites outside of the United States. These sites may not meet safety standards of the Food and Drug Administration (FDA). In addition, the FDA warns patients never to buy certain medications online because of their inherent dangers. Advise patients to use *www.fda.gov/cder/consumerinfo/buyonlineGuide_text.htm* for consumer safety tips. Box 3-5 lists medications that the FDA warns people never to purchase online.

Some sites offer virtual prescribing. This means that the Internet user provides some information and asks for a prescription. For example, the patient may type in, "My cholesterol is too high. What medication will get it down?" The site will then ask the patient a few questions and select a medication. In other cases, the patient may simply request a medication: "I want some amoxicillin." In either case, the prescription is filled and mailed to the patient. Warn patients about the dangers of self-prescribing medications. Serious health risks can arise.

Checkpoint Question

6. Name three safety tips to teach patients about buying medications on the Internet.

Financial Assistance for Medications

Patients who are having trouble paying for their prescription medications can find many financial resources on the Web. You should advise patients to search the drug company's home page, for example, *www.Pfizer.com*.

Health Records

Patients may choose to create their own "health records" and store personal health information on sites. Patients who travel frequently may opt for this. Patients can store information about their medications, immunizations, laboratory tests, surgeries, and so on. For their own protection, patients should be discouraged from doing this. Instead, advise patients to download medical record forms, complete the printed copy, and store them safely.

Some websites provide forms online for patients to record their health histories. Parents can sign an emergency consent form giving permission for another person to give consent for their child to be treated in case of an emergency. This is valuable for parents who travel on business and have their child stay with a relative or friend.

Advance directives and legal forms for medical power of attorney are also available online. Patients should be advised to seek legal counsel and speak to a physician before completing these forms. The federal government does have cards available online for patients to complete and carry with them regarding their wishes to be an organ and tissue donor at *www.organdonor.gov*.

Box 3-5

MEDICATIONS THAT SHOULD NEVER BE BOUGHT ON THE INTERNET

According to the Federal Drug Administration, certain drugs should never be purchased on the Internet. These medications can cause serious harm if they are not prescribed correctly and the patient is not closely monitored.

- Accutane (isotretinoin)
- Actiq (fentanyl citrate)
- Clozaril (clozapine)
- Humatrope (somatropin [rDNA origin])
- Lotronex (alosetron hydrochloride)
- Mifeprex (mifepristone or RU-486)
- Thalomid (thalidomide)
- Tikosyn (dofetilide)
- Tracleer (bosentan)
- Trovan (trovafloxacin mesylate or alatrofloxacin mesylate injection)
- Xyrem (sodium oxybate)

WHAT IF

Parents ask you how to keep their child safe on the Internet. What should you say?

First and foremost, explain to the parent that direct parental observation is the best method. Encourage parents to have an open and honest discussion with their child regarding the dangers on the Internet. Computers should be kept in living rooms or family rooms. Advise parents not to let children have a computer with Internet access in their bedroom. Parents can require a password to be entered for Internet access. This prevents access when the parent is not present. Most Web browser programs let the parent allow access only to "safe" sites. A few sites can add filters or safety nets to a child's computer.

Injury Prevention

Injuries are a leading cause of death for children. The American Academy of Pediatrics (*www.aap.org*) has reference materials that can help parents with safety tips. The federal government sites (*www.cdc.gov and www.nih.gov*) also have good information that you can direct parents to search. Safe Kids Worldwide is another excellent resource (*www.safekids.org*).

INTRANET

An **intranet** is a private network of computers that share data. Intranets, sometimes called internal webs, are used in large facilities. The only people with access to an intranet home page are people with an affiliation to the facility. Access may be limited to those within the offices or may allow for access from home computer systems. The benefits of an intranet are enhanced communication, quick access to needed information, and increased productivity. Common examples of data found on an intranet are:

- policy and procedure manuals
- marketing information
- minutes from meetings and upcoming agendas
- staff schedules
- local hospital announcements or information
- commonly used forms
- internal newsletters
- internal job postings
- phone lists
- video conference support
- links to specialty sites.

Checkpoint Question

7. How does an intranet differ from the Internet?

MEDICAL SOFTWARE APPLICATIONS

The types of medical applications and their possibilities are endless. Every day, thousands of new software packages are released into the market. Upgrades and new versions of existing packages are also released daily. Each type of software program will have good benefits and will lack some features. The type of software that you will use will vary among different facilities. The selection of software is based on the size of the facility and specialty. Other factors include how many users can use software at one time, whether the software can be used with multiple windows open, and how often does the company plans to update it.

Never buy or install a new software program or update an existing version without permission.

Learning to use a particular software program and navigate quickly and efficiently through its features takes time. Most programs come with a tutorial program. On-site training is often included in the purchase price of major software applications. Training options will be discussed later in the chapter.

Medical software applications can be divided into two main groups: clinical and administrative. Clinical software packages help the health care professional provide the best possible health care to patients. Administrative software packages focus on tasks to keep the office flowing efficiently and financially strong. The next sections introduce you to what types of software capabilities are available and most commonly used. Keep in mind that new technologies are emerging every day.

Clinical Applications

Clinical software is designed to help the health care professional provide the most efficient, safest, and most reliable health care available. Here are some examples of the benefits that clinical software programs can bring into the health care facility:

1. Create a **virtual** patient chart. A virtual chart is a paperless chart in which all documentation is stored on computer. Some offices create dual charts (virtual and paper), and other offices will keep one or the other. The advantages to a virtual charting system are that it saves filing space, increases access to patients' charts for all staff members, eliminates hunting for misplaced charts, and keeps the charts better organized and neater. Since the charting is done through keyboarding, the notes are always readable.

2. Clinical software can maintain an up-to-date list of clinical tasks organized by employee's name. For example, suppose you just saw a patient and made a note on his chart that you need to check his laboratory tests tomorrow. The task manager would automatically assign this task to your list of duties for tomorrow. This

promotes organization and decreases the potential for tasks to get overlooked or forgotten.

3. The software available for prescription management and drug information is tremendous. A good program that focuses on pharmaceutical information will decrease medication errors, increase patient satisfaction, and provide better patient care, and it can be financially beneficial to the patient and to the facility. At minimum, the software should enable the doctor to find the patient's name in a database, virtually write the prescription, and download it directly to the patient's pharmacy. This allows the pharmacist to fill the prescription before the patient arrives. Thus the patient gets the medication much faster. More important, since most prescription filling errors are due to doctor's poor handwriting, this potentially lethal error is prevented. Most medication software packages red-flag the physician if the prescription is contraindicated for the patient. Medications can be contraindicated because of a particular disease (e.g., asthma or diabetes), interaction with other medications the patient is taking, or an allergy.

4. Computer programs can insert laboratory reports directly into the patient's records. This is more time efficient than faxing or manually recording the results. It also eliminates transcription errors. Most software will alert the doctor when a new laboratory report has been received. Laboratory reports of serious or life-threatening findings will still be telephoned to the office.

5. Perhaps one of the greatest technologies is the importing of the actual imaging study into a patient's chart. Some software allows the doctor to see the radiograph or computed tomograph from the office.

Checkpoint Question

8. What is a virtual chart?

Administrative Applications

There are hundreds of administrative software packages available for health care facilities. Most systems have a combination of features. Some examples of benefits administrative software can bring to the facility follow:

1. Appointment making and tracking are more efficient with a computer program than with a book format. Good appointment software will allow you to enter appointments quickly and make changes more easily. It should allow for an unlimited comment area near the patient's name. The comment area allows you to add special notes. Appointment software can keep a waiting list of patients who are looking for appointments or wanting to move their appointment date and time to the first available. Appointment software can also automatically print notices to remind patients of the need to make appointments.

2. Software can allow you or the office manager to track patient flows. This can be helpful to adjust staff scheduling needs, with more help at the busiest hours or days and less staff on slower days. It can alert managers to the productivity of staff members. This allows you to schedule appointments at various intervals and thus promotes patient flow. It can track the time patients wait in the waiting room or examination room. Examining such information allows the staff to change the office flow to decrease waiting times or to indicate the need for additional staff. It can also highlight the days when patients are most likely to cancel their appointments. Patient demographics can be obtained, used for marketing, and allow the office to apply for special funding based on patient demographics.

3. Software programs are needed to send insurance claims electronically. You will be able to send claims and track their progress. This allows for faster reimbursement to the practice and can identify problems of reimbursement earlier. The programs that you will use should have access to numerous plans and can be updated frequently and easily.

4. Software programs can allow integration with insurance companies and other businesses to allow for automatic quick payment and posting. This saves time and is less complicated to use than traditional accounting books.

5. Health care facilities should have software that allows for credit card authorization. A variety of card types should be available (Visa, MasterCard, American Express).

6. Insurance software can allow you to check for patient eligibility. Most programs have enough room for the addresses and phone numbers of the primary, secondary, and tertiary providers. Case manager names should be added when available. Software can also allow for preadmission certifications to be completed and electronically submitted. Preadmission or preauthorization allows you and the patient to verify that the insurance company will cover the procedure or admission. Some software programs come with codes (ICD-9, CPT, HCPCS) and anesthesia codes preinstalled.

7. Some programs aim to comply with the Health Insurance Portability and Accountability Act (HIPAA). HIPAA is a federal act that requires all health care professionals to follow a variety of privacy and confidentiality rules; these programs allow you to document your adherence to these rules and regulations. For more information on HIPAA, visit *www.hipaa.org*.

8. Other programs alert you to send collection letters. These programs have a variety of template collection letters. Always double-check the information before sending a collection letter.

9. A variety of financial software programs track accounts receivable and accounts payable. You may need to adjust the billing cycles to meet the needs of

the office in which you are working. Software programs can also automate the tickler system.

10. Automated payroll software can automatically calculate tax deductions and other deductions. You will be able to arrange for direct deposit of employee checks through these software programs.

11. A medical office can't effectively run without a word processing system. These systems help you write letters and other types of documentation.

12. An important part of any administrative software is the section that handles the personnel records. Contracts, disciplinary reports, performance evaluations, and so on can all be stored in a virtual personnel record.

Meeting Maker

Meeting Maker is a common package that promotes internal coordination of meetings and calendars. This system is primarily used in large facilities with multiple offices and multiple administrative personnel. This is how the system works: Everyone is listed as user. Each user enters his or her schedule into a personal calendar. Calendars can be seen daily, weekly, or monthly. For example, you may type in, "Monday, Middletown office, 8 A.M.–4 P.M.; Tuesday, Southside office, 10 A.M.–5 P.M." The system allows you to view other people's calendars. It is possible to allow other people to enter data to your calendar. You can also maintain a list of tasks and print your schedule. If you are asked to arrange a staff meeting, you enter the names of the people who should come, and the computer will select a date and time that is convenient for everyone.

HANDHELD COMPUTERS

A handheld device, or personal digital assistant (PDA), can do almost anything that your desktop computer can do. Companies that make PDA software can be found at these three Web addresses: *www.pdacortex.com, www.skyscape.com,* and *www.handheldmed.com.* At minimum, handheld computers come with software that can do these functions:

- Address book
- Calendar
- Memo pad
- E-mail
- Word processing

Information can be entered into the handheld device either with a stylus (pen) or on a small keyboard. It is possible to attach a regular-size keyboard to a PDA. Information can be sent back and forth between a PDA and a desktop computer in either of two ways. The PDA can be placed in a cradle that is connected via a cable to the desktop ("hot sync"), or information can be sent via e-mail. PDAs can beam information among themselves (business cards, memos) and can attach their modem through a cellular phone for Internet access.

TRAINING OPTIONS

To achieve the optimal benefit from any computer or software package, you must be trained in its use. There are a number of ways that this can be accomplished:

- the company from which the computer was purchased may provide personnel to train you and other staff members
- a user manual will come with your system. You can refer to it when you have problems
- help screens installed with every software package allow the user to self-teach. The disadvantage of this method is that it is often time consuming
- most software packages come with a tutorial. This is an on-screen short course on the use of the software
- most computer manufacturers and software programs will have a service called a help desk, which provides technical support. It is usually accessed by calling a toll-free number and is manned by computer professionals who can answer your questions concerning the system.

A combination of these methods is the best approach to learning about your computer and software.

COMPUTER ETHICS

The computer is a must in all health care facilities. Its capabilities are endless. It can, however, lead to invasion of patients' privacy and unethical behavior. Some key points to keep in mind are:

- never give out your login password. New employees must be issued their own password
- never leave a screen open with patient information and walk away from the computer. Exit the file
- only key people need access to sensitive patient information. Some programs, such as those with laboratory results, should have individual passwords
- do not use the office Internet access for your own pleasure. It is inappropriate to surf the Internet for personal reasons while at work
- e-mails should be read only by the person to whom they were sent. To avoid conflicts, each health care professional should have his or her own e-mail account, and the facility should have a generic e-mail address. It is never appropriate for you to receive personal e-mail messages on the office's e-mail address. It is also inappropriate to access your personal e-mail while at work
- sensitive patient data should not be sent via e-mail from one facility to the other unless it is clearly known that the recipient of the e-mail is the only one with access to it
- do not take advantage of your position in the medical field. Remember, you have a legal and ethical responsibility to protect patient information.

Procedure 3-1

Searching on the Internet

Equipment/Supplies

- Computer with Web browser software
- Modem
- Active Internet connection account

Steps	Purpose
1. Connect your computer to the Internet.	An Internet connection is necessary to search the Internet.
2. Locate a search engine.	A search engine is necessary to find information on the Internet.
3. Select two or three key words and type them at the appropriate place on the Web page.	Key words tell the search engine what to look for.
4. View the number of search results. If no sites were found, check spelling and retype or choose new key words.	The search engine was unable to find sites that can provide the information you requested.
5. If the search produced a long list, do an advanced search and refine your key words.	Reading through numerous sites is not time efficient.
6. Select an appropriate site and open its home page.	This allows you to view the information on the website.
7. If you are satisfied with the site's information, either download the material or bookmark the page. If you are unsatisfied with its information, either visit a site listed on the results page or return to the search engine.	Downloading or bookmarking the information gives you access to it in the future.
8. Complete this task within 10 minutes.	Quickly and effectively searching the Internet is necessary for good time management.

Summary

Computers are an essential piece of technology in the health care facility. As an allied health professional you will use the computer for both clinical and administrative tasks. Computers will help you perform your job more efficiently, timely, and professionally. Computers also promote good patient care. You will be able to communicate with various health care professionals by using electronic mail. The Internet plays a key role in medicine. Patients and health care professionals use the Internet to find new medical cures and for seeking current information about various health topics. You will need to be able to navigate the Web quickly and safely. It is essential that you stay abreast of computer technology, as it changes and improves daily.

Critical Thinking Challenges

1. Log on to the Internet and locate a search engine. Search for a medical topic. It can be administrative or clinical. What are your key words? How many sites are listed? Now, using the same key words, use the advanced search engine. How many sites are listed? What are the benefits of using the advanced search method?
2. Select any five Web addresses listed in this chapter. View their home page. What benefits did the sites offer? What information or topics were missing or appeared inaccurate?
3. Review Box 3-2 about how to select a site safely. Find three websites that use these types of phrases or words. Do you think these sites are misleading? Do you think they pose a danger to patients?

4. Create a patient education pamphlet about the Internet. The pamphlet may focus on a particular disease process or contain broad information. Make sure you provide at least six Web addresses.

Answers to Checkpoint Questions

1. The two types of Internet connections that are recommended for downloading large files are DSL and cable.
2. The encryption feature scrambles messages as they leave your site and unscrambles them when they arrive at the receiver's site.
3. You cannot be 100% guaranteed that your e-mail messages are secure, but you can take many steps to safeguard them.
4. A search engine allows you to find the sites that will have the information that you need quickly and efficiently.
5. A literary search is different because it is searching for a professional journal article that addresses a topic versus searching for general information.
6. Three safety tips that you need to teach patients about buying medications online are: (1) buy medications only from a site with a VIPPS certification; (2) buy only medications for which they have prescriptions; and (3) buy medications only from sites within the United States.
7. An intranet is a private network of computers; the Internet is a global network of computers.
8. A virtual chart is a paperless chart that holds all necessary documents on the computer.

 Websites

OSHA ergonomics
www.osha-slc.gov/SLTC/ergonomics/index.html
Websites that offer additional information
www.tifaq.com
www.healthfinder.gov
www.medlineplus.gov
www.healthcentral.com
www.Mayoclinic.com
www.familydoctor.org
www.raredisease.org (this site has a database of over 1,000 rare diseases and over 900 drugs that can be used to treat rare diseases)

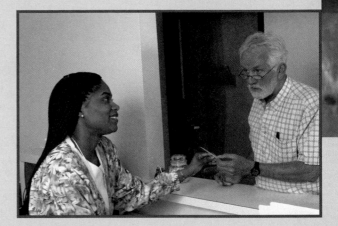

Anatomy and Physiology with Medical Terminology

4

Basic Medical Terminology Components

CHAPTER OBJECTIVES

In this chapter, you'll learn:

1. To describe the origin of medical language.
2. To analyze the component parts of a medical term.
3. To list basic prefixes, suffixes, and combining forms.
4. To use basic prefixes, suffixes, and combining forms to build medical terms.
5. To explain common rules for proper medical term formation, pronunciation, and spelling.

MOST MEDICAL TERMS STEM from Greek or Latin origins. These date to the founding of modern medicine by the Greeks and the influence of Latin when it was the universal language in the Western world. Other languages, such as German and French, have also influenced medical terms, and many new terms are derived from English, which is considered the universal language. Most terms related to diagnosis and surgery have Greek origin, and most anatomical terms can be traced to Latin.

> ## ETYMOLOGY
>
> The Greek root *etymon* refers to that which is true or genuine. Etymology is the study of the origin and development of words from the source language, original meaning, and history of usage.

Once you learn the basic medical term structure and memorize the most common term components (prefixes, suffixes, and combining forms), you can get the meaning of most medical terms by defining their parts. Those mysterious words, which are almost frightening at first, will soon no longer be a concern. You will analyze each term with your newly acquired knowledge and the help of a good medical dictionary.

This chapter lists common prefixes, suffixes, and a selected number of common combining forms. The basic rules for proper medical term formation, pronunciation, and spelling are also presented here.

The key to success in building a medical vocabulary is the groundwork you do now by making flash cards and memorizing the basic term components in this chapter. The work will pay big dividends if you do.

ANALYSIS OF TERM COMPONENTS

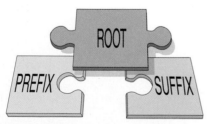

Most medical terms have three components: root, suffix, and prefix.

Root and Suffix

Each term is formed by combining at least one root, the foundation or subject of the word, and a suffix, the ending that modifies and gives essential meaning to the root. For example, in lipemia,

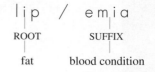

lip / emia
ROOT   SUFFIX
fat   blood condition

Lip (fat), the root, is the subject. It is modified by the suffix (emia) to indicate a condition of fat in the blood. Note that each component is dependent on the other to express meaning.

Note: lipemia is synonymous with lipidemia (formed from lip, oid, and emia)

Prefix

The prefix is a word structure placed at the beginning of a term when needed to further modify the root or roots. For example, in hyperlipemia

hyper / lip / emia
PREFIX   ROOT   SUFFIX
excessive   fat   blood condition

The addition of the prefix, hyper, modifies the root to denote excessive fat in the blood.

Additional Roots

Often a medical term is formed of two or more roots. For example, in hyperlipoproteinemia

hyper / lip / o / protein / emia
PREFIX   ROOT   VOWEL   ROOT   SUFFIX
excessive   fat   protein   blood condition

In this term, the additional root, protein (joined to lip by the vowel "o"), further defines the word to indicate an excessive amount of fat and protein in the blood.

Combining Vowels and Combining Forms

When a medical term has more than one root, each is joined by a vowel, usually an o. As shown in the term hyper/lip/o/protein/emia, the o links the two roots and fosters easier pronunciation. This vowel is known as a *combining vowel;* o is the most common combining vowel (i is the second most common) and is used so frequently to join root to root or root to suffix that it is routinely attached to the root and presented as a *combining form:*

l i p   ROOT

l i p / o   COMBINING FORM (ROOT WITH COMBINING VOWEL ATTACHED)

This text lists combining forms for easier term formation and analysis.

QUICK REVIEW

Complete the following sentences:

1. Most medical terms have three basic parts: the _____ *root*, *suffix*, and *prefix*.
2. The root is the *foundation or subject* of the term.
3. The *suffix* is the word ending that modifies and gives essential meaning to the root.
4. The *prefix* is a word structure at the beginning of a term that further modifies the root.
5. Often a medical term is formed of *two* _____ or more roots.
6. When a medical term has more than one root, it is joined together by a *combining vowel* (usually an *o*).
7. A combining form is a *root* with a *vowel* attached.

QUICK REVIEW ANSWERS

1. root, suffix, prefix
2. foundation or subject
3. suffix
4. prefix
5. two
6. combining vowel, o
7. root, vowel

RULES FOR FORMING AND SPELLING MEDICAL TERMS

Memorizing and spelling basic medical word components are the first steps for learning how to form medical terms. The next step is to construct the words using the following rules:

1. A combining vowel is used to join root to root as well as root to any suffix beginning with a consonant:

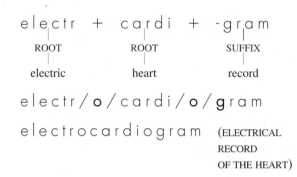

electr + cardi + -gram
ROOT   ROOT   SUFFIX
electric heart   record

electr/o/cardi/o/gram

electrocardiogram (ELECTRICAL RECORD OF THE HEART)

2. A combining vowel is *not* used before a suffix that begins with a vowel:

vas + ectomy
ROOT   SUFFIX
vessel excision

vas/ectomy

vasectomy (EXCISION OF A VESSEL)

3. If the root ends in a vowel and the suffix begins with the same vowel, drop the final vowel from the root and do not use a combining vowel:

cardi + itis
ROOT   SUFFIX
heart   inflammation

card/itis

carditis (INFLAMMATION OF THE HEART)

4. Most often, a combining vowel is inserted between two roots even when the second root begins with a vowel:

cardi + esophag + eal

| ROOT | ROOT | SUFFIX |
| heart | esophagus | pertaining to |

cardi/o/esophageal

cardioesophageal   (PERTAINING TO THE HEART AND ESOPHAGUS)

5. Occasionally, when a prefix ends in a vowel and the root begins with a vowel, the final vowel is dropped from the prefix:

para + enter + al

| PREFIX | ROOT | SUFFIX |
| alongside of | intestine | pertaining to |

par/enter/al

parenteral   (PERTAINING TO ALONGSIDE OF THE INTESTINE)

Breaking down and defining the components in a term often clues you to its meaning. Frequently, however, you must consult a medical dictionary to obtain a precise definition. Take a moment to look up *parenteral,* so you understand the complete meaning.

Note: There are many exceptions to these rules. Follow the basic guidelines, but be prepared to accept exceptions as you encounter them. Rely on your medical dictionary for additional guidance.

DEFINING MEDICAL TERMS THROUGH WORD STRUCTURE ANALYSIS

You can usually define a term by interpreting the suffix first, then the prefix (if present), then the succeeding root or roots. For example, in pericarditis,

peri / card / itis

PREFIX	ROOT	SUFFIX
2	3	1
around	heart	inflammation

pericarditis   (INFLAMMATION AROUND THE HEART)

You sense the basic meaning of this term by understanding its components; however, the dictionary clarifies that the term refers to inflammation of the pericardium, the sac that encloses the heart.

Note: Beginning students often have difficulty differentiating between prefixes and roots (or combining forms) because the root appears first in a medical term when a prefix is not used. It is important to memorize the most common prefixes so that you can tell the difference. Also, keep in mind that a prefix is only used as needed to further modify the root or roots.

QUICK REVIEW

1. A combining vowel is used to join root to root as well as root to any suffix beginning with a consonant.
2. A combining vowel is not used before a suffix that begins with a vowel.
3. If the root ends in a vowel and the suffix begins with the same vowel, drop the final vowel from the root and do not use a combining vowel.
4. Most often, a combining vowel is inserted between two roots even when the second root begins with a vowel.
5. Occasionally, when a prefix ends in a vowel and the root begins with a vowel, the final vowel is dropped from the prefix.

Identify which of the rules listed above were applied when forming the following terms:

1. angi + -ectasis = angi/ectasis *2*

2. hemat + -logy = hemato/logy *1*

3. oste + -ectomy = ost/ectomy *3*

4. electr + encephal + -gram = electro/encephalo/gram *4, 1*

5. para- + umbilic + -al = par/umbilic/al *5, 2*

6. vas + -ectomy = vas/ectomy *2*

7. arteri + -itis = arter/itis *3*

8. gastr + enter + -cele = gastro/entero/cele *1, 4*

9. gastr + -tomy = gastro/tomy *1*

10. hypo + ox + -ia = hyp/ox/ia *5, 2*

QUICK REVIEW ANSWERS

1. 2	5. 5, 2	9. 1
2. 1	6. 2	10. 5, 2
3. 3	7. 3	
4. 4, 1	8. 4, 1	

FORMATION OF MEDICAL TERMS

Most medical terms build from the root. Prefixes and suffixes are attached to the root to modify its meaning. Often two or more roots are linked before being modified. The following are examples of the various patterns of medical term formation using the root cardi (heart) as a base. Note the rules used for forming each term.

Root/Suffix

cardi / ac

HEART   PERTAINING TO
(pertaining to the heart)

Prefix/Root/Suffix

epi / card / ium

UPON   HEART   TISSUE
(tissue upon the heart, i.e., external lining of the heart)

Prefix/Prefix/Root/Suffix

sub / endo / cardi / al

BENEATH   WITHIN   HEART   PERTAINING TO
(pertaining to beneath and within the heart)

Root/Combining Vowel/Suffix

cardi / o / logy

HEART   STUDY OF
(study of the heart)

Root/Combining Vowel/Root/Suffix

cardi / o / pulmon / ary

HEART   LUNG   PERTAINING TO
(pertaining to the heart and lungs)

Root/Combining Vowel/Suffix (symptomatic)

cardi / o / dynia

HEART   PAIN
(pain in the heart)

Root/Combining Vowel/Suffix (diagnostic)

cardi / o / rrhexis

HEART   RUPTURE
(a rupture of the heart)

Root/Combining Vowel/Suffix (operative)

cardi / o / rrhaphy

HEART   SUTURE
(a suture of the heart)

A Few Exceptions

As noted above, most medical terms are formed by the combination of a root or roots modified by suffixes and prefixes. Occasionally, terms are formed by a root alone or a combination of roots.

EXAMPLES

duct

ROOT

to lead

ovi / duct

ROOT   ROOT

egg   to lead

Oviduct refers to the uterine tube.

Sometimes, you will find a term formed from the combination of a prefix and a suffix.

EXAMPLE

meta   /   stasis

PREFIX   SUFFIX

beyond, after,   stop or stand
or change

Metastasis refers to the spread of a disease, such as cancer, from one location to another.

QUICK REVIEW

Analyze the following terms by separating each component, and then define the individual elements:

1. gastric _____ *gastr/ic* _____

2. epigastric _____ *epi/gastr/ic* _____

3. gastrocardiac _____ *gastr/o/cardi/ac* _____

4. epigastralgia _____ *epi/gastr/algia* _____

5. gastroscopy _____ *gastr/o/scopy* _____

6. epigastrocele _____ *epi/gastr/o/cele* _____

7. gastrotomy _____ *gastr/o/tomy* _____

8. epigastrorrhaphy _____ *epi/gastr/o/rrhaphy* _____

QUICK REVIEW ANSWERS

1. gastr/ic   pertaining to the stomach
2. epi/gastr/ic   pertaining to upon the stomach
3. gastr/o/cardi/ac or gastro/cardi/ac   pertaining to the stomach and heart
4. epi/gastr/algia   pain upon the stomach
5. gastr/o/scopy or gastro/scopy   examination of the stomach
6. epi/gastr/o/cele or epi/gastro/cele   pouching or hernia upon the stomach
7. gastr/o/tomy or gastro/tomy   incision in the stomach
8. epi/gastr/o/rrhaphy or epi/gastro/rrhaphy   suture upon the stomach

SPELLING MEDICAL TERMS

Correct spelling of medical terms is crucial for communication among health care professionals. Careless spelling causes misunderstandings that can have serious consequences. The following are some of the pitfalls to avoid.

1. Some words sound exactly the same but are spelled differently and have different meanings. Context is the clue to spelling. For example,

   i l e u m   (PART OF THE INTESTINE)

   i l i u m   (PART OF THE HIP BONE)

   s i t o l o g y   (STUDY OF FOOD)

   c y t o l o g y   (STUDY OF CELLS)

2. Other words sound similar but are spelled differently and have different meanings. For example,

   a b d u c t i o n   (TO DRAW AWAY FROM)

   a d d u c t i o n   (TO DRAW TOWARD)

   h e p a t o m a   (LIVER TUMOR)

   h e m a t o m a   (BLOOD TUMOR)

   a p h a g i a   (INABILITY TO SWALLOW)

   a p h a s i a   (INABILITY TO SPEAK)

3. When letters are silent in a term, they risk being omitted when spelling the word. For example,

   pt has a "t" sound if found at the beginning of a term [e.g., pterygium, but both the "p" and "t" are pronounced when found within a term [e.g., nephroptosis (nef-rop-tō'sis)]

   ph has an "f" sound (e.g., diaphragm)

   ps has an "s" sound (e.g., psychology)

4. Some words have more than one accepted spelling. For example,

   o r t h o p e d i c   ORTHOPAEDIC (BRITISH)

   l e u k o c y t e   LEUCOCYTE (BRITISH)

5. Some combining forms have the same meaning but different origins that compete for usage. For example, there are three combining forms referring to the uterus:

   h y s t e r / o   (GREEK)

   m e t r / o   (GREEK)

   u t e r / o   (LATIN)

Acceptable Term Formations

As you learn medical terms, you can have fun experimenting with creating words, such as glyco (sweet) + cardio (heart) = sweetheart! However, in the real medical world, the word is formed when the term is coined. Often there seems to be no reason why a particular word form became acceptable. That is why you should check your medical dictionary when in doubt about the spelling, formation, or precise meaning.

RULES OF PRONUNCIATION

When you first learn to pronounce medical terms, the task can seem insurmountable. The first time you open your mouth to say a term is a tense moment for those who want to get it right! The best preparation is to study the basic rules of pronunciation, repeat the words after hearing them pronounced on the CD-ROM accompanying this text and/or after your instructor has said them, and try to keep the company of others who use medical language. There is nothing like the validation you get from the fact that no one laughed or snarled at you when you said something "medical" for the very first time! Your confidence will build with every word you use.

Following are some helpful shortcuts:

Shortcuts to Pronunciation

Consonant	Example
c (before a, o, u) = k	cavity colon cure
c (before e, i) = s	cephalic cirrhosis
ch = k	cholesterol
g (before a, o, u) = g	gallstone gonad gurney

Consonant	Example
g (before e, i) = j	generic giant
ph = f	phase
pn = n	pneumonia
ps = s	psychology
pt = t	ptosis pterygium
rh = r	rhythm
rrh = r	hemorrhoid
x = z (as first letter)	xerosis

The Phonetic System

Phonetic spelling for pronunciation of most medical terms in this text is in parentheses below the term. The phonetic system used is basic and has only a few standard rules. The macron and breve are the two diacritical marks used. The macron (¯) is placed over vowels that have a long sound:

ā	day
ē	be
ī	kite
ō	no
ū	unit

The breve (˘) is placed over vowels that have a short sound:

ă	alone
ĕ	ever
ĭ	pit
ŏ	ton
ŭ	sun

The primary accent (´) is placed after the syllable that is stressed when saying the word. Monosyllables do not have a stress mark. Other syllables are separated by hyphens.

QUICK REVIEW

1. The *pt* in *pterygium* has a/an __t__ sound.

2. The *ch* in the word *chronic* has a/an __k__ sound.

3. The *c* in the word *cirrhosis* has a/an __s__ sound.

4. The *x* in *xerosis* has a/an __z__ sound.

5. The *g* in *genital* has a/an __j__ sound.

6. The *pn* in *pneumatic* has a/an __n__ sound.

QUICK REVIEW ANSWERS

1. t	4. z
2. k	5. j
3. s	6. n

SINGULAR AND PLURAL FORMS

Most often, plurals are formed by adding -s or -es to the end of a singular form. The following are common exceptions.

Singular		Plural	
Ending	**Example**	**Ending**	**Example**
-a	vertebra	-ae	vertebrae
-is	diagnosis	-es	diagnoses
-ma	condyloma	-mata	condylomata
-on	phenomenon	-a	phenomena
-um	bacterium	-a	bacteria
-us[a]	fungus	-i	fungi
-ax	thorax	-aces	thoraces
-ex	apex	-ices	apices
-ix	appendix	-ices	appendices
-y	myopathy	-ies	myopathies

[a]Viruses and sinuses are not exceptions.

QUICK REVIEW

Convert the following singular forms to plural:

1. bulla _bullae_

2. speculum _specula_

3. fungus _fungi_

4. stoma _stomata_

5. anomaly _anomalies_

6. prognosis _prognoses_

QUICK REVIEW ANSWERS

1. bullae	4. stomata
2. specula	5. anomalies
3. fungi	6. prognoses

COMMON PREFIXES

Following is a list of commonly used prefixes organized within categories. A hyphen is placed after each prefix to indicate its link at the beginning of a medical term. Each includes a term example. Appendix A includes a summary list of prefixes in alphabetical order.

Prefix	Meaning	Example
NEGATION		
a-, an-	without	aphonia (*without* voice or sound)
		anaerobic (pertaining to *without* air)
anti-, contra-	against or opposed to	anticoagulant (*against* clotting)
		contraception (*opposed* to becoming pregnant)
de-	from, down, or not	decapitate [separation of the head (caput) *from* the body]
POSITION/DIRECTION		
ab-	away from	abnormal (pertaining to *away from* normal)
ad-	to, toward, or near	adhesion (*to* stick to)
circum-, peri-	around	circumvascular (pertaining to *around* a vessel)
		periosteum (pertaining to *around* bone)
dia-, trans-	across or through	dialysis [dissolution *across* or *through* (a membrane)]
		transmission (to send *across* or *through*)
e-, ec-, ex-	out or away	edentia (condition of teeth *out*) [dent/o=teeth]
		eccentric (pertaining to *away* from center)
		excise (to cut *out*) [cis/o=to cut]
ecto-, exo-, extra-	outside	ectopic (pertaining to a place *outside*)
		exocrine (denoting secretion *outside*)
		extravascular (pertaining to *outside* a vessel)
en-, endo-, intra-	within	encapsulate (*within* little box)
		endoscope (instrument for examination *within*)
		intradermal (pertaining to *within* skin)
epi-	upon	epidermal (pertaining to *upon* the skin)
inter-	between	intercostal (pertaining to *between* the ribs) [cost/o=rib]
meso-	middle	mesomorphic (pertaining to *middle* form)
meta-	beyond, after, or change	metastasis [*beyond* stopping or standing (spread of disease from one part of the body to another)]
		metamorphosis (condition of *change* in form)
para-	alongside of or abnormal	paramedic (pertaining to *alongside of* medicine)
		paranoia (condition of *abnormal* thinking)
retro-	backward or behind	retrograde (going *backward*)
sub-, infra-	below or under	infraumbilical (pertaining to *below* the navel) [umbilic/o=navel]
		sublingual (pertaining to *under* the tongue) [lingu/o=tongue]
QUANTITY OR MEASUREMENT		
bi-	two or both	bilateral (pertaining to *two or both* sides)
hemi-, semi-	half	hemicephalic (pertaining to *half* of the head)
		semilunar (pertaining to *half* moon) [luna=moon]

Prefix	Meaning	Example
hyper-	above or excessive	hyperlipemia (*excessive* fat in blood)
hypo-	below or deficient	hypothermia (condition of *below* normal temperature) [therm/o=heat]
macro-	large or long	macrocyte (*large* cell)
micro-	small	microlith (*small* stone)
mono-, uni-	one	monochromatic (pertaining to *one* color) [chromat/o=color]
		unilateral (pertaining to *one* side)
oligo-	few or deficient	oliguria (condition of *deficient* urine)
pan-	all	panacea (a cure-*all*)
poly-, multi-	many	polyphobia (condition of *many* fears)
		multicellular (pertaining to *many* cells)
quadr-	four	quadriplegia (paralysis of all *four* limbs)
super-, supra-	above or excessive	suprarenal (pertaining to *above* the kidney)
		supernumerary [*excessive* numbers (too many to count)]
tri-	three	triangle (*three* angles)
ultra-	beyond or excessive	ultrasonic (pertaining to *beyond* sound)
TIME		
ante-, pre-, pro-	before	antepartum (*before* labor)
		premature (*before* ripe)
		prognosis [*before* knowing (prediction of course and outcome of a disease)]
brady-	slow	bradycardia (condition of *slow* heart)
tachy-	fast	tachycardia (condition of *fast* heart)
post-	after or behind	postoperative [*after* operation (surgery)]
re-	again or back	reactivate (to make active *again*)
GENERAL		
con-, syn-, sym-	together or with	syndactylism (webbing *together* of toes or fingers) [dactyl/o=finger or toe]
		symbiosis (presence of life *together*) [bio=life]
		congenital (pertaining to being born *with*)
dys-	painful, difficult, or faulty	dysphonia [condition of *difficult* voice or sound (hoarseness)]
eu-	good or normal	eugenic (pertaining to *good* production)
neo-	new	neoplasia [a *new* (abnormal) formation]

COMMON COMBINING FORMS

Following are selected combining forms (roots with combining vowels attached) to give you a start toward building medical terms. Each is presented with a slash between the root and the combining vowel along with a term example.

Combining Forms

Combining Form	Meaning	Example
abdomin/o **lapar/o**	abdomen	abdominal (pertaining to *abdomen*) laparotomy (incision into the *abdomen*)
acr/o	extremity or topmost	acrodynia (pain in an *extremity*) acrophobia [exaggerated fear of *topmost* places (heights)]
aden/o	gland	adenoma (*gland* tumor)
aer/o	air or gas	aerobic (pertaining to *air*)
angi/o **vas/o** **vascul/o**	vessel	angioplasty (surgical repair of a blood *vessel*) vasectomy (excision of a *vessel*) vascular (pertaining to a *vessel*)
carcin/o	cancer	carcinogenic (pertaining to production of *cancer*)
cardi/o	heart	cardiologist (one who specializes in treatment of the *heart*)
cephal/o	head	cephalic (pertaining to the *head*)
cyan/o	blue	cyanotic (pertaining to *blue*)
cyt/o	cell	cytology (study of *cells*)
derm/o **dermat/o** **cutane/o**	skin	dermal (pertaining to the *skin*) dermatology (study of the *skin*) cutaneous (pertaining to the *skin*)
dextr/o	right or on the right side	dextrocardia (condition of the heart *on the right side*)
erythr/o	red	erythrocyte (*red* cell)
fibr/o	fiber	fibroma (*fiber* tumor)
gastr/o	stomach	gastric (pertaining to the *stomach*)
gen/o	origin or production	osteogenic (pertaining to *origin or production* in bone)
gluc/o **glucos/o** **glyc/o**	sugar	glucogenesis (origin or production of *sugar*) glucose (*sugar*) glycolysis (breakdown or dissolution of *sugar*)
hem/o **hemat/o**	blood	hemogram (record of *blood*) hematology (study of *blood*)
hepat/o	liver	hepatoma (tumor of the *liver*)
hydr/o	water	hydrophobia (exaggerated fear of *water*)
leuk/o	white	leukocyte (*white* cell)
lip/o	fat	lipoid (resembling *fat*)
lith/o	stone	lithiasis (formation or presence of a *stone*)
melan/o	black	melanoma (*black* tumor)
morph/o	form	morphology (study of *form*)
my/o **myos/o**	muscle	myocardium (heart *muscle*) myositis (inflammation of *muscle*)
nas/o **rhin/o**	nose	nasal (pertaining to the *nose*) rhinitis (inflammation of the *nose*)

Combining Form	Meaning	Example
necr/o	death	necrocytosis (condition or increase of cell *death*)
or/o	mouth	oral (pertaining to the *mouth*)
orth/o	straight, normal, or correct	orthostatic (pertaining to standing *straight*)
oste/o	bone	osteal (pertaining to *bone*)
path/o	disease	pathology (study of *disease*)
ped/o	child or foot	pediatrics (treatment of *child*) pedal (pertaining to the *foot*)
phob/o	exaggerated fear or sensitivity	hydrophobia (*exaggerated fear* of water) photophobia (*sensitivity* to light)
phon/o	voice or sound	phonic (pertaining to *voice* or sound)
plas/o	formation	dysplasia (condition of faulty *formation*)
pod/o	foot	podiatry (treatment of the *foot*)
psych/o	mind	psychology (study of the *mind*)
py/o	pus	pyopoiesis (formation of *pus*)
ren/o **nephr/o**	kidney	renal (pertaining to the *kidney*) nephrosis (condition of the *kidney*)
scler/o	hard	sclerosis (a condition of *hardness*)
sinistr/o	left or on the left side	sinistropedal (pertaining to the *left* foot)
son/o	sound	sonometer (an instrument to measure *sound*)
sten/o	narrow	stenosis (a condition of *narrow*)
therm/o	heat	thermometer (instrument for measuring *heat*)
tox/o **toxic/o**	poison	toxemia (*poison* in blood) toxicology (study of *poison*)
troph/o	nourishment or development	trophocyte (a cell that provides *nourishment*) hypertrophy (condition of excessive *development*)
ur/o **urin/o**	urine	urology (study of *urine*) urinary (pertaining to *urine*)

CANCER

Cancer is Latin for *crab*. The word is derived from the Greek word *karkinos* that was used by Hippocrates and other early writers and also means *crab*. Some authorities say the word was used because it describes the appearance of the disease; i.e., just as the crab's feet extend in all directions from its body, so can the disease extend in the human. Other authorities relate the term to the obstinacy of a crab in pursuing prey.

TOXIN

The Greek root *toxicon* means *arrow poison* and is derived from the word for the archer's bow. The Greeks often used darts and arrows coated with a poisonous substance.

COMMON SUFFIXES

Suffixes are endings that modify the root. They give the root essential meaning by forming a noun, verb, or adjective.

There are two types of suffixes: simple and compound. Simple suffixes form basic terms. For example, ic (pertaining to), a simple suffix, combined with the root gastr (stomach) forms the term gastric (pertaining to the stomach). Compound suffixes are formed by a combination of basic term components. For example, the root tom (to cut) combined with the simple suffix y (denoting a process of) forms the compound suffix tomy (incision); the compound suffix ectomy (excision or removal) is formed by a combination of the prefix ec (out) with the root tom (to cut) and the simple suffix y (a process of). Compound suffixes are added to the roots to provide a specific meaning. For example, hyster (a root meaning uterus) combined with ectomy forms hysterectomy (excision of the uterus). Noting the differences between simple and compound suffixes will help you analyze medical terms.

Suffixes in this text are divided into four categories:

- Symptomatic suffixes, which describe the evidence of illness
- Diagnostic suffixes, which provide the name of a medical condition
- Operative (surgical) suffixes, which describe a surgical treatment
- General suffixes, which have general applications

Commonly used suffixes follow in alphabetical order except for groups with the same meaning. A hyphen is placed before each to indicate their link at the end of a term.

Suffix	Meaning	Example
SYMPTOMATIC SUFFIXES (WORD ENDINGS THAT DESCRIBE EVIDENCE OF ILLNESS)		
-algia	pain	cephalalgia [*pain* in the head (headache)]
-dynia		cephalodynia [*pain* in the head (headache)]
-genesis	origin or production	pathogenesis (*origin or production* of disease)
-lysis	breaking down or dissolution	hemolysis (*breakdown* of blood)
-megaly	enlargement	hepatomegaly (*enlargement* of the liver)
-oid	resembling	lipoid (*resembling* fat)
-penia	abnormal reduction	leukopenia [*abnormal reduction* of white (blood cells)]
-rrhea	discharge	rhinorrhea (runny *discharge* from nose)
-spasm	involuntary contraction	vasospasm (*involuntary contraction* of a blood vessel)
DIAGNOSTIC SUFFIXES (WORD ENDINGS THAT DESCRIBE A CONDITION OR DISEASE)		
-cele	pouching or hernia	gastrocele (*pouching* of the stomach)
-ectasis	expansion or dilation	angiectasis (*expansion or dilation* of a blood vessel)
-emia	blood condition	hyperlipemia (*blood condition* of excessive fat)
-iasis	formation or presence of	lithiasis (*formation or presence of* a stone or stones)
-itis	inflammation	hepatitis (*inflammation* of the liver)
-malacia	softening	osteomalacia (*softening* of bone)
-oma	tumor	carcinoma (cancer *tumor*)
-osis	condition or increase	sclerosis (*condition* of being hard) leukocytosis (*increase* of white cells)
-phil **-philia**	attraction for	basophil (cell with an *attraction for* basic dyes) pneumophilia (condition that has an *attraction for* the lungs)

Suffix	Meaning	Example
-ptosis	falling or downward displacement	gastroptosis (*downward displacement* of the stomach)
-rrhage **-rrhagia**	to burst forth (usually blood)	hemorrhage (*to burst forth* blood)
-rrhexis	rupture	hepatorrhexis (*rupture* of the liver)

OPERATIVE SUFFIXES [WORD ENDINGS THAT DESCRIBE A SURGICAL (OPERATIVE) TREATMENT]

Suffix	Meaning	Example
-centesis	puncture for aspiration	abdominocentesis (*puncture for aspiration* of the abdomen)
-desis	binding	arthrodesis (*binding* together of a joint) [arthr/o=joint]
-ectomy	excision or removal	nephrectomy (*excision or removal* of a kidney)
-pexy	suspension or fixation	gastropexy [*fixation* of the stomach (to the abdominal wall)]
-plasty	surgical repair or reconstruction	rhinoplasty (*surgical repair* of the nose)
-rrhaphy	suture	osteorrhaphy (*suture* of bone)
-stomy	creation of an opening	gastrostomy (*creation of an opening* in the stomach)
-tomy	incision	laparotomy (*incision* into the abdomen)
-tripsy	crushing	lithotripsy (*crushing* of stone)

GENERAL SUFFIXES (SUFFIXES THAT HAVE GENERAL APPLICATIONS)

Noun Endings (suffixes that form a noun when combined with a root)

Suffix	Meaning	Example
-e	noun marker	erythrocyte (a red blood cell)
-ia **-ism**	condition of	phobia (*condition of* an exaggerated fear or sensitivity) alcoholism (*condition of* alcohol abuse)
-ium	structure or tissue	epigastrium [*structure* upon the stomach (region in the abdomen)] pericardium [*tissue* around the heart (sac enclosing the heart)]
-ation **-y**	condition or process of	starvation (*condition or process of* starving) adenopathy (*condition or process of* gland disease)

Adjective Endings (suffixes that mean "pertaining to" and form an adjective when combined with a root)

Suffix		Example
-ac		cardiac (*pertaining to* the heart)
-al	*or*	pedal (*pertaining to* the foot)
-ar		glandular (*pertaining to* a gland)
-ary		pulmonary (*pertaining to* the lung)
-eal		esophageal (*pertaining to* the esophagus)
-ic		toxic (*pertaining to* poison)
-ous		fibrous (*pertaining to* fiber)
-tic		cyanotic (*pertaining to* blue)

Diminutive Endings (suffixes meaning "small")

Suffix		Example
-icle		ventricle (*small* belly or pouch)
-ole		bronchiole (*small* airway)
-ula		macula (*small* spot)
-ule		pustule (*small* pimple)

Suffix	Meaning	Example
Other General Suffixes		
-gram	record	sonogram (*record* of sound)
-graph	instrument for recording	sonograph (*instrument for recording* sound)
-graphy	process of recording	sonography (*process of recording* sound)
-iatrics **-iatry**	treatment	pediatrics (*treatment* of children) psychiatry (*treatment* of the mind)
-ist	one who specializes in	pharmacist (*one who specializes in* drugs)
-logist	one who specializes in the study or treatment of	psychologist (*one who specializes in the study or treatment of* the mind)
-logy	study of	cytology (*study of* cells)
-meter	instrument for measuring	spirometer (*instrument for measuring* breathing) [spir/o= breathing]
-metry	process of measuring	spirometry (*process of measuring* breathing)
-poiesis	formation	hemopoiesis (*formation* of blood)
-scope	instrument for examination	endoscope (*instrument for examination* within)
-scopy	examination	endoscopy (*examination* within)
-stasis	stop or stand	hemostasis (*stop* blood) orthostasis (*stand* straight)

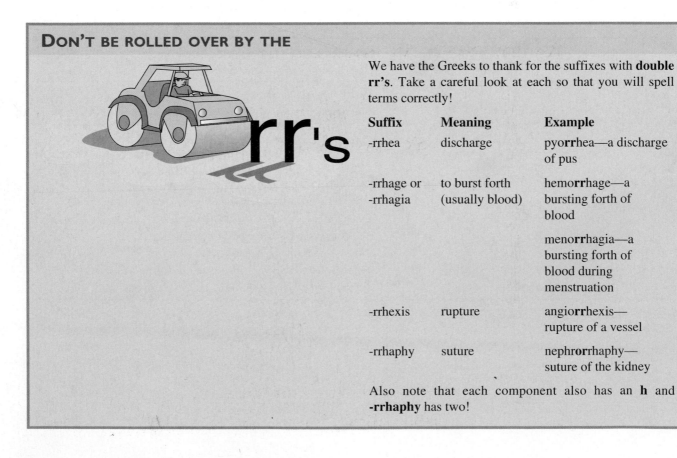

DON'T BE ROLLED OVER BY THE rr's

We have the Greeks to thank for the suffixes with **double rr's**. Take a careful look at each so that you will spell terms correctly!

Suffix	Meaning	Example
-rrhea	discharge	pyo**rr**hea—a discharge of pus
-rrhage or -rrhagia	to burst forth (usually blood)	hemo**rr**hage—a bursting forth of blood meno**rr**hagia—a bursting forth of blood during menstruation
-rrhexis	rupture	angio**rr**hexis— rupture of a vessel
-rrhaphy	suture	nephr**orr**haphy— suture of the kidney

Also note that each component also has an **h** and **-rrhaphy** has two!

PRACTICE EXERCISES

Kathi L. Sloat

For the following words, draw a line or lines to separate prefixes, roots, combining forms, and suffixes. Then define the word according to the meaning of: **P=prefix; R=root; CF=combining form; S=suffix.**

EXAMPLE

hyperlipemia

_____ / _____ / _____
P   R   S

hyper/lip/emia
P   R   S

DEFINITION: above or excessive/fat/blood condition

1. pancytopenia

pan / cyto / penia
P   CF   S

DEFINITION: all/cell/abnormal reduction

2. leukemia

leuk / emia
R   S

DEFINITION: white / blood condition

3. toxoid

tox / oid
R   S

DEFINITION: poison/resembling

4. mesomorphic

meso / morph / ic
P   R   S

DEFINITION: middle/form/pertaining to

5. acrodynia

acro / dynia
CF   S

DEFINITION: extremity/pain

6. metastasis

meta / stasis
P   S

DEFINITION: beyond /stop or stand

7. ultrasonography

ultra / sono / graphy
P   CF   S

DEFINITION: beyond or excessive/ sound/process of recording

8. tachycardia

tachy , _card_ , _ia_
  P   R   S

DEFINITION: _fast/heart/condition of_

9. pyopoiesis

pyo , _poiesis_
  CF   S

DEFINITION: _pus/formation_

10. adenitis

aden , _itis_
  R   S

DEFINITION: _gland/inflamation_

11. macrocephalous

macro , _cephal_ , _ous_
  P   R   S

DEFINITION: _large or long/head/pertaining to_

12. paracentesis

para , _centesis_
  P   S

DEFINITION: _alongside of or abnormal/puncture for aspiration_

13. microlithiasis

micro , _lith_ , _iasis_
  P   R   S

DEFINITION: _small/stone/formation or presence of_

14. orthopedic

ortho , _ped_ , _ic_
  CF   R   S

DEFINITION: _straight, normal or correct/foot/pertaining to_

15. angiomegaly

angio , _megaly_
  CF   S

DEFINITION: _vessel/enlargement_

16. psychiatry

psych , _iatry_
  R   S

DEFINITION: _mind/treatment_

17. carcinogenesis

carcino , _genesis_
  CF   S

DEFINITION: _cancer/origin or production_

18. nephrologist

nephro / _logist_
CF / S

DEFINITION: _kidney / one who specializes in the study or treatment of_

19. rhinostenosis

rhino / _sten_ / _osis_
CF / R / S

DEFINITION: _nose / narrow / condition or increase_

20. hypohydration

hypo / _hydr_ / _ation_
P / R / S

DEFINITION: _below or deficient / water / condition or process of_

21. aerogastralgia

aero / _gastr_ / _algia_
CF / R / S

DEFINITION: _air or gas / stomach / pain_

22. fibroma

fibr / _oma_
R / S

DEFINITION: _fiber / tumor_

23. necrophilia

necro / _philia_
CF / S

DEFINITION: _death / attraction for_

24. sclerosis

sclero / _osis_
R / S

DEFINITION: _hard / condition_

25. hemolysis

hemo / _lysis_
CF / S

DEFINITION: _blood / breaking down or dissolution_

26. acrophobia

acro / _phob_ / _ia_
CF / R / S

DEFINITION: _extremity / topmost / exaggerated fear or sensitivity / condition of_

27. cytometer

cyto / _meter_
CF / S

DEFINITION: _cell / instrument for measuring_

28. cyanotic

___cyano___ / ___tic___
    CF   S

DEFINITION: ___blue / pertaining to___

29. extravascular

___extra___ / ___vascul___ / ___ar___
    P   R   S

DEFINITION: ___outside / vessel / pertaining to___

30. hypertrophy

___hyper___ / ___troph___ / ___y___
    P   R   S

DEFINITION: ___above or excessive / nourishment or development / condition or process of___

Write in the appropriate prefix to complete the following terms:

31. __c__ nasal = *above* the nose
   a. para   b. peri   c. supra   d. infra   e. sub

32. __d__ activate = make active *again*
   a. de   b. retro   c. pro   d. re   e. hyper

33. __c__ operative = *before* surgery
   a. intra   b. post   c. pre   d. peri   e. circum

34. __b__ hydrated = *not* watered
   a. anti   b. de   c. ec   d. dys   e. contra

35. __e__ dermal = *across or through* the skin
   a. ecto   b. endo   c. intra   d. epi   e. trans

36. __c__ acute = *excessively* severe
   a. sub   b. hypo   c. super   d. oligo   e. pan

37. __b__ umbilical = *below or under* the navel
   a. hyper   b. infra   c. peri   d. para   e. pre

38. __a__ cardia = *outside* the heart
   a. exo   b. endo   c. retro   d. para   e. peri

39. __b__ phonia = *difficult* voice
   a. ab   b. dys   c. a   d. eu   e. para

40. __b__ duction = to turn *away from*
   a. ad   b. ab   c. ecto   d. pro   e. ante

41. __b__ phylaxis = to guard *before*
   a. retro   b. pro   c. post   d. peri   e. anti

42. __d__ vascular = *around* a blood vessel
   a. intra   b. inter   c. para   d. circum   e. endo

43. __c__ plegia = *half* paralysis
   a. quadri   b. peri   c. hemi   d. bi   e. mono

Match the following:

44. _f_ away from   a. retro-

45. _g_ between   b. peri-

46. _h_ alongside of   c. anti-

47. _b_ around   d. ecto-

48. _a_ behind   e. dia-

49. _j_ within   f. ab-

50. _c_ against or opposed to   g. inter-

51. _i_ without   h. para-

52. _d_ outside   i. an-

53. _e_ across or through   j. intra-

Give the meaning of the following prefixes:

54. poly- _many_   60. bi- _2 or both_

55. hypo- _below_   61. quadri- _four_

56. oligo- _few_   62. semi- _half_

57. mono- _one_   63. infra- _below or under_

58. pan- _all_   64. hyper- _above_

59. ultra- _beyond_

Match the following:

65. _c_ before   a. brady-

66. _d_ after   b. re-

67. _e_ fast   c. ante-

68. _a_ slow   d. post-

69. _b_ again   e. tachy-

Circle the correct meaning for the following term components:

70. a-
    a. double   b. both   c. two   (d.) without   e. against

71. pod/o
    a. child   (b.) foot   c. voice   d. sound   e. pus

72. or/o
    a. lip   b. nourishment   c. gland   (d.) mouth   e. normal

73. neo-
    a. birth   b. death   c. origin   (d.) new   e. disease

74. -plasty
    (a.) surgical repair   b. cancer   c. tumor   d. excision   e. incision

75. -ation
    a. measure   b. disease   c. tissue   d. pain   (e.) process

76. -tripsy
    a. nourishment   b. poison   (c.) crushing   d. incision   e. stone

77. -ectasis
    a. blood condition   b. formation of   (c.) expansion d. rupture   e. discharge

78. dextr/o
    a. hard   b. straight   (c.) right   d. left   e. long

Match the following:

79. __f__ black   a. tri-

80. __a__ three   b. leuk/o

81. __j__ red   c. cyan/o

82. __g__ four   d. dextr/o

83. __b__ white   e. uni-

84. __e__ one   f. melan/o

85. __c__ blue   g. quadri-

86. __k__ two   h. sinistr/o

87. __i__ few   i. oligo-

88. __d__ right   j. erythr/o

89. __h__ left   k. bi-

Circle the appropriate suffix for each of the following meanings:

90. record
    a. -meter   b. -metry   (c.) -gram   d. -graph   e. graphy

91. condition or increase
    a. -itis   b. -iasis   (c.) -osis   d. -ium   e. -ous

92. excision
    a. -tomy   b. -stomy   (c.) -ectomy   d. -centesis e. cele

93. pertaining to
    a. -ia   b. -ar   c. -ism   d. -ium   e. -icle

94. rupture
    a. -rrhagia   b. -rrhea   c. -rrhagia   d. -rrhexis   e. -megaly

95. small
    a. -ous   b. -eal   c. -ula   d. -ia   e. -ary

96. condition of
    a. -ism   b. -ium   c. -ule   d. -ic   e. al

Match the following terms related to the kidney with the definitions listed below:

nephrolysis   nephrostomy   nephroptosis   nephrotomy
nephritis   nephropexy   nephroma   nephrocele
nephrogenous   nephrolithiasis   nephrorrhaphy   nephrectomy

97. inflammation of the kidney _____ *nephritis* _____

98. dissolution or breakdown of the kidney _____ *nephrolysis* _____

99. incision in the kidney _____ *nephrotomy* _____

100. developing from the kidney _____ *nephrogenous* _____

101. surgical fixation of the kidney _____ *nephropexy* _____

102. creation of an opening in the kidney _____ *nephrostomy* _____

103. excision of the kidney _____ *nephrectomy* _____

104. presence of kidney stones _____ *nephrolithiasis* _____

105. kidney tumor _____ *nephroma* _____

106. hernia of the kidney _____ *nephrocele* _____

107. suture of the kidney _____ *nephrorrhaphy* _____

108. downward displacement of the kidney _____ *nephroptosis* _____

Circle the operative term in each of the following lists:

109. a. nephroptosis   b. hemolysis   c. angiectasis   d. colostomy   e. necrosis

110. a. vasorrhaphy   b. hematoma   c. gastrocele   d. endoscope   e. cardiorrhexis

111. a. morphologic   b. adenolysis   c. abdominocentesis   d. osteomalacia   e. polyrrhea

Fill in the blanks for the following regarding singular/plural forms:

112. An ovum is an egg produced by an ovary. There are two *ovaries* in the

female that produce eggs or *ova* .

113. The spread of cancer to a distant organ is called metastasis. The spread of cancer to more than one organ is _metastases_.

114. A verruca is a wart. The term for several warts is _verrucae_.

115. Condylomata are genital warts. One genital wart is a _condyloma_.

116. Indices is a plural form of _index_.

117. A thrombus is a clot. Several clots are termed _thrombi_.

Circle the correct spelling:

118. a. nephoraphy   b. nephorrapy   c. nephrorrhaphy   d. nephorrhapy

119. a. abdominoscopy   b. abdemenoscopi   c. abdomenscopy   d. abdominoschope

120. a. perrycardium   b. pericardium   c. periocardium   d. parcardium

5

Organization of the Human Body

CHAPTER OBJECTIVES

In this chapter, you'll learn:

1. To define the terms *anatomy* and *physiology*.
2. To describe the organization of the body from chemicals to the whole organism.
3. To list 11 body systems and give the general function of each.
4. To define *metabolism* and name the two phases of metabolism.
5. To briefly explain the role of ATP in the body.
6. To differentiate between extracellular and intracellular fluids.
7. To define and give examples of homeostasis.
8. To compare negative feedback and positive feedback.
9. To list and define the main directional terms for the body.
10. To list and define the three planes of division of the body.
11. To name the subdivisions of the dorsal and ventral cavities.
12. To name and locate subdivisions of the abdomen.
13. To name the basic units of length, weight, and volume in the metric system.
14. To define the metric prefixes *kilo-, centi-, milli-,* and *micro-*.
15. To show how word parts are used to build words related to the body's organization (see Word Anatomy at the end of the chapter).

KEY TERMS

anabolism	cell	homeostasis	organ
anatomy	dissect	liter	physiology
ATP	feedback	metabolism	system
catabolism	gram	meter	tissue

STUDIES OF the normal structure and functions of the body are the basis for all medical sciences. It is only from understanding the normal that one can analyze what is going wrong in cases of disease. These studies give one an appreciation for the design and balance of the human body and for living organisms in general.

STUDIES OF THE HUMAN BODY

The scientific term for the study of body structure is **anatomy** (ah-NAT-o-me). The *–tomy* part of this word in Latin means "cutting," because a fundamental way to learn about the human body is to cut it apart, or **dissect** (dis-sekt) it. **Physiology** (fiz-e-OL-o-je) is the term for the study of how the body functions, and is based on a Latin term meaning "nature." Anatomy and physiology are closely related— that is, form and function are intertwined. The stomach, for example, has a pouch-like shape because it stores food during digestion. The cells in the lining of the stomach are tightly packed to prevent strong digestive juices from harming underlying tissue.

Levels of Organization

All living things are organized from very simple levels to more complex levels (Fig. 5-1). Living matter is derived from simple chemicals. These chemicals are formed into the complex substances that make living **cells**—the basic units of all life. Specialized groups of cells form **tissues,** and tissues may function together as **organs.** Organs working together for the same general purpose make up the body **systems.** All of the systems work together to maintain the body as a whole organism.

 Checkpoint Question

1. In studying the human body, one may concentrate on its structure or its function. What are these two studies called?

BODY SYSTEMS

Most studies of the human body are organized according to the individual systems, as listed below, grouped according to their general functions.

- Protection, support, and movement
  - The **integumentary** (in-teg-u-MEN-tar-e) **system.** The word *integument* (in-TEG-u-ment*)* means skin. The skin with its associated structures is considered a separate body system. The structures associated with the skin include the hair, the nails, and the sweat and oil glands.
  - The **skeletal system.** The basic framework of the body is a system of 206 bones and the joints between them, collectively known as the **skeleton.**

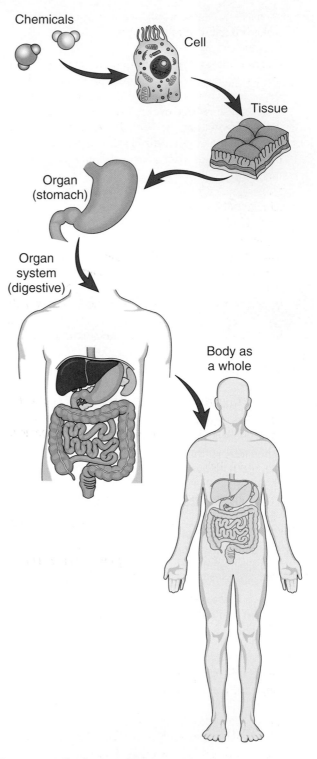

FIGURE 5-1. Levels of organization. The organ shown is the stomach, which is part of the digestive system.

- The **muscular system.** The muscles in this system are attached to the bones and produce movement of the skeleton. These skeletal muscles also give the body structure, protect organs, and maintain posture. The two other types of muscles are smooth muscle, present in the walls of body organs, such as the stomach and intestine, and cardiac muscle, which makes up the wall of the heart.

- Coordination and control
  - The **nervous system.** The brain, the spinal cord, and the nerves make up this complex system by which the body is controlled and coordinated. The organs of special sense (the eyes, ears, taste buds, and organs of smell), together with the receptors for pain, touch, and other generalized senses, receive stimuli from the outside world. These stimuli are converted into impulses that are transmitted to the brain. The brain directs the body's responses to these outside stimuli and also to stimuli coming from within the body. Such higher functions as memory and reasoning also occur in the brain.
  - The **endocrine** (EN-do-krin) **system.** The scattered organs known as endocrine glands are grouped together because they share a similar function. All produce special substances called hormones, which regulate such body activities as growth, food utilization within the cells, and reproduction. Examples of endocrine glands are the thyroid, pituitary, and adrenal glands.
- Circulation
  - The **cardiovascular system.** The heart and blood vessels make up the system that pumps blood to all the body tissues, bringing with it nutrients, oxygen, and other needed substances. This system then carries waste materials away from the tissues to points where they can be eliminated.
  - The **lymphatic system.** Lymphatic vessels assist in circulation by bringing fluids from the tissues back to the blood. Organs of the lymphatic system, such as the tonsils, thymus gland, and the spleen, play a role in immunity, protecting against disease. The lymphatic system also aids in the absorption of digested fats through special vessels in the intestine. The fluid that circulates in the lymphatic system is called lymph. The lymphatic and cardiovascular systems together make up the circulatory system.
- Nutrition and fluid balance
  - The **respiratory system.** This system includes the lungs and the passages leading to and from the lungs. The purpose of this system is to take in air and conduct it to the areas designed for gas exchange. Oxygen passes from the air into the blood and is carried to all tissues by the cardiovascular system. In like manner, carbon dioxide, a gaseous waste product, is taken by the circulation from the tissues back to the lungs to be expelled.
  - The **digestive system.** This system comprises all the organs that are involved with taking in nutrients (foods), converting them into a form that body cells can use, and absorbing these nutrients into the circulation. Organs of the digestive system include the mouth, esophagus, stomach, intestine, liver, and pancreas.

- The **urinary system.** The chief purpose of the urinary system is to rid the body of waste products and excess water. The main components of this system are the kidneys, the ureters, the bladder, and the urethra. (Note that some waste products are also eliminated by the digestive and respiratory systems and by the skin.)
- Production of offspring
  - The **reproductive system.** This system includes the external sex organs and all related internal structures that are concerned with the production of offspring.

The number of systems may vary in different lists. Some, for example, show the sensory system as separate from the nervous system. Others have a separate entry for the immune system, which protects the body from foreign matter and invading organisms. The immune system is identified by its function rather than its structure and includes elements of both the cardiovascular and lymphatic systems. Bear in mind that even though the systems are studied as separate units, they are interrelated and must cooperate to maintain health.

METABOLISM AND ITS REGULATION

All the life-sustaining reactions that go on within the body systems together make up **metabolism** (meh-TAB-o-lizm). Metabolism can be divided into two types of activities:

- In **catabolism** (kah-TAB-o-lizm), complex substances are broken down into simpler compounds (Fig. 5-2) The breakdown of the nutrients in food yields simple chemical building blocks and energy to power cell activities.
- In **anabolism** (ah-NAB-o-lizm), simple compounds are used to manufacture materials needed for growth, function, and repair of tissues. Anabolism is the building phase of metabolism.

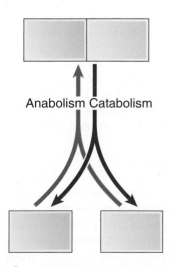

Anabolism Catabolism

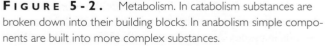

FIGURE 5-2. Metabolism. In catabolism substances are broken down into their building blocks. In anabolism simple components are built into more complex substances.

CLINICAL PERSPECTIVES

Homeostatic Imbalance: When Feedback Fails

Each body structure contributes in some way to homeostasis, often through feedback mechanisms. The nervous and endocrine systems are particularly important in feedback. The nervous system's electrical signals react quickly to changes in homeostasis, while the endocrine system's chemical signals (hormones) react more slowly but over a longer time. Often both systems work together to maintain homeostasis.

As long as feedback keeps conditions within normal limits, the body remains healthy, but if feedback cannot maintain these conditions, the body enters a state of *homeostatic imbalance*. Moderate imbalance causes illness and disease, while severe imbalance causes death. At some level, all illnesses and diseases can be linked to homeostatic imbalance.

For example, feedback mechanisms closely monitor and maintain normal blood pressure. When blood pressure rises, negative feedback mechanisms lower it to normal limits. If these mechanisms fail, *hypertension* (high blood pressure) develops. Hypertension further damages the cardiovascular system and, if untreated, may lead to death. With mild hypertension, lifestyle changes in diet, exercise, and stress management may lower blood pressure sufficiently, whereas severe hypertension often requires drug therapy. The various types of antihypertensive medication all help negative feedback mechanisms lower blood pressure.

Feedback mechanisms also regulate body temperature. When body temperature falls, negative feedback mechanisms raise it back to normal limits, but if these mechanisms fail and body temperature continues to drop, *hypothermia* develops. Its main effects are uncontrolled shivering, lack of coordination, decreased heart and respiratory rates, and, if left untreated, death. Cardiac surgeons use hypothermia to their advantage during open-heart surgery by cooling the body. This stops the heart and decreases its blood flow, creating a motionless and bloodless surgical field.

The energy obtained from the breakdown of nutrients is used to form a compound often described as the "energy currency" of the cell. It has the long name of **adenosine triphosphate** (ah-DEN-o-sene tri-FOS-fate), but is commonly abbreviated **ATP.** Chapter 8 has more information on metabolism and ATP.

Homeostasis

Normal body function maintains a state of internal balance, an important characteristic of all living things. Such conditions as body temperature, the composition of body fluids, heart rate, respiration rate, and blood pressure must be kept within set limits to maintain health. (See Box 5-1, Homeostatic Imbalance: When Feedback Fails.) This steady state within the organism is called **homeostasis** (ho-me-o-STA-sis), which literally means "staying (stasis) the same (homeo)."

Fluid Balance

Our bodies are composed of large amounts of fluids. The amount and composition of these fluids must be regulated at all times. One type of fluid bathes the cells, carries nutrient substances to and from the cells, and transports the nutrients into and out of the cells. This type is called **extracellular fluid** because it includes all body fluids outside the cells. Examples of extracellular fluids are blood, lymph, and the fluid between the cells in tissues. A second type of fluid, **intracellular fluid,** is contained within the cells. Extracellular and intracellular fluids account for about 60% of an adult's weight.

Feedback

The main method for maintaining homeostasis is **feedback,** a control system based on information returning to a source. We are all accustomed to getting feedback about the results of our actions and using that information to regulate our behavior. Grades on tests and assignments, for example, may inspire us to work harder if they're not so great or "keep up the good work" if they are good.

Most feedback systems keep body conditions within a set normal range by reversing any upward or downward shift. This form of feedback is called **negative feedback,** because actions are reversed. A familiar example of negative feedback is the thermostat in a house (Fig. 5-3) When the house temperature falls, the thermostat triggers the furnace to turn on and increase the temperature; when the house temperature reaches an upper limit, the furnace is shut off. In the body, a center in the brain detects changes in temperature and starts mechanisms for cooling or warming if the temperature is above or below the average set point of 37°C (98.6° F) (Fig. 5-4).

As another example, when glucose (a sugar) increases in the blood, the pancreas secretes insulin, which causes body cells to use more glucose. Increased uptake of glucose and the subsequent drop in blood sugar level serves as a signal to

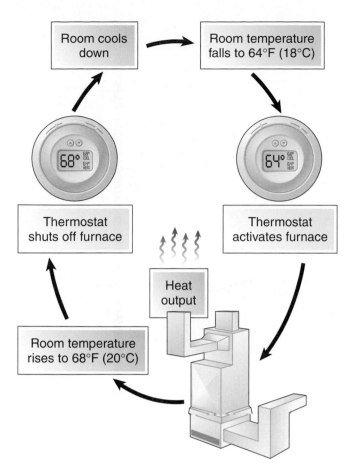

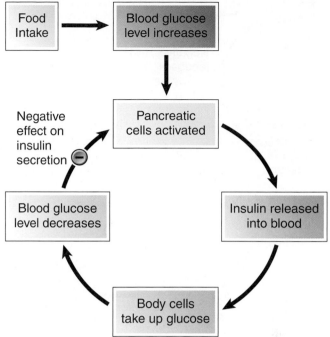

FIGURE 5-5. Negative feedback in the endocrine system. Glucose utilization regulates insulin production by means of negative feedback.

FIGURE 5-3. Negative feedback. A home thermostat illustrates how this type of feedback keeps temperature within a set range.

release the hormone oxytocin into the blood. This hormone stimulates further contractions of the uterus. As contractions increase in force, the uterine muscles are stretched even more, causing further release of oxytocin. The escalating contractions and hormone release continue until the baby is born. In positive feedback, activity continues until the stimulus is removed or some outside force interrupts the activity. Positive and negative feedback are compared in Figure 5-6.

The Effects of Aging

With age, changes occur gradually in all body systems. Some of these changes, such as wrinkles and gray hair, are obvious. Others, such as decreased kidney function, loss of bone mass, and formation of deposits within blood vessels,

the pancreas to reduce insulin secretion (Fig. 5-5). As a result of insulin's action, the secretion of insulin is reversed. This type of self-regulating feedback loop is used in the endocrine system to maintain proper levels of hormones.

A few activities involve **positive feedback**, in which a given action promotes more of the same. The process of childbirth illustrates positive feedback. As the contractions of labor begin, the muscles of the uterus are stretched. The stretching sends nervous signals to the pituitary gland to

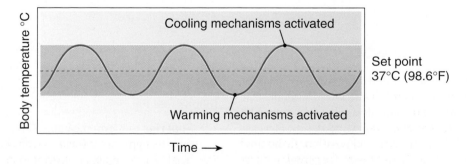

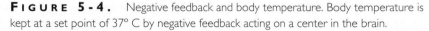

FIGURE 5-4. Negative feedback and body temperature. Body temperature is kept at a set point of 37° C by negative feedback acting on a center in the brain.

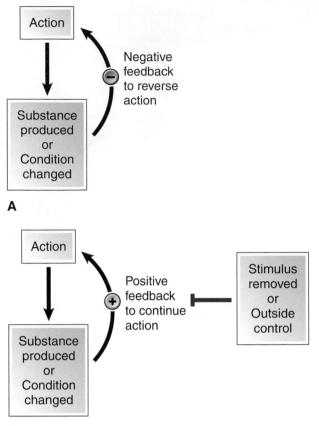

A

B

 FIGURE 5-6. Comparison of positive and negative feedback. **(A)** In negative feedback, the result of an action reverses the action. **(B)** In positive feedback, the result of an action stimulates further action. Positive feedback continues until the stimulus is removed or an outside force stops the cycle.

are not visible. However, they may make a person more subject to injury and disease.

Checkpoint Questions

2. Metabolism is divided into a breakdown phase and a building phase. What are these two phases called?

3. What type of system is used primarily to maintain homeostasis?

DIRECTIONS IN THE BODY

Because it would be awkward and inaccurate to speak of bandaging the "southwest part" of the chest, a number of terms are used universally to designate position and directions in the body. For consistency, all descriptions assume that the body is in the **anatomical position.** In this posture, the subject is standing upright with face front, arms at the sides with palms forward, and feet parallel, as shown by the smaller illustration in Figure 5-7.

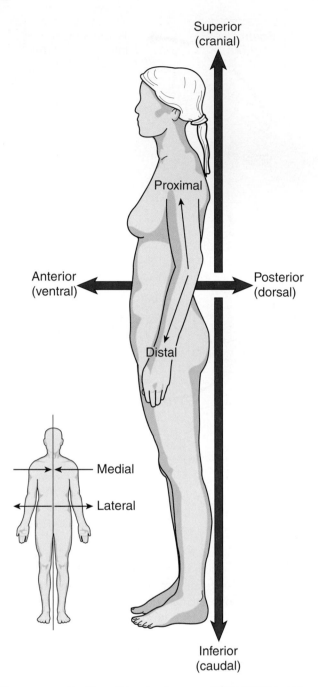

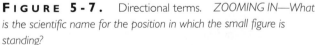 **FIGURE 5-7.** Directional terms. *ZOOMING IN—What is the scientific name for the position in which the small figure is standing?*

Directional Terms

The main terms for describing directions in the body are as follows (see Fig. 5-7):

- **Superior** is a term meaning above, or in a higher position. Its opposite, **inferior,** means below, or lower. The heart, for example, is superior to the intestine.
- **Ventral** and **anterior** have the same meaning in humans: located toward the belly surface or front of the

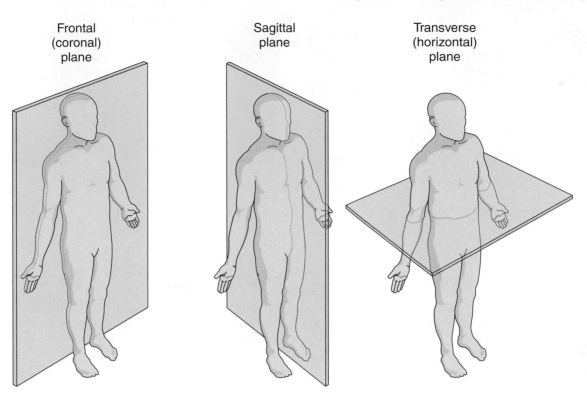

Frontal (coronal) plane

Sagittal plane

Transverse (horizontal) plane

FIGURE 5-8. Planes of division. *ZOOMING IN—Which plane divides the body into superior and inferior parts? Which plane divides the body into anterior and posterior parts?*

body. Their corresponding opposites, **dorsal** and **posterior,** refer to locations nearer the back.
- **Cranial** means nearer to the head. **Caudal** means nearer to the sacral region of the spinal column (*i.e.,* where the tail is located in lower animals), or, in humans, in an inferior direction.
- **Medial** means nearer to an imaginary plane that passes through the midline of the body, dividing it into left and right portions. **Lateral,** its opposite, means farther away from the midline, toward the side.
- **Proximal** means nearer the origin of a structure; **distal,** farther from that point. For example, the part of your thumb where it joins your hand is its proximal region; the tip of the thumb is its distal region.

Planes of Division

To visualize the various internal structures in relation to each other, anatomists can divide the body along three planes, each of which is a cut through the body in a different direction (Fig. 5-8).

- The **frontal plane**. If the cut were made in line with the ears and then down the middle of the body, you would see an anterior, or ventral (front), section and a posterior, or dorsal (back), section. Another name for this plane is *coronal plane.*
- The **sagittal** (SAJ-ih-tal) **plane**. If you were to cut the body in two from front to back, separating it into right and left portions, the sections you would see would be

sagittal sections. A cut exactly down the midline of the body, separating it into equal right and left halves, is a **midsagittal** section.
- The **transverse plane.** If the cut were made horizontally, across the other two planes, it would divide the body into a superior (upper) part and an inferior (lower) part. There could be many such cross-sections, each of which would be on a transverse plane, also called a *horizontal plane.*

Tissue Sections

Some additional terms are used to describe sections (cuts) of tissues, as used to prepare them for study under the microscope (Fig. 5-9) A cross section (see figure) is a cut made perpendicular to the long axis of an organ, such as a cut made across a banana to give a small round slice. A longitudinal section is made parallel to the long axis, as in cutting a banana from tip to tip to make a slice for a banana split. An oblique section is made at an angle. The type of section used will determine what is seen under the microscope, as shown with a blood vessel in Figure 5-9.

These same terms are used for images taken by techniques such as computed tomography (CT) or magnetic resonance imaging (MRI). (See Box 5-2, Medical Imaging: Seeing Without Making a Cut). In imaging studies, the term cross section is used more generally to mean any two-dimensional view of an internal structure obtained by imaging, as shown in Figure 5-10.

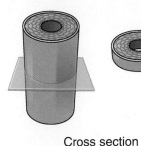
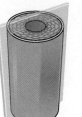
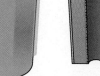
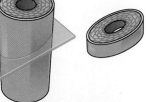

Cross section   Longitudinal section   Oblique section

FIGURE 5-9.   Tissue sections.

 Checkpoint Question

4. What are the three planes in which the body can be cut? What kind of a plane divides the body into two equal halves?

BODY CAVITIES

Internally, the body is divided into a few large spaces, or **cavities,** which contain the organs. The two main cavities are the **dorsal cavity** and **ventral cavity** (Fig. 5-11).

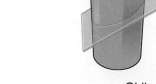 **Box 5-2**

HOT TOPICS

Medical Imaging: Seeing Without Making a Cut

Three imaging techniques that have revolutionized medicine are radiography, computed tomography, and magnetic resonance imaging. With them, physicians today can "see" inside the body without making a single cut. Each technique is so important that its inventor received a Nobel Prize.

The oldest is radiography (ra-de-OG-rah-fe), in which a machine beams x-rays (a form of radiation) through the body onto a piece of film. Like other forms of radiation, x-rays damage body tissues, but modern equipment uses extremely low doses. The resulting picture is called a radiograph. Dark areas indicate where the beam passed through the body and exposed the film, whereas light areas show where the beam did not pass through. Dense tissues (bone, teeth) absorb most of the x-rays, preventing them from exposing the film. For this reason, radiography is commonly used to visualize bone fractures and tooth decay as well as abnormally dense tissues like tumors. Radiography does not provide clear pictures of soft tissues because most of the beam passes through and exposes the film, but contrast media can help make structures like blood vessels and hollow organs more visible. For example, barium sulfate (which absorbs x-rays) coats the digestive tract when ingested.

Computed tomography (CT) is based on radiography and also uses very low doses of radiation. During a CT scan, a machine revolves around the patient, beaming x-rays through the body onto a detector. The detector takes numerous pictures of the beam and a computer assembles them into transverse sections, or "slices." Unlike conventional radiography, CT produces clear images of soft structures such as the brain, liver, and lungs. It is commonly used to visualize brain injuries and tumors, and even blood vessels when used with contrast media.

Magnetic resonance imaging uses a strong magnetic field and radiowaves. So far, there is no evidence to suggest that MRI causes tissue damage. The MRI patient lies inside a chamber within a very powerful magnet. The molecules in the patient's soft tissues align with the magnetic field inside the chamber. When radiowaves beamed at the region to be imaged hit the soft tissue, the aligned molecules emit energy that the MRI machine detects, and a computer converts these signals into a picture. MRI produces even clearer images of soft tissue than does computed tomography and can create detailed pictures of blood vessels without contrast media. MRI can visualize brain injuries and tumors that might be missed using CT.

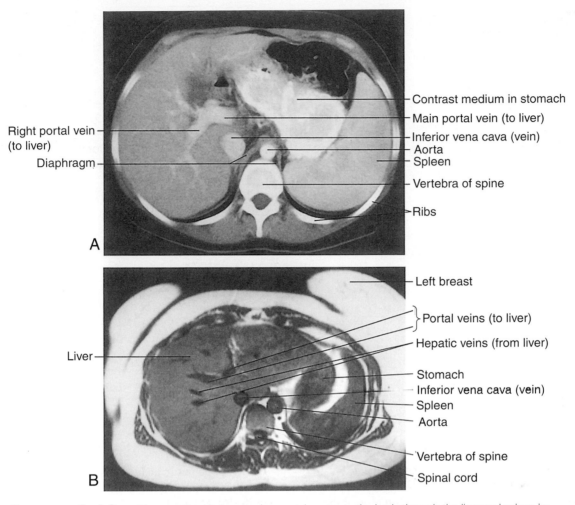

Right portal vein (to liver)

Diaphragm

A

Contrast medium in stomach

Main portal vein (to liver)

Inferior vena cava (vein)

Aorta

Spleen

Vertebra of spine

Ribs

Left breast

Portal veins (to liver)

Hepatic veins (from liver)

Liver

Stomach

Inferior vena cava (vein)

Spleen

Aorta

Vertebra of spine

Spinal cord

B

FIGURE 5-10. Cross-sections in imaging. Images taken across the body through the liver and spleen by **(A)** computed tomography (CT) and **(B)** magnetic resonance imaging (MRI). (Reprinted with permission from Erkonen WE. Radiology 101: Basics and Fundamentals of Imaging. Philadelphia: Lippincott Williams & Wilkins, 1998.)

Dorsal Cavity

The dorsal body cavity has two subdivisions: the **cranial cavity,** containing the brain, and the **spinal cavity (canal),** enclosing the spinal cord. These two areas form one continuous space.

Ventral Cavity

The ventral cavity is much larger than the dorsal cavity. It has two main subdivisions, which are separated by the **diaphragm** (DI-ah-fram), a muscle used in breathing. The **thoracic** (tho-RAS-ik) **cavity** is located superior to (above) the diaphragm. Its contents include the heart, the lungs, and the large blood vessels that join the heart. The heart is contained in the pericardial cavity, formed by the pericardial sac; the lungs are in the pleural cavity, formed by the pleurae, the membranes that enclose the lungs (Fig. 5-12) The **mediastinum** (me-de-as-TI-num) is the space between the lungs, including the organs and vessels contained in that space.

The **abdominopelvic** (ab-dom-ih-no-PEL-vik) **cavity** (see Fig. 5-11) is located inferior to (below) the diaphragm. This space is further subdivided into two regions. The superior portion, the **abdominal cavity,** contains the stomach, most of the intestine, the liver, the gallbladder, the pancreas, and the spleen. The inferior portion, set off by an imaginary line across the top of the hip bones, is the **pelvic cavity.** This cavity contains the urinary bladder, the rectum, and the internal parts of the reproductive system.

 Checkpoint Question

5. There are two main body cavities, one posterior and one anterior. Name these two cavities.

Regions of the Abdomen

It is helpful to divide the abdomen for examination and reference into nine regions (Fig. 5-13).

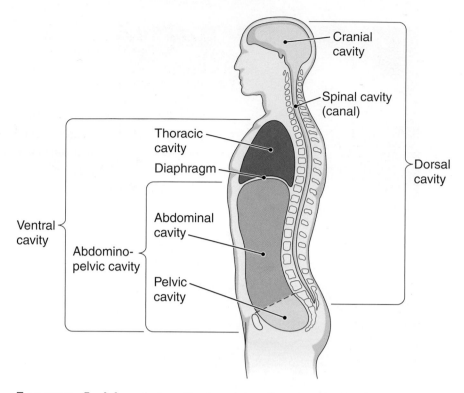

FIGURE 5-11. Body cavities, lateral view. Shown are the dorsal and ventral cavities with their subdivisions. *ZOOMING IN—What cavity contains the diaphragm?*

The three central regions, from superior to inferior are:

- the **epigastric** (ep-ih-GAS-trik) **region,** located just inferior to the breastbone
- the **umbilical** (um-BIL-ih-kal) **region** around the umbilicus (um-BIL-ih-kus), commonly called the *navel*
- the **hypogastric** (hi-po-GAS-trik) **region,** the most inferior of all the midline regions

The regions on the right and left, from superior to inferior, are:

- the **hypochondriac** (hi-po-KON-dre-ak) **regions,** just inferior to the ribs
- the **lumbar regions,** which are on a level with the lumbar regions of the spine
- the iliac, or **inguinal** (IN-gwih-nal), **regions,** named for the upper crest of the hipbone and the groin region, respectively

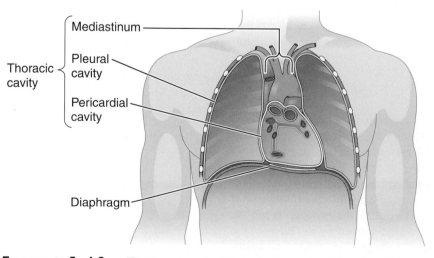

FIGURE 5-12. The thoracic cavity. Shown are the pericardial cavity, which contains the heart, and the pleural cavity, which contains the lungs.

The metric system is like the monetary system in the United States. Both are decimal systems based on multiples of the number 10. One hundred cents equal one dollar; one hundred centimeters equal one meter. Each multiple in the decimal system is indicated by a prefix:

kilo = 1000

centi = 1/100

milli = 1/1000

micro = 1/1,000,000

Units of Length

The basic unit of length in the metric system is the **meter** (m). Using the prefixes above, 1 kilometer is equal to 1000 meters. A centimeter is 1/100 of a meter; stated another way, there are 100 centimeters in 1 meter. The United States has not changed over to the metric system, as was once expected. Often, measurements on packages, bottles, and yard goods are now given according to both scales. In this

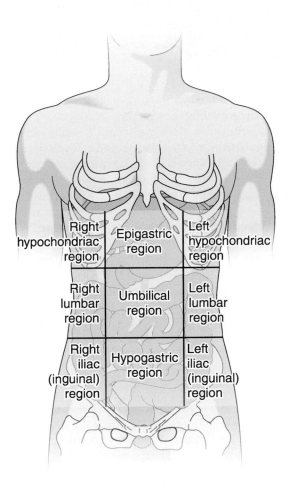

FIGURE 5-13. The nine regions of the abdomen.

A simpler but less precise division into four quadrants is sometimes used. These regions are the right upper quadrant (RUQ), left upper quadrant (LUQ), right lower quadrant (RLQ), and left lower quadrant (LLQ) (Fig. 5-14) (See Box 5-3, Health Information Technicians, for a description of a profession that uses anatomical, physiological, and medical terms.)

Checkpoint Question

6. Name the three central regions and the three left and right lateral regions of the abdomen.

THE METRIC SYSTEM

Now that we have set the stage for further study of the body's structure and function, we should take a look at the metric system, because this system is used for all scientific measurements. The drug industry and the health-care industry already have converted to the metric system, so anyone who plans a career in healthcare should be acquainted with metrics.

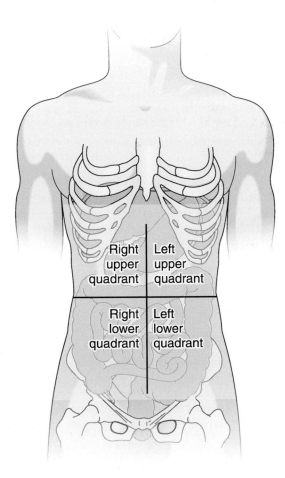

FIGURE 5-14. Quadrants of the abdomen. The organs within each quadrant are shown.

Box 5-3

HEALTH PROFESSIONS

Health Information Technicians

Every time a patient receives medical treatment, information is added to the patient's medical record, which includes data about symptoms, medical history, test results, diagnoses, and treatment. **Health information technicians** organize and manage these records, working closely with physicians, nurses, and other health professionals to ensure that medical records provide a complete, accurate basis for quality patient care.

Accurate medical records are also essential for administrative purposes. Health information technicians assign a **code** to each diagnosis and procedure a patient receives, and this information is used for accurate patient billing. In addition, health information technicians analyze medical records to discover trends in health and disease. This research can be used to improve patient care, manage costs, and help establish new medical treatments.

Health information technicians need a strong clinical knowledge base. A thorough background in medical terminology is essential when reading and interpreting medical records. Anatomy and physiology are definitely required!

Most health information technologists work in hospitals and long-term care facilities. Others work in medical clinics, government agencies, insurance companies, and consulting firms. Job prospects are promising because of the growing need for healthcare. In fact, health information technology is projected to be one of the fastest growing careers in the United States. For more information about this profession, contact the American Health Information Management Association.

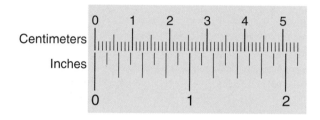

FIGURE 5-15. Comparison of centimeters and inches.

text, equivalents in the more familiar units of inches and feet are included along with the metric units for comparison. There are 2.5 centimeters (cm) or 25 millimeters (mm) in 1 inch, as shown in Figure 5-15. Some equivalents that may help you to appreciate the size of various body parts are as follows:

1 mm = 0.04 inch, or 1 inch = 25 mm

1 cm = 0.4 inch, or 1 inch = 2.5 cm

1 m = 3.3 feet, or 1 foot = 30 cm

Units of Weight

The same prefixes used for linear measurements are used for weights and volumes. The **gram** (g) is the basic unit of weight. Thirty grams are about equal to 1 ounce, and 1 kilogram to 2.2 pounds. Drug dosages are usually stated in grams or milligrams. One thousand milligrams equal 1 gram; a 500-milligram (mg) dose would be the equivalent of 0.5 gram (g), and 250 mg is equal to 0.25 g.

Units of Volume

The dosages of liquid medications are given in units of volume. The basic metric measurement for volume is the **liter** (L) (LE-ter). There are 1000 milliliters (mL) in a liter. A liter is slightly greater than a quart, a liter being equal to 1.06 quarts. For smaller quantities, the milliliter is used most of the time. There are 5 mL in a teaspoon and 15 mL in a tablespoon. A fluid ounce contains 30 mL.

Temperature

The Celsius (centigrade) temperature scale, now in use by most countries and by scientists in this country, is discussed in Chapter 8.

 Checkpoint Question

7. Name the basic units of length, weight, and volume in the metric system.

Word Anatomy

Medical terms are built from standardized word parts (prefixes, roots, and suffixes). Learning the meanings of these parts can help you remember words and interpret unfamiliar terms.

Word part	Meaning	Example
Studies of the Human Body		
-tomy	cutting, incision of	**Anatomy** can be revealed by making incisions in the body.
dis-	apart, away from	To **dissect** is to cut apart.
physi/o	nature, physical	**Physiology** is the study of how the body functions.
Body Processes		
cata-	down	**Catabolism** is the breakdown of complex substances into simpler ones.
ana-	upward, again, back	**Anabolism** is the building up of simple compounds into more complex substances.
home/o-	same	**Homeostasis** is the steady state (sameness) within an organism.
stat	stand, stoppage, constancy	In **homeostasis**, "-stasis" refers to constancy

Summary

I. Studies of the human body
  1. Anatomy—study of structure
  2. Physiology—study of function
  A. Levels of organization—chemicals, cell, tissue, organ, organ system, whole organism

II. Body systems
  1. Integumentary system—skin and associated structures
  2. Skeletal system—support
  3. Muscular system—movement
  4. Nervous system—reception of stimuli and control of responses
  5. Endocrine system—production of hormones for regulation of growth, metabolism, reproduction
  6. Cardiovascular system—movement of blood for transport
  7. Lymphatic system—aids in circulation, immunity, and absorption of digested fats
  8. Respiratory system—intake of oxygen and release of carbon dioxide
  9. Digestive system—intake, breakdown, and absorption of nutrients
  10. Urinary system—elimination of waste and water
  11. Reproductive system—production of offspring

III. Metabolism and its regulation
  1. Metabolism—all the chemical reactions needed to sustain life
    a. Catabolism—breakdown of complex substances into simpler substances; release of energy from nutrients

      (1) ATP (adenosine triphosphate)—energy compound of cells
    b. Anabolism—building of body materials
  A. Homeostasis—steady state of body conditions
    1. Fluid balance
      a. Extracellular fluid—outside the cells
      b. Intracellular fluid—inside the cells
    2. Feedback—regulation by return of information within a system
      a. Negative feedback—reverses an action
      b. Positive feedback—promotes continued activity
  B. Effects of aging—changes in all systems

IV. Directions in the body
  1. Anatomical position—upright, palms forward, face front, feet parallel
  A. Directional terms
    1. Superior—above or higher; inferior—below or lower
    2. Ventral (anterior)—toward belly or front surface; dorsal (posterior)—nearer to back surface
    3. Cranial—nearer to head; caudal—nearer to sacrum
    4. Medial—toward midline; lateral—toward side
    5. Proximal—nearer to point of origin; distal—farther from point of origin
  B. Planes of division
    1. Body divisions
      a. Sagittal—from front to back, dividing the body into left and right parts
        (1) Midsagittal—exactly down the midline
      b. Frontal (coronal)—from left to right, dividing the body into anterior and posterior parts

c. Transverse—horizontally, dividing the body into superior and inferior parts

2. Tissue sections
   a. Cross section—perpendicular to long axis
   b. Transverse section—parallel to long axis
   c. Oblique section—at an angle

V. Body cavities

A. Dorsal cavity—contains cranial and spinal cavities for brain and spinal cord

B. Ventral cavity
   1. Thoracic—chest cavity
      a. Divided from abdominal cavity by diaphragm
      b. Contains heart and lungs
      c. Mediastinum—space between lungs and the organs contained in that space
   2. Abdominopelvic cavity
      a. Abdominal cavity—upper region containing stomach, most of intestine, pancreas, liver, spleen, and others
      b. Pelvic cavity—lower region containing reproductive organs, urinary bladder, rectum

3. Nine regions of the abdomen
   a. Central—epigastric, umbilical, hypogastric
   b. Lateral (right and left)—hypochondriac, lumbar, iliac (inguinal)
4. Quadrants—abdomen divided into four regions

VI. The metric system—based on multiples of 10

1. Basic units
   a. Meter—length
   b. Gram—weight
   c. Liter—volume
2. Prefixes—indicate multiples of 10
   a. Kilo—1000 times
   b. Centi—1/100th (0.01)
   c. Milli—1/1000th (0.001)
   d. Micro—1/1,000,000 (0.000001)
A. Units of length
B. Units of weight
C. Units of volume
D. Temperature—measured in Celsius (centigrade) scale

Questions for Study and Review

Building Understanding

Fill in the blanks
1. Tissues may function together as _____.
2. Glands that produce hormones belong to the _____ system.
3. The eyes are located _____ to the nose.
4. Normal body function maintains a state of internal balance called _____.
5. The basic unit of volume in the metric system is the _____.

Matching
Match each numbered item with the most closely related lettered item.

____ 6. One of two systems that control and coordinate other systems

    a. nervous system

____ 7. The system that brings needed substances to the body tissues

    b. abdominal cavity

____ 8. The system that converts foods into a form that body cells can use

    c. cardiovascular system

____ 9. The cavity that contains the liver

    d. pelvic cavity

____ 10. The cavity that contains the urinary bladder

    e. digestive system

Multiple choice
____ 11. The study of normal body structure is
   a. homeostasis
   b. anatomy
   c. physiology
   d. metabolism
____ 12. Fluids contained within cells are described as
   a. intracellular
   b. ventral
   c. extracellular
   d. dorsal
____ 13. A type of feedback in which a given action promotes more of the same is called
   a. homeostasis
   b. biofeedback
   c. positive feedback
   d. negative feedback
____ 14. The cavity that contains the mediastinum is the
   a. dorsal
   b. ventral
   c. abdominal
   d. pelvic
____ 15. The foot is located _____ to the knee.
   a. superior
   b. inferior
   c. proximal
   d. distal

Understanding Concepts

16. Compare and contrast the studies of anatomy and physiology. Would it be wise to study one without the other?
17. List in sequence the levels of organization in the body from simplest to most complex. Give an example for each level.

18. Compare and contrast the anatomy and physiology of the nervous system with that of the endocrine system.
19. What is ATP? What type of metabolic activity releases the energy used to make ATP?
20. Compare and contrast intracellular and extracellular fluids.
21. Explain how an internal state of balance is maintained in the body.
22. List the subdivisions of the dorsal and ventral cavities. Name some organs found in each subdivision.

Conceptual Thinking

23. The human body is organized from very simple levels to more complex levels. With this in mind describe why a disease at the chemical level can have an effect on organ system function.
24. When glucose levels in the blood drop below normal the pancreas releases a hormone called glucagon. Using your understanding of negative feedback, discuss the possible role of glucagon in blood glucose homeostasis.
25. Your patient's chart reads: "Patient reports pain in right lower quadrant of abdomen. X-ray reveals mass in right iliac region." Locate this region on yourself and explain why it is important for health professionals to use anatomical terminology when describing the human body.

6

Tissues, Glands, and Membranes

CHAPTER OBJECTIVES

In this chapter, you'll learn:

1. To name the four main groups of tissues and give the location and general characteristics of each.
2. To describe the difference between exocrine and endocrine glands and give examples of each.
3. To give examples of liquid, soft, fibrous, and hard connective tissues.
4. To describe three types of epithelial membranes.
5. To list several types of connective tissue membranes.
6. To show how word parts are used to build words related to tissues, glands, and membranes (see Word Anatomy at the end of the chapter).

KEY TERMS

adipose	epithelium	membrane	parietal
areolar	exocrine	mucosa	serosa
cartilage	fascia	myelin	visceral
collagen	histology	neuroglia	
endocrine	matrix	neuron	

TISSUES ARE GROUPS OF CELLS similar in structure, arranged in a characteristic pattern, and specialized for the performance of specific tasks. The study of tissues is known as **histology** (his-TOL-o-je). This study shows that the form, arrangement, and composition of cells in different tissues account for their properties. For a description of the health professional who prepares tissues for study, see Box 6-1, Histotechnologist.

The tissues in our bodies might be compared with the different materials used to construct a building. Think for a moment of the great variety of building materials used according to need—wood, stone, steel, plaster, insulation, and others. Each of these has different properties, but together they contribute to the building as a whole. The same may be said of tissues.

TISSUE CLASSIFICATION

The four main groups of tissue are the following:

- **Epithelial** (ep-ih-THE-le-al) **tissue** covers surfaces, lines cavities, and forms glands.
- **Connective tissue** supports and forms the framework of all parts of the body.
- **Muscle tissue** contracts and produces movement.
- **Nervous tissue** conducts nerve impulses.

EPITHELIAL TISSUE

Epithelial tissue, or **epithelium** (ep-ih-THE-le-um), forms a protective covering for the body. It is the main tissue of the skin's outer layer. It also forms membranes, ducts, and the lining of body cavities and hollow organs, such as the organs of the digestive, respiratory, and urinary tracts.

Structure of Epithelial Tissue

Epithelial cells are tightly packed to better protect underlying tissue or form barriers between systems. The cells vary in shape and arrangement according to their function. Epithelial tissue is classified on the basis of these characteristics. In shape, the cells may be described as follows:

- **Squamous** (SKWA-mus)—flat and irregular
- **Cuboidal**—square
- **Columnar**—long and narrow

The cells may be arranged in a single layer, in which case it is described as **simple** (Fig. 6-1). Simple epithelium functions as a thin barrier through which materials can pass fairly easily. For example, simple epithelium allows for absorption of materials from the lining of the digestive tract into the blood and allows for passage of oxygen from the blood to body tissues. Areas subject to wear-and-tear that require protection are covered with epithelial cells in multiple layers, an arrangement described as **stratified** (Fig. 6-2). If the cells are staggered so that they appear to be in multiple layers but really are not, they are termed *pseudostratified*. Terms for both shape and arrangement are used to describe epithelial tissue. Thus, a single layer of flat, irregular cells would be described as *simple squamous epithelium,* whereas tissue with many layers of these same cells would be described as *stratified squamous epithelium.*

Some organs, such as the urinary bladder, must vary a great deal in size as they work. These organs are lined with **transitional epithelium**, which is capable of great expansion but returns to its original form once tension is relaxed—as when, in this case, the bladder is emptied.

Special Functions of Epithelial Tissue

The cells of some epithelium produce secretions, including **mucus** (MU-kus) (a clear, sticky fluid), digestive juices,

---

Box 6-1

HEALTH PROFESSIONS

Histotechnologist

In the clinical laboratory, the histotechnologist is the health care professional who prepares tissue samples for microscopic examination. When a tissue sample arrives at the laboratory, the histotechnologist cuts it into very thin slices, called sections, mounts the sections on glass slides, and treats them with various chemicals to preserve and prepare them for staining. The histotechnologist then stains the preserved sections with specific dyes to emphasize cellular details that a pathologist might look for. To perform these tasks, histotechnologists require a strong clinical background and a thorough understanding of chemistry, anatomy, and physiology.

Most histotechnologists work in hospital and medical clinic laboratories, although some find employment in research laboratories, pharmaceutical companies, and government agencies. Job prospects are promising because of the growing need for health care and the development of new laboratory tests and technologies. For more information about careers in histotechnology, contact the American Society for Clinical Laboratory Science.

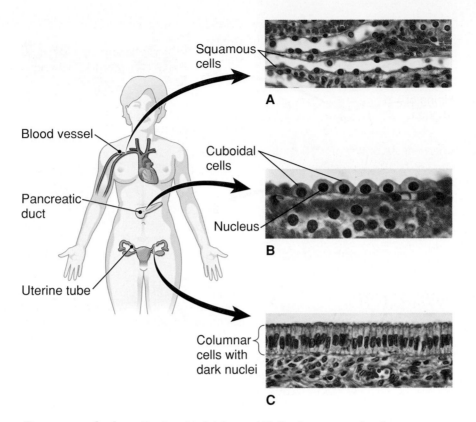

FIGURE 6-1. Simple epithelial tissues. **(A)** Simple squamous has flat, irregular cells. **(B)** Cuboidal cells are square in shape with darkly staining round nuclei. **(C)** Columnar cells are long and narrow with darkly staining nuclei. (A, B, and C, Reprinted with permission from Cormack DH. Essential Histology. 2nd ed. Philadelphia: Lippincott Williams & Wilkins, 2001.) *ZOOMING IN—In how many layers are these epithelial cells?*

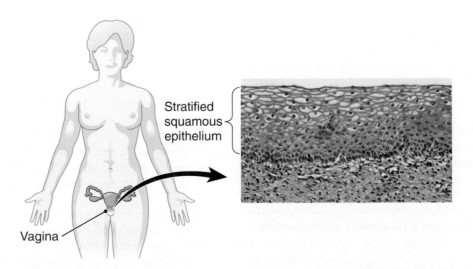

FIGURE 6-2. Stratified squamous epithelium. Cells are arranged in multiple layers. (Reprinted with permission from Cormack DH. Essential Histology. 2nd ed. Philadelphia: Lippincott Williams & Wilkins, 2001.)

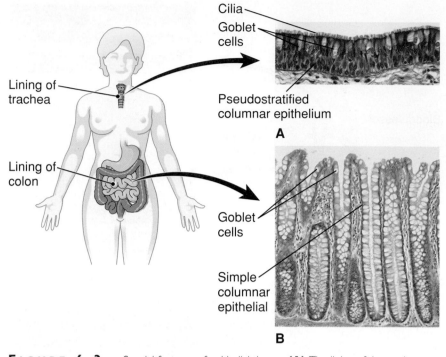

FIGURE 6-3. Special features of epithelial tissues. **(A)** The lining of the trachea showing cilia and goblet cells that secrete mucus. **(B)** The lining of the intestine showing goblet cells. (A and B, Reprinted with permission from Cormack DH. Essential Histology. 2nd ed. Philadelphia: Lippincott Williams & Wilkins, 2001.)

sweat, and other substances. The air that we breathe passes over epithelium that lines the passageways of the respiratory (breathing) system. Mucus-secreting **goblet cells**, named for their shape, are scattered among the pseudostratified epithelial cells (Fig. 6-3A). The epithelial cells also have tiny hairlike projections called **cilia**. Together, the mucus and the cilia help trap bits of dust and other foreign particles that could otherwise reach the lungs and damage them. The digestive tract is lined with simple columnar epithelium that also contains goblet cells. They secrete mucus that protects the lining of the digestive organs (Fig. 6-3B).

Epithelium repairs itself quickly after it is injured. In areas of the body subject to normal wear and tear, such as the skin, the inside of the mouth, and the lining of the intestinal tract, epithelial cells reproduce frequently, replacing damaged tissue. Certain areas of the epithelium that form the outer layer of the skin are capable of modifying themselves for greater strength whenever they are subjected to unusual wear and tear; the growth of calluses is a good example of this response.

Checkpoint Question

1. Epithelium is classified according to cell shape. What are the three basic shapes?

Glands

The active cells of many glands are epithelial cells. A gland is an organ specialized to produce a substance that is sent out to other parts of the body. The gland manufactures these secretions from materials removed from the blood. Glands are divided into two categories based on how they release their secretions:

- **Exocrine** (EK-so-krin) **glands** have ducts or tubes to carry secretions away from the gland. The secretions may be carried to another organ, to a body cavity, or to the body surface. They are effective in a limited area near their source. Examples of exocrine glands include the glands in the gastrointestinal tract that secrete digestive juices, the sebaceous (oil) glands of the skin, and the lacrimal glands that produce tears. These and other exocrine glands are discussed in the chapters on specific systems.

  In structure, an exocrine gland may consist of a single cell, such as the cells that secrete mucus into the digestive tract. Most, however, are composed of multiple cells in various arrangements (Fig. 6-4). They may be tubular, in a simple straight form, or in a branched formation, as are found in the digestive tract. They may also be coiled, as are the sweat glands of the skin.

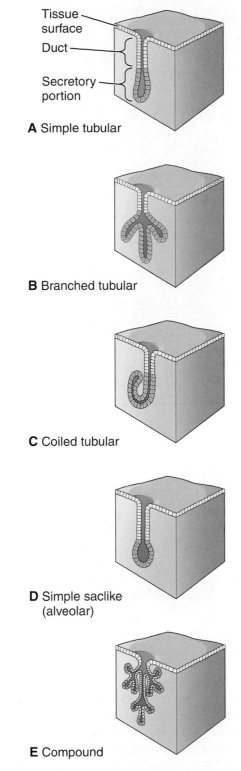

A Simple tubular

B Branched tubular

C Coiled tubular

D Simple saclike (alveolar)

E Compound

F I G U R E   6 - 4 .   Some structural types of exocrine glands. **(A)** Simple tubular, as found in the intestine. **(B)** Branched tubular, as found in the stomach. **(C)** Coiled tubular, such as the sweat glands of the skin. **(D)** Simple saclike (alveolar), such as the oil glands of the skin. **(E)** Compound, with tubes and sacs, such as the salivary glands.

They may be saclike, as are the sebaceous (oil) glands of the skin, or compound formations of tubes and sacs, as are the salivary glands in the mouth.

- **Endocrine** (EN-do-krin) **glands** secrete directly into the blood, which then carries their secretions to another area of the body. These secretions, called **hormones**, have effects on specific tissues known as the *target tissues.* Endocrine glands have an extensive network of blood vessels.

Checkpoint Question

2. Glands are classified according to whether they secrete through ducts or secrete directly into the bloodstream. What are these two categories of glands?

CONNECTIVE TISSUE

The supporting fabric of all parts of the body is connective tissue. This is so extensive and widely distributed that if we were able to dissolve all the tissues except connective tissue, we would still be able to recognize the contours of the entire body. Connective tissue has large amounts of nonliving material between the cells. This intercellular background material or **matrix** (MA-trix) contains varying amounts of water, fibers, and hard minerals.

There are several ways of classifying connective tissue. Some is considered more generalized because it occurs throughout the body wherever structure and protection are needed. Others, such as bone and blood, have a more specialized function. Based on the composition of the matrix, the various connective tissues also differ in their degree of hardness. For simplicity, we will categorize them according to these physical properties:

- Liquid connective tissue—blood and lymph (the fluid that circulates in the lymphatic system) are examples of liquid connective tissues (Fig. 6-5). The cells in liquid connective tissue are suspended in a fluid environment.
- Soft connective tissue—loosely held together with semi-liquid material between the cells; includes adipose (fat) tissue and areolar (loose) connective tissue.
- Fibrous connective tissue—most connective tissue contains some fibers, but this type is densely packed with them. Cells called *fibroblasts* produce the fibers in connective tissue. (The word ending *-blast* refers to a young and active cell). Examples of structures composed of fibrous connective tissue are ligaments, tendons, and the capsules (coverings) around certain organs.
- Hard connective tissue—has a very firm consistency, as in **cartilage**, or is hardened by minerals in the matrix, as in bone.

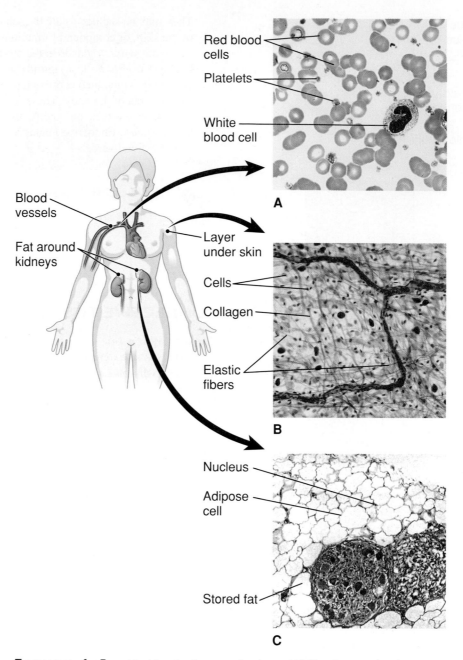

FIGURE 6-5. Liquid and soft connective tissue. **(A)** Blood smear showing various blood cells in a liquid matrix. **(B)** Areolar (loose) connective tissue, a mixture of cells and fibers in a jellylike matrix. **(C)** Adipose tissue showing stored fat. The nuclei are at the edges of the cells. (A, Reprinted with permission from McClatchey KD. Clinical Laboratory Medicine. 2nd ed. Philadelphia: Lippincott Williams & Wilkins, 2001; B, reprinted with permission from Cormack DH. Essential Histology. 2nd ed. Philadelphia: Lippincott Williams & Wilkins, 2001; C, reprinted with permission from Mills, SE. Histology for Pathologists. 3rd ed. Philadelphia: Lippincott Williams & Wilkins, 2006.) *ZOOMING IN—Which of these tissues has the most fibers? Which of these tissues is modified for storage?*

 Checkpoint Question

3. Connective tissue varies according to the composition of the material that is between the cells. What is the general name for this intercellular material?

Soft Connective Tissue

The **areolar** (ah-RE-o-lar), or loose, form of connective tissue (see Fig. 6-5) is found in membranes around vessels and organs, between muscles, and under the skin. It is the most common type of connective tissue in the body. It contains cells and fibers in a very loose, jellylike background material.

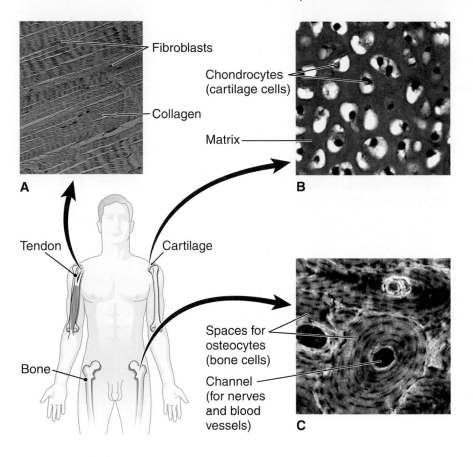

Fibroblasts

Chondrocytes
(cartilage cells)

Collagen

Matrix

Tendon

Cartilage

Bone

Spaces for
osteocytes
(bone cells)

Channel
(for nerves
and blood
vessels)

A

B

C

FIGURE 6-6. Fibrous and hard connective tissue. **(A)** Fibrous connective tissue. In tendons and ligaments, the fibers are arranged in the same direction. **(B)** In cartilage, the cells (chondrocytes) are enclosed in a firm matrix. **(C)** Bone is the hardest connective tissue. The cells (osteocytes) are within the hard matrix. (A and B, Reprinted with permission from Mills SE. Histology for Pathologists. 3rd ed. Philadelphia: Lippincott Williams & Wilkins, 2006; C, reprinted with permission from Gartner LP, Hiatt JL. Color Atlas of Histology. 4th ed. Philadelphia: Lippincott Williams & Wilkins, 2005.)

Adipose (AD-ih-pose) **tissue** (see Fig. 6-5) contains cells that are able to store large amounts of fat. The fat in this tissue is used as a reserve energy supply for the body. Adipose tissue also serves as a heat insulator and as protective padding for organs and joints.

Fibrous Connective Tissue

Fibrous connective tissue (Fig. 6-6A) is very dense and has large numbers of fibers that give it strength and flexibility. The main type of fiber in this and other connective tissues is **collagen** (KOL-ah-jen), a flexible white protein. (see Box 6-2, Collagen: The Body's Scaffolding).

Some fibrous connective tissue contains large amounts of elastic fibers that allow the tissue to stretch and then return to its original length. This type of elastic connective tissue appears in the vocal cords, the passageways of the respiratory tract, and the walls of the large arteries (blood vessels).

Fibrous connective tissue makes up the fibrous membranes that cover various organs, as described later in this chapter. Particularly strong forms make up the tough **capsules** around certain organs, such as the kidneys, the liver, and some glands. If the fibers in the connective tissue are all arranged in the same direction, like the strands of a cable, the tissue can pull in one direction. Examples are the cordlike **tendons**, which connect muscles to bones, and the **ligaments**, which connect bones to other bones.

Hard Connective Tissue

The hard connective tissues, cartilage and bone, are more solid than the other groups.

Cartilage

Because of its strength and flexibility, cartilage is used as a structural material and as reinforcement. It is also used as a shock absorber and as a bearing surface that reduces friction between moving parts, as at joints. A common form of cartilage known as **hyaline** (HI-ah-lin) **cartilage** forms the

Box 6-2

A CLOSER LOOK
Collagen: The Body's Scaffolding

The most abundant protein in the body, making up about 25% of total protein, is collagen. Its name, derived from a Greek word meaning "glue," reveals its role as the main structural protein in connective tissue.

Fibroblasts secrete collagen molecules into the surrounding matrix, where the molecules are then assembled into fibers. These fibers give the matrix its strength and its flexibility. Collagen fibers' high tensile strength makes them stronger than steel fibers of the same size, and their flexibility confers resilience on the tissues that contain them. For example, collagen in skin, bone, tendons, and ligaments resists pulling forces, whereas collagen found in joint cartilage and between vertebrae resists compression. Based on amino acid structure, there are at least 19 types of collagen, each of which imparts a different property to the connective tissue containing it.

The arrangement of collagen fibers in the matrix reveals much about the tissue's function. In the skin and membranes covering muscles and organs, collagen fibers are arranged irregularly, with fibers running in all directions. The result is a tissue that can resist stretching forces in many different directions. In tendons and ligaments, collagen fibers have a parallel arrangement, forming strong ropelike cords that can resist longitudinal pulling forces. In bone tissue, collagen fibers' meshlike arrangement promotes deposition of calcium salts into the tissue, which gives bone strength while also providing flexibility.

Collagen's varied properties are also evident in the preparation of a gelatin dessert. Gelatin is a collagen extract made by boiling animal bones and other connective tissue. It is a viscous liquid in hot water but forms a semisolid gel on cooling.

---

tough, translucent material, popularly called *gristle*, seen over the ends of the long bones (see Fig. 6-6B). Hyaline cartilage is also found at the tip of the nose and in parts of the larynx ("voicebox") and the trachea ("windpipe").

Another form of cartilage, **fibrocartilage** (fi-bro-KAR-tih-laj), is found between segments of the spine, at the anterior joint between the pubic bones of the hip, and in the knee joint. **Elastic cartilage** can spring back into shape after it is bent. An easy place to observe the properties of elastic cartilage is in the outer portion of the ear. It is also located in the larynx.

The cells that produce cartilage are **chondrocytes** (KON-dro-sites), a name derived from the word root *chondro,* meaning "cartilage" and the root *cyto,* meaning "cell."

Bone

The tissue of which bones are made, called **osseous** (OS-e-us) **tissue**, is much like cartilage in its cellular structure (see Fig. 6-6C). In fact, the skeleton of the fetus in the early stages of development is made almost entirely of cartilage. This tissue gradually becomes impregnated with salts of calcium and phosphorus that make bone characteristically solid and hard. The cells that form bone are called **osteoblasts** (OS-te-o-blasts), a name that combines the root for bone (*osteo*) with a root (*blast*) that means an immature cell. As these cells mature, they are referred to as **osteocytes** (OS-te-o-sites). Within the osseous tissue are nerves and blood vessels. Enclosed within bones is a specialized type of tissue, the bone marrow. The red bone marrow contained in certain bone regions produces blood cells.

Checkpoint Question

4. Connective tissue is the supportive and protective material found throughout the body. What are some examples of liquid, soft, fibrous, and hard connective tissue?

MUSCLE TISSUE

Muscle tissue is designed to produce movement by contraction of its cells, which are called **muscle fibers** because most of them are long and threadlike. If a piece of well-cooked meat is pulled apart, small groups of these muscle fibers may be seen. Muscle tissue is usually classified as follows:

- **Skeletal muscle,** which works with tendons and bones to move the body (Fig. 6-7A). This type of tissue is described as **voluntary muscle** because it can be made to contract by conscious thought. The cells in skeletal muscle are very large and are remarkable in having multiple nuclei and a pattern of dark and light banding described as **striations**. This type of muscle is also called striated muscle.
- **Cardiac muscle,** which forms the bulk of the heart wall and is known also as **myocardium** (mi-o-KAR-de-um) (see Fig. 6-7B). This is the muscle that produces the regular contractions known as *heartbeats.* Cardiac muscle is described as **involuntary muscle** because it typically contracts independently of thought. Most of the time we are not aware of its actions at all. Cardiac muscle has branching cells and specialized

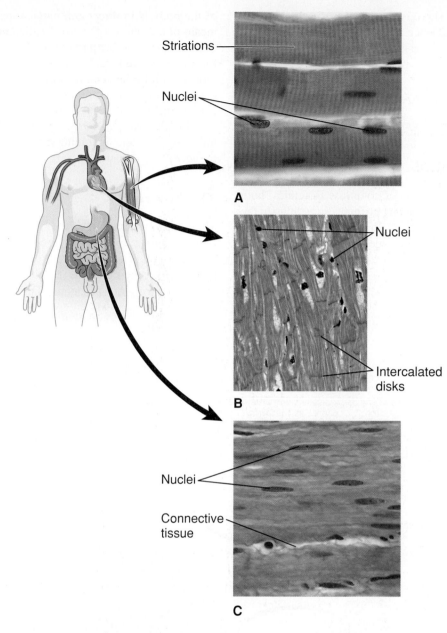

FIGURE 6-7. Muscle tissue. **(A)** Skeletal muscle cells have bands (striations) and multiple nuclei. **(B)** Cardiac muscle makes up the wall of the heart. **(C)** Smooth muscle is found in soft body organs and in vessels. (A and C, Reprinted with permission from Cormack DH. Essential Histology, 2nd ed. Philadelphia: Lippincott Williams & Wilkins, 2001; B, reprinted with permission from Gartner LP, Hiatt JL. Color Atlas of Histology, 4th ed. Philadelphia: Lippincott Williams & Wilkins, 2005.)

membranes between the cells that appear as dark lines under the microscope. Their technical name is *interca-lated* (in-TER-cal-a-ted) *disks*.

• **Smooth muscle** is also involuntary muscle (see Fig. 6-7C). It forms the walls of the hollow organs in the ventral body cavities, including the stomach, intestines, gallbladder, and urinary bladder. Together these organs are known as viscera (VIS-eh-rah), so smooth muscle is

sometimes referred to as *visceral muscle*. Smooth muscle is also found in the walls of many tubular structures, such as the blood vessels and the tubes that carry urine from the kidneys. A smooth muscle is attached to the base of each body hair. Contraction of these muscles causes the condition of the skin that we call *gooseflesh*. Smooth muscle cells are of a typical size and taper at each end. They are not striated and have only one nucleus per cell.

Muscle tissue, like nervous tissue, repairs itself only with difficulty or not at all once an injury has been sustained. When injured, muscle tissue is frequently replaced with connective tissue.

Checkpoint Question

5. What are the three types of muscle tissue?

NERVOUS TISSUE

The human body is made up of countless structures, both large and small, each of which contributes something to the action of the whole organism. This aggregation of structures might be compared to a large corporation. For all the workers in the corporation to coordinate their efforts, there must be some central control, such as the president or CEO. In the body, this central agent is the **brain**. Each structure of the body is in direct communication with the brain by means of its own set of "wires," called **nerves**. Nerves from even the most remote parts of the body come together and form a great trunk cable called the **spinal cord**, which in turn leads into the central switchboard of the brain. Here, messages come in and orders go out 24 hours a day. Some nerves, the cranial nerves, connect directly with the brain and do not form part of the spinal cord. This entire communication system, including the brain, is made of nervous tissue.

The Neuron

The basic unit of nervous tissue is the **neuron** (NU-ron), or nerve cell (Fig. 6-8A). A neuron consists of a nerve cell body plus small branches from the cell called *fibers*. One type of fiber, the **dendrite** (DEN-drite), is generally short and forms tree-like branches. This type of fiber carries

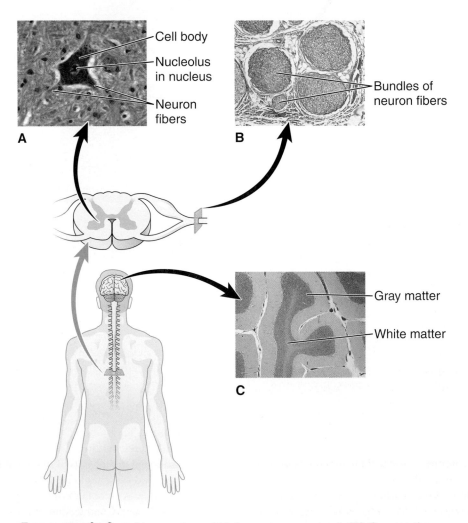

Cell body
Nucleolus in nucleus
Neuron fibers
A

Bundles of neuron fibers
B

Gray matter
White matter
C

FIGURE 6-8. Nervous tissue. **(A)** A neuron, or nerve cell. **(B)** Cross-section of a nerve. **(C)** Brain tissue. (Reprinted with permission from Cormack DH. Essential Histology. 2nd ed. Philadelphia: Lippincott Williams & Wilkins, 2001.)

Box 6-3

HOT TOPICS

Stem Cells: So Much Potential

At least 200 different types of cells are found in the human body, each with its own unique structure and function. All originate from unspecialized precursors called **stem cells**, which exhibit two important characteristics: they can divide repeatedly and have the potential to become specialized cells.

Stem cells come in two types. **Embryonic stem cells**, found in early embryos, are the source of all body cells and potentially can differentiate into any type of cell. **Adult stem cells**, found in babies and children as well as adults, are stem cells that remain in the body after birth and can differentiate into only a few cell types. They assist with tissue growth and repair. For example, in red bone marrow, these cells differentiate into blood cells, whereas in the skin, they differentiate into new skin cells after a cut or scrape.

The potential healthcare applications of stem cell research are numerous. In the near future, stem cell trans-

plants may be used to repair damaged tissues in treating illnesses such as diabetes, cancer, heart disease, Parkinson disease, and spinal cord injury. This research may also help explain how cells develop and why some cells develop abnormally, causing birth defects and cancer. Stem cells may also be used to test drugs before trying them on animals and humans.

But stem cell research is controversial. Some argue that it is unethical to use embryonic stem cells because they are obtained from aborted fetuses or fertilized eggs left over from in vitro fertilization. Others argue that these cells would be discarded anyway and have the potential to improve lives. A possible solution is the use of adult stem cells. However, adult stem cells are less abundant and lack embryonic stem cells' potential to differentiate, so more research is needed to make this a viable option.

---

messages in the form of nerve impulses to the nerve cell body. A single fiber, the **axon** (AK-son), carries impulses away from the nerve cell body. Neurons may be quite long; their fibers can extend for several feet. A **nerve** is a bundle of such nerve cell fibers held together with connective tissue (see Fig. 6-8B).

Just as wires are insulated to keep them from being short-circuited, some axons are insulated and protected by a coating of material called **myelin** (MI-eh-lin). Groups of myelinated fibers form "white matter," so called because of the color of the myelin, which is much like fat in appearance and consistency.

Not all neurons have myelin, however; some axons are unmyelinated, as are all dendrites and all cell bodies. These areas appear gray in color. Because the outer layer of the brain has large collections of cell bodies and unmyelinated fibers, the brain is popularly termed *gray matter,* even though its interior is composed of white matter (see Fig. 6-8C).

Neuroglia

Nervous tissue is supported by specialized cells known as **neuroglia** (nu-ROG-le-ah) or *glial* (GLI-al) *cells*, which are named from the Greek word *glia* meaning "glue." Some of these cells protect the brain from harmful substances; others get rid of foreign organisms and cellular debris; still others form the myelin sheath around axons. They do not, however, transmit nerve impulses.

 Checkpoint Questions

6. What is the basic cellular unit of the nervous system and what is its function?

7. What are the nonconducting support cells of the nervous system called?

All of the various tissues discussed previously develop from primitive cells. Read about these cells in Box 6-3, Stem Cells: So Much Potential.

MEMBRANES

Membranes are thin sheets of tissue. Their properties vary: some are fragile, others tough; some are transparent, others opaque (*i.e.,* they cannot be seen through). Membranes may cover a surface, may serve as a dividing partition, may line a hollow organ or body cavity, or may anchor an organ. They may contain cells that secrete lubricants to ease the movement of organs, such as the heart and lung, and the movement of joints. Epithelial membranes and connective tissue membranes are described below.

Epithelial Membranes

An **epithelial membrane** is so named because its outer surface is made of epithelium. Underneath, however, there is a layer of connective tissue that strengthens the membrane, and in some cases, there is a thin layer of smooth muscle under that. Epithelial membranes are made of closely packed active cells that manufacture lubricants and protect the deeper tissues from invasion by microorganisms. Epithelial membranes are of several types:

- **Serous** (SE-rus), **membranes** line the walls of body cavities and are folded back onto the surface of internal organs, forming their outermost layer.
- **Mucous** (MU-kus) **membranes** line tubes and other spaces that open to the outside of the body.
- The **cutaneous** (ku-TA-ne-us) **membrane**, commonly known as the *skin*, has an outer layer of epithelium.

Serous Membranes

Serous membranes line the closed ventral body cavities and do not connect with the outside of the body. They secrete a thin, watery lubricant, known as serous fluid, that allows organs to move with a minimum of friction. The thin epithelium of serous membranes is a smooth, glistening kind of tissue called **mesothelium** (mes-o-THE-le-um). The membrane itself may be referred to as the **serosa** (se-RO-sah).

There are three serous membranes:

- **The pleurae** (PLU-re), or **pleuras** (PLU-rahs), line the thoracic cavity and cover each lung.
- The **serous pericardium** (per-ih-KAR-de-um) forms part of a sac that encloses the heart, which is located in the chest between the lungs.
- The **peritoneum** (per-ih-to-NE-um) is the largest serous membrane. It lines the walls of the abdominal cavity, covers the organs of the abdomen, and forms supporting and protective structures within the abdomen.

Serous membranes are arranged so that one portion forms the lining of a closed cavity, while another part folds back to cover the surface of the organ contained in that cavity. The relationship between an organ and the serous membrane around it can be visualized by imagining your fist punching into a large, soft balloon (Fig. 6-9). Your fist is the organ and the serous membrane around it is in two layers, one against your fist and one folded back to form an outer layer. Although in two layers, each serous membrane is continuous.

The portion of the serous membrane attached to the wall of a cavity or sac is known as the **parietal** (pah-RI-eh-tal) **layer**; the word *parietal* refers to a wall. In the example above, the parietal layer is represented by the outermost layer of the balloon. Parietal pleura lines the thoracic (chest) cavity, and parietal pericardium lines the fibrous sac (the fibrous pericardium) that encloses the heart (see Fig. 6-9).

Because internal organs are called *viscera*, the portion of the serous membrane attached to an organ is the **visceral layer**. Visceral pericardium is on the surface of the heart, and each lung surface is covered by visceral pleura. Portions of the peritoneum that cover organs in the ab-

domen are named according to the particular organ involved. The visceral layer in our balloon example is in direct contact with your fist.

The visceral and parietal layers of a serous membrane normally are in direct contact with a minimal amount of lubricant between them. The area between the two layers of the membrane forms a **potential space**. That is, it is *possible* for a space to exist there, although normally one does not. Only if substances accumulate between the layers, as when inflammation causes the production of excessive amounts of fluid, is there an actual space.

Mucous Membranes

Mucous membranes are so named because they produce a thick and sticky substance called **mucus** (MU-kus). (Note that the adjective *mucous* contains an "o," whereas the noun *mucus* does not.) These membranes form extensive continuous linings in the digestive, respiratory, urinary, and reproductive systems, all of which are connected with the outside of the body. These membranes vary somewhat in both structure and function. The cells that line the nasal cavities and the passageways of the respiratory tract are supplied with tiny, hairlike extensions called *cilia*. The microscopic cilia move in waves that force secretions outward. In this way, foreign particles, such as bacteria, dust, and other impurities trapped in the sticky mucus, are prevented from entering the lungs and causing harm. Ciliated epithelium is also found in certain tubes of both the male and the female reproductive systems.

The mucous membranes that line the digestive tract have special functions. For example, the mucous membrane of the stomach serves to protect the deeper tissues from the action of powerful digestive juices. If for some reason a portion of this membrane is injured, these juices begin to digest a part of the stomach itself—as happens in cases of peptic ulcers. Mucous membranes located farther along in the digestive system are designed to absorb nutrients, which the blood then transports to all body cells.

The noun **mucosa** (mu-KO-sah) is used in referring to the mucous membrane of an organ.

 Checkpoint Question

8. Epithelial membranes have an outer layer of epithelium. What are the three types of epithelial membranes?

Connective Tissue Membranes

The following list is an overview of membranes that consist of connective tissue with no epithelium.

- **Synovial** (sin-O-ve-al) **membranes** are thin connective tissue membranes that line the joint cavities. They secrete a lubricating fluid that reduces friction between the ends of bones, thus permitting

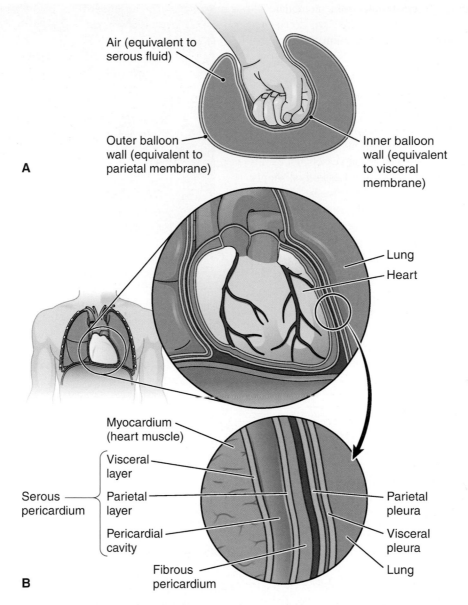

A

Air (equivalent to serous fluid)

Outer balloon wall (equivalent to parietal membrane)

Inner balloon wall (equivalent to visceral membrane)

Lung

Heart

Myocardium (heart muscle)

Serous pericardium

Visceral layer

Parietal layer

Pericardial cavity

Parietal pleura

Visceral pleura

Lung

Fibrous pericardium

B

FIGURE 6-9. Organization of serous membranes. **(A)** An organ fits into a serous membrane like a fist punching into a soft balloon. **(B)** The outer layer of a serous membrane is the parietal layer. The inner layer is the visceral layer. The fibrous pericardium reinforces the parietal pericardium.

free movement of the joints. Synovial membranes also line small cushioning sacs near the joints called **bursae** (BUR-se).
- The **meninges** (men-IN-jeze) are several layers of membranes covering the brain and the spinal cord.

Fascia (FASH-e-ah) refers to fibrous bands or sheets that support organs and hold them in place. Fascia is found in two regions:

- **Superficial fascia** is the continuous sheet of tissue that underlies the skin and contains adipose (fat) tissue that insulates the body and protects the skin. This tissue is

also called *subcutaneous fascia,* because it is located beneath the skin.
- **Deep fascia** covers, separates, and protects skeletal muscles.

Finally, there are membranes whose names all start with the prefix *peri-* because they are around organs:

- The **fibrous pericardium** (per-e-KAR-de-um) forms the cavity that encloses the heart, the pericardial cavity. This fibrous sac and the serous pericardial membranes described above are often referred to together as the pericardium (see Fig. 6-9B).

- The **periosteum** (per-e-OS-te-um) is the membrane around a bone.
- The **perichondrium** (per-e-KON-dre-um) is the membrane around cartilage.

TISSUES AND AGING

With aging, tissues lose elasticity and collagen becomes less flexible. These changes affect the skin most noticeably, but internal changes occur as well. The blood vessels, for example, have a reduced capacity to expand. Less blood supply and lower metabolism slow the healing process. Tendons and ligaments stretch, causing a stooped posture and joint instability. Bones may lose calcium salts, becoming brittle and prone to fracture. With age, muscles and other tissues waste from loss of cells, a process termed *atrophy* (AT-ro-fe) (Fig. 6-10).

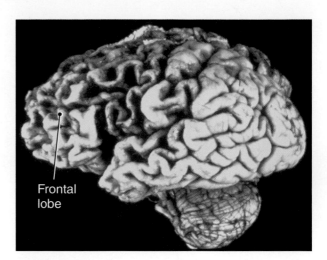

Frontal lobe

FIGURE 6-10. Atrophy of the brain. Brain tissue has thinned and larger spaces appear between sections of tissue, especially in the frontal lobe. (Reprinted with permission from Okazaki H, Scheithauer BW. Atlas of neuropathology. New York: Gower Medical Publishing, 1988. By permission of the author.)

Word Anatomy

Medical terms are built from standardized word parts (prefixes, roots, and suffixes). Learning the meanings of these parts can help you remember words and interpret unfamiliar terms.

Word part	Meaning	Example
hist/o	tissue	*Histology* is the study of tissues.
Epithelial Tissue		
epi-	on, upon	*Epithelial* tissue covers body surfaces.
pseud/o-	false	*Pseudostratified* epithelium appears to be in multiple layers, but is not.
Connective Tissue		
-blast	immature cell, early stage of cell	A *fibroblast* is a cell that produces fibers.
chondr/o	cartilage	A *chondrocyte* is a cartilage cell.
oss, osse/o	bone, bone tissue	*Osseous* tissue is bone tissue.
oste/o	bone, bone tissue	An *osteocyte* is a mature bone cell.
Muscle Tissue		
my/o	muscle	The *myocardium* is the heart muscle.
cardi/o	heart	
Nervous Tissue		
neur/o	nerve, nervous system	A *neuron* is a nerve cell.
Membranes		
pleur/o	side, rib	The *pleurae* are membranes that line the chest cavity.
peri-	around	The *peritoneum* wraps around the abdominal organs.

Summary

I. Tissue classification—epithelial tissue, connective tissue, muscle tissue, nervous tissue

II. Epithelial tissue—covers surfaces; lines cavities, organs, and ducts
    A. Structure of epithelial tissue
        1. Cells—squamous, cuboidal, columnar
        2. Arrangement—simple or stratified
    B. Special functions of epithelial tissue
        1. Produces secretions, *e.g.,* mucus, digestive juices, sweat
        2. Filters impurities using cilia
    C. Glands—active cells are epithelial cells
        1. Exocrine
            a. Secrete through ducts
            b. Examples: digestive glands, tear glands, sweat and oil glands of skin
        2. Endocrine
            a. Secrete into bloodstream
            b. Produce hormones

III. Connective tissue—supports, binds, forms framework of body
    A. Liquid
        1. Blood
        2. Lymph
    B. Soft—jellylike intercellular material (matrix)
        1. Areolar (loose)
        2. Adipose—stores fat
    C. Fibrous—dense tissue with collagenous or elastic fibers between cells
        1. Examples
            a. Tendons—attach muscle to bone
            b. Ligaments—connect bones
            c. Capsules—around organs
            d. Fascia—bands or sheets that support organs
    D. Hard—firm and solid
        1. Cartilage—found at joints and ends of bones, nose, outer ear, trachea, etc.
            a. Types—hyaline, elastic, fibrocartilage
            b. Cells—chondrocytes
        2. Bone
            a. Contains mineral salts

            b. Cells
                (1) Osteoblasts—produce bone
                (2) Osteocytes—mature cells

IV. Muscle tissue—contracts to produce movement
    1. Skeletal muscle—voluntary; moves skeleton
    2. Cardiac muscle—forms main part of the heart
    3. Smooth muscle—involuntary; forms visceral organs

V. Nervous tissue
    A. Neuron—nerve cell
        1. Cell body—contains nucleus
        2. Dendrite—fiber carrying impulses toward cell body
        3. Axon—fiber carrying impulses away from cell body
            a. Myelin—fatty material that insulates some axons
                (1) Myelinated fibers—make up white matter
                (2) Unmyelinated cells and fibers—make up gray matter
    B. Neuroglia—support and protect nervous tissue

VI. Membranes—thin sheets of tissue
    A. Epithelial membranes—outer layer epithelium
        1. Serous membrane—secretes watery fluid
            a. Parietal layer—lines body cavity
            b. Visceral layer—covers internal organs
            c. Examples—pleurae, pericardium, peritoneum
        2. Mucous membrane
            a. Secretes mucus
            b. Lines tube or space that opens to the outside (*e.g.,* respiratory, digestive, reproductive tracts)
        3. Cutaneous membrane—skin
    B. Connective tissue membranes
        1. Synovial membrane—lines joint cavity
        2. Meninges—around brain and spinal cord
        3. Fascia—under skin and around muscles
        4. Pericardium—around heart; periosteum—around bone; perichondrium—around cartilage

VII. Tissues and aging—atrophy

Questions for Study and Review

Building Understanding

Fill in the blanks
1. A group of similar cells arranged in a characteristic pattern is called a(n) _____.
2. Glands that secrete their products directly into the blood are called _____ glands.
3. Tissue that supports and forms the framework of the body is called _____ tissue.
4. Skeletal muscle is also described as _____ muscle.
5. Nervous tissue is supported by specialized cells known as _____.

Matching

Match each numbered item with the most closely related lettered item.

_____ 6. Membrane around the heart   a. perichondrium
_____ 7. Membrane around each lung   b. pericardium
_____ 8. Membrane around bone   c. peritoneum
_____ 9. Membrane around cartilage   d. periosteum
_____10. Membrane around abdominal   e. pleura
        organs

Multiple choice

_____11. Epithelium composed of a single layer of long and narrow cells is called
    a. simple cuboidal epithelium
    b. simple columnar epithelium
    c. stratified cuboidal epithelium
    d. stratified columnar epithelium

_____12. Tendons and ligaments are examples of
    a. liquid connective tissue
    b. soft connective tissue
    c. fibrous connective tissue
    d. hard connective tissue

_____13. A tissue composed of long striated cells with multiple nuclei is
    a. smooth muscle tissue
    b. cardiac muscle tissue
    c. skeletal muscle tissue
    d. nervous tissue

_____14. A bundle of nerve cell fibers held together with connective tissue is called a(n)
    a. dendrite
    b. axon
    c. nerve
    d. myelin

_____15. All of the following are types of epithelial membranes except
    a. cutaneous membrane
    b. mucous membrane
    c. serous membrane
    d. synovial membrane

Understanding Concepts

16. Explain how epithelium is classified and discuss at least three functions of this tissue type.
17. Compare the structure and function of exocrine and endocrine glands and give two examples of each type.
18. Describe the functions of connective tissue. Name two kinds of fibers found in connective tissue and discuss how their presence affects tissue function.
19. Compare and contrast the three different types of muscle tissue.
20. Compare serous and mucous membranes.

Conceptual Thinking

21. Prolonged exposure to cigarette smoke causes damage to ciliated epithelium that lines portions of the respiratory tract. Discuss the implications of this damage.
22. The middle ear is connected to the throat by a tube called the eustachian (auditory) tube. All are lined by a continuous mucous membrane. Using this information, describe why a throat infection (pharyngitis) may lead to an ear infection (otitis media).
23. Osteogenesis imperfecta is a connective tissue disease characterized by abnormal collagen fiber synthesis. Based on the fact that collagen is the predominant fiber type in connective tissue, list some possible symptoms of this disease.

7

Anatomy and Physiology of the Body Systems

CHAPTER OBJECTIVES

In this chapter, you'll learn:

1. To identify major anatomical regions and cavities.
2. To describe the structure and physiological functions of the following organ systems: circulatory, immune, lymphatic, respiratory, digestive, urinary, reproductive, nervous, endocrine, integumentary, and musculoskeletal.

KEY TERMS

absorption
acetylcholine
afferent
alveolus (pl., alveoli)
angiotensin
aorta
arrector pili
arteriole
artery
atrium
autonomic nervous system
axon
brain stem
bronchiole
bronchus (pl., bronchi)
capillary
cerebrospinal fluid (CSF)
cerebrum
choroid
chyle
cochlea
conjunctiva
dendrite
dermis
diaphragm
diaphysis

diencephalon
digestion
effector
efferent
endocardium
endosteum
epicardium
epidermis
epiglottis
epiphysis
erythropoietin
excretion
fascicle
gamete
hilum
hormone
integument
interneuron
keratin
kidney
lacrimal
larynx
lung
lymph
mediastinum
medulla oblongata

melanin
meninges
midbrain
motor
motor unit
myocardium
neurotransmitter
ossicle
osteon
ovary
ovulation
ovum (pl., ova)
parasympathetic nervous
   system
pericardium
periosteum
peristalsis
peritoneum
pharynx
pleura
receptor
retina
sclera
sebaceous
sebum
sensory

septum
skeleton
somatic nervous system
spermatozoon
   (pl., spermatozoa)
steroid
stratum
subcutaneous
sudoriferous
surfactant
sympathetic nervous
   system
synapse
target tissue
tendon
testis (pl., testes)
trachea
tympanic membrane
urea
ureter
urinary bladder
uterus
vein
ventricle
venule
vestibule

THE SKIN is the one system that can be inspected in its entirety without requiring specialized medical imaging techniques. The skin not only gives clues to its own health but also reflects the health of other body systems. Although the skin may be viewed simply as a membrane enveloping the body, it is far more complex than the other epithelial membranes described.

The skin is associated with accessory structures, also known as appendages, which include glands, hair, and nails. Together with blood vessels, nerves, and sensory organs, the skin and its associated structures form the **integumentary** (in-teg-u-MEN-tar-e) **system**. This name is from the word **integument** (in-TEG-u-ment), which means "covering." The term cutaneous (ku-TA-ne-us) also refers to the skin. The functions of this system are discussed later in the chapter after a description of its structure.

STRUCTURE OF THE SKIN

The skin consists of two layers (Fig. 7-1):

- The **epidermis** (ep-ih-DER-mis), the outermost portion, which itself is subdivided into thin layers called

strata (STRA-tah) (sing. stratum). The epidermis is composed entirely of epithelial cells and contains no blood vessels.
- The **dermis**, or true skin, which has a framework of connective tissue and contains many blood vessels, nerve endings, and glands.

Figure 7-2 is a photograph of the skin as seen through a microscope showing the layers and some accessory structures.

Epidermis

The epidermis is the surface portion of the skin, the outermost cells of which are constantly lost through wear and tear. Because there are no blood vessels in the epidermis, the cells must be nourished by capillaries in the underlying dermis. New epidermal cells are produced in the deepest layer, which is closest to the dermis. The cells in this layer, the **stratum basale** (bas-A-le), or **stratum germinativum** (jermin-a-TI-vum), are constantly dividing and producing daughter cells, which are then pushed upward toward the surface of the skin. As the epidermal cells die from the gradual

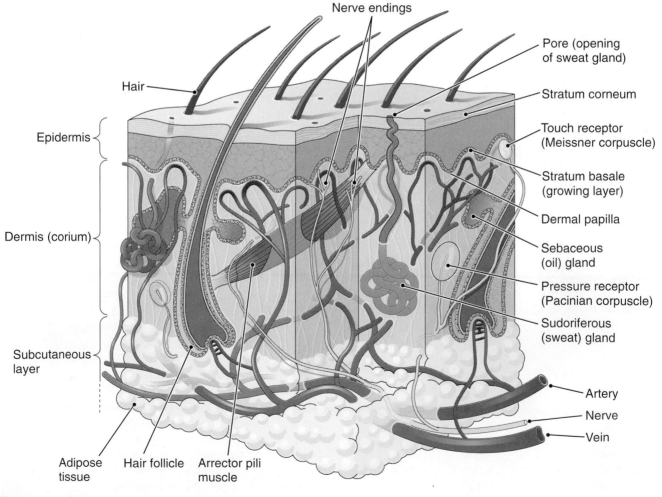

FIGURE 7-1. Cross-section of the skin.

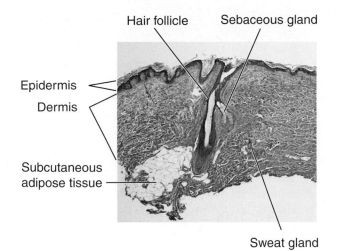

Hair follicle   Sebaceous gland

Epidermis

Dermis

Subcutaneous
adipose tissue

Sweat gland

FIGURE 7-2. Microscopic view of thin skin. Tissue layers and some accessory structures are labeled. (Reprinted with permission from Cormack DH. *Essential Histology*. 2nd ed. Philadelphia: Lippincott Williams & Wilkins, 2001.)

loss of nourishment, they undergo changes. Mainly, their cytoplasm is replaced by large amounts of a protein called **keratin** (KER-ah-tin), which serves to thicken and protect the skin (Fig. 7-3).

By the time epidermal cells approach the surface, they have become flat, filled with keratin, and horny, forming the uppermost layer of the epidermis, the **stratum corneum** (KOR-ne-um). The stratum corneum is a protective layer and is deeper in thick skin than in thin skin. Cells at the surface are constantly being lost and replaced from below, especially in areas of the skin that are subject to wear and tear, as on the scalp, face, soles of the feet, and palms of the hands. Although this process of **exfoliation** (eks-fo-le-A-shun) occurs naturally at all times, many cosmetics companies sell products to promote exfoliation, presumably to "enliven" and "refresh" the skin.

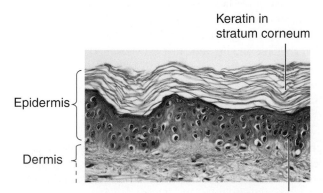

Keratin in
stratum corneum

Epidermis

Dermis

Stratum basale

FIGURE 7-3. Upper portion of the skin. Layers of keratin in the stratum corneum are visible at the surface. Below are layers of stratified squamous epithelium making up the remainder of the epidermis. (Reprinted with permission from Cormack DH. *Essential Histology*. 2nd ed. Philadelphia: Lippincott Williams & Wilkins, 2001.)

Between the stratum basale and the stratum corneum there are additional layers of stratified epithelium that vary in number and quantity depending on the thickness of the skin.

Cells in the deepest layer of the epidermis produce **melanin** (MEL-ah-nin), a dark pigment that colors the skin and protects it from the harmful rays of sunlight. The cells that produce this pigment are the **melanocytes** (MEL-ah-no-sites). Irregular patches of melanin are called freckles.

Dermis

The **dermis**, the so-called "true skin," has a framework of elastic connective tissue and is well supplied with blood vessels and nerves. Because of its elasticity, the skin can stretch, even dramatically as in pregnancy, with little damage. Most of the accessory structures of the skin, including the sweat glands, the oil glands, and the hair, are located in the dermis and may extend into the subcutaneous layer under the skin.

The thickness of the dermis also varies in different areas. Some places, such as the soles of the feet and the palms of the hands, are covered with very thick layers of skin, whereas others, such as the eyelids, are covered with very thin and delicate layers. (See Box 7-1, Thick and Thin Skin: Getting a Grip on Their Differences.)

Portions of the dermis extend upward into the epidermis, allowing blood vessels to get closer to the surface cells (see Figs. 7-1 and 7-2). These extensions, or **dermal papillae**, can be seen on the surface of thick skin, such as at the tips of the fingers and toes. Here they form a distinct pattern of ridges that help to prevent slipping, such as when grasping an object. The unchanging patterns of the ridges are determined by heredity. Because they are unique to each person, fingerprints and footprints can be used for identification.

Checkpoint Questions

1. The skin and all its associated structures comprise a body system. What is the name of this system?

2. The skin itself is composed of two layers. Moving from the superficial to the deeper layer, what are the names of these two layers?

Subcutaneous Layer

The dermis rests on the **subcutaneous** (sub-ku-TA-ne-us) layer, sometimes referred to as the hypodermis or the superficial fascia (see Fig. 7-1). This layer connects the skin to the surface muscles. It consists of loose connective tissue and large amounts of adipose (fat) tissue. The fat serves as insulation and as a reserve supply for energy. Continuous bundles of elastic fibers connect the subcutaneous tissue with the dermis, so there is no clear boundary between the two.

The blood vessels that supply the skin with nutrients and oxygen and help to regulate body temperature run through the subcutaneous layer. This tissue is also rich in nerves and

Box 7-1

A CLOSER LOOK

Thick and Thin Skin: Getting a Grip on Their Differences

The skin is the largest organ in the body, weighing about 4 kg. Though it appears uniform in structure and function, its thickness in fact varies, from less than 1 mm covering the eyelids to more than 5 mm on the upper back. Many of the functional differences between skin regions reflect the thickness of the epidermis and not the skin's overall thickness. Based on epidermal thickness, skin can be categorized as thick (about 1 mm deep) or thin (about 0.1 mm deep).

Areas of the body exposed to significant wear and tear (the palms, fingertips, and bottoms of the feet and toes) are covered with thick skin. It is composed of a thick stratum corneum and an extra layer not found in thin skin, the stratum lucidum, both of which make thick skin resistant to abrasion. Thick skin is also characterized by epidermal

ridges (*e.g.,* fingerprints) and numerous sweat glands, but lacks hair and sebaceous (oil) glands. These adaptations make the thick skin covering the hands and feet effective for grasping or gripping. Thick skin's dermis also contains many sensory receptors, giving the hands and feet a superior sense of touch.

Thin skin covers areas of the body not exposed to much wear and tear. It has a very thin stratum corneum and lacks a distinct stratum lucidum. Though thin skin lacks epidermal ridges and has fewer sensory receptors than thick skin, it has several specializations that thick skin does not. Thin skin is covered with hair, which may help prevent heat loss from the body. In fact, hair is most densely distributed in skin that covers regions of great heat loss — the head, axillae (armpits), and groin. Thin skin also contains numerous sebaceous glands, making it supple and free of cracks that may let infectious organisms enter.

---

nerve endings, including those that supply nerve impulses to and from the dermis and epidermis. The thickness of the subcutaneous layer varies in different parts of the body; it is thinnest on the eyelids and thickest on the abdomen.

Checkpoint Question

3. What is the composition of the subcutaneous layer?

ACCESSORY STRUCTURES OF THE SKIN

The integumentary system includes some structures associated with the skin—glands, hair, and nails—that not only protect the skin itself but have some more generalized functions as well.

Sebaceous (Oil) Glands

The **sebaceous** glands are saclike in structure, and their oily secretion, **sebum** (SE-bum), lubricates the skin and hair and prevents drying. The ducts of the sebaceous glands open into the hair follicles (Fig. 7-4A).

Babies are born with a covering produced by these glands that resembles cream cheese; this secretion is called the **vernix caseosa** (VER-niks ka-se-O-sah), which literally means "cheesy varnish." Modified sebaceous glands, **meibomian** (mi-BO-me-an) **glands**, are associated with the eyelashes and produce a secretion that lubricates the eyes.

Blackheads consist of a mixture of dried sebum and keratin that may collect at the openings of the sebaceous glands.

If these glands become infected, pimples result. If a sebaceous gland becomes blocked, a sac of accumulated sebum may form and gradually increase in size. Such a sac is referred to as a sebaceous cyst. Usually, it is not difficult to remove such tumorlike cysts by surgery.

Sudoriferous (Sweat) Glands

The **sudoriferous** (su-do-RIF-er-us) glands, or sweat glands, are coiled, tubelike structures located in the dermis and the subcutaneous tissue (see Fig. 7-4B). Most of the sudoriferous glands function to cool the body. They release sweat, or perspiration, that draws heat from the skin as the moisture evaporates at the surface. These **eccrine** (EK-rin) type sweat glands are distributed throughout the skin. Each gland has a secretory portion and an excretory tube that extends directly to the surface and opens at a pore (see also Fig. 7-2). Because sweat contains small amounts of dissolved salts and other wastes in addition to water, these glands also serve a minor excretory function.

Present in smaller number, the **apocrine** (AP-o-krin) sweat glands are located mainly in the armpits (axillae) and groin area. These glands become active at puberty and release their secretions through the hair follicles in response to emotional stress and sexual stimulation. The apocrine glands release some cellular material in their secretions. Body odor develops from the action of bacteria in breaking down these organic cellular materials.

Several types of glands associated with the skin are modified sweat glands. These are the ceruminous (seh-RU-min-us) glands in the ear canal that produce ear wax, or **cerumen**; the ciliary glands at the edges of the eyelids; and the **mammary glands**.

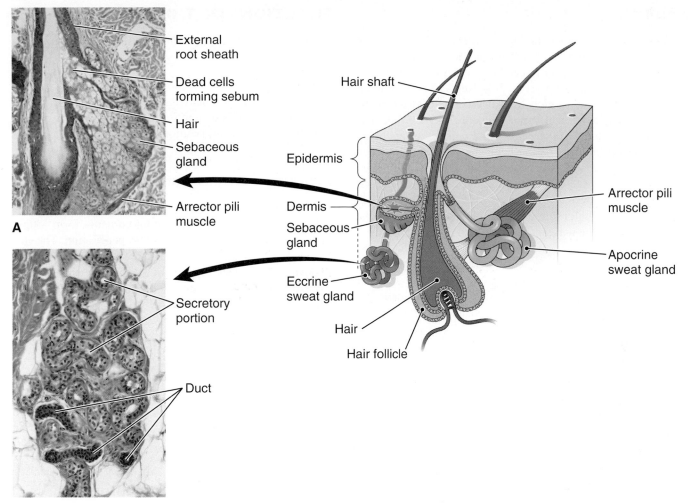

External root sheath

Dead cells forming sebum

Hair

Sebaceous gland

Arrector pili muscle

A

Secretory portion

Duct

B

Hair shaft

Epidermis

Dermis

Sebaceous gland

Eccrine sweat gland

Hair

Hair follicle

Arrector pili muscle

Apocrine sweat gland

FIGURE 7-4. Portion of skin showing associated glands and hair. **(A)** A sebaceous (oil) gland and its associated hair follicle. **(B)** An eccrine (temperature-regulating) sweat gland. (A and B, Reprinted with permission from Cormack DH. *Essential Histology.* 2nd ed. Philadelphia: Lippincott Williams & Wilkins, 2001.) *ZOOMING IN—How do the sebaceous glands and apocrine sweat glands secrete to the outside? What kind of epithelium makes up the sweat glands?*

 Checkpoint Questions

4. Some skin glands produce an oily secretion called sebum. What is the name of these glands?
5. What is the scientific name for the sweat glands?

Hair

Almost all of the body is covered with hair, which in most areas is soft and fine. Hairless regions are the palms of the hands, soles of the feet, lips, nipples, and parts of the external genital areas. Hair is composed mainly of keratin and is not living. Each hair develops, however, from living cells located in a bulb at the base of the hair **follicle**, a sheath of epithelial and connective tissue that encloses the hair (see Fig. 7-4). Melanocytes in this growth region add pigment to the developing hair. Different shades of melanin produce the

various hair colors we see in the population. The part of the hair that projects above the skin is the shaft; the portion below the skin is the root of the hair.

Attached to most hair follicles is a thin band of involuntary muscle (see Fig. 7-1). When this muscle contracts, the hair is raised, forming "goose bumps" on the skin. The name of this muscle is **arrector pili** (ah-REK-tor PI-li), which literally means "hair raiser." This response is of no importance to humans but helps animals with furry coats to conserve heat. As the arrector pili contracts, it presses on the sebaceous gland associated with the hair follicle, causing the release of sebum to lubricate the skin.

 Checkpoint Question

6. Each hair develops within a sheath. What is this sheath called?

Nails

Nails protect the fingers and toes and also help in grasping small objects with the hands. They are made of hard keratin produced by cells that originate in the outer layer of the epidermis (stratum corneum) (Fig. 7-5). New cells form continuously in a growth region (nail matrix) located under the proximal end of the nail, a portion called the nail root. The remainder of the nail plate rests on a nail bed of epithelial tissue. The color of the dermis below the nail bed can be seen through the clear nail. The pale **lunula** (LU-nu-lah), literally "little moon," at the proximal end of the nail appears lighter because it lies over the thicker growing region of the nail. The **cuticle**, an extension of the stratum corneum, seals the space between the nail plate and the skin above the root.

Nails of both the toes and the fingers are affected by general health. Changes in nails, including abnormal color, thickness, shape, or texture (*e.g.*, grooves or splitting), occur in patients with chronic diseases such as heart disease, peripheral vascular disease, malnutrition, and anemia.

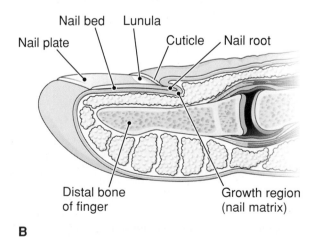

A

B

F I G U R E 7 - 5 .   Nail structure. **(A)** Photograph of a nail, superior view. **(B)** Midsagittal section of a fingertip. (A, Reprinted with permission from Bickley LS. Bates' Guide to Physical Examination and History Taking. 8th ed. Philadelphia: Lippincott Williams & Wilkins, 2003.)

FUNCTIONS OF THE SKIN

Although the skin has many functions, the following are its four major functions:

- Protection against infection.
- Protection against dehydration (drying).
- Regulation of body temperature.
- Collection of sensory information.

Protection Against Infection

Intact skin forms a primary barrier against invasion of pathogens. The cells of the stratum corneum form a tight interlocking pattern that is resistant to penetration. The surface cells are constantly being shed, causing the mechanical removal of pathogens. Rupture of this barrier, as in cases of wounds or burns, invites infection of deep tissues. The skin also protects against bacterial toxins (poisons) and some harmful chemicals in the environment.

Protection Against Dehydration

Both keratin in the epidermis and the oily sebum released to the surface of the skin from the sebaceous glands help to waterproof the skin and prevent water loss by evaporation from the surface.

Regulation of Body Temperature

Both the loss of excess heat and protection from cold are important functions of the skin. Indeed, most of the blood supply to the skin is concerned with temperature regulation. In cold conditions, vessels in the skin constrict (become narrower) to reduce the flow of blood to the surface and diminish heat loss. The skin may become visibly pale under these conditions. Special vessels that directly connect arteries and veins in the skin of the ears, nose, and other exposed locations provide the volume of blood flow needed to prevent freezing.

To cool the body, the skin forms a large surface for radiating body heat to the surrounding air. When the blood vessels dilate (widen), more blood is brought to the surface so that heat can be dissipated.

The other mechanism for cooling the body involves the sweat glands, as noted above. The evaporation of perspiration draws heat from the skin. A person feels uncomfortable on a hot and humid day because water does not evaporate as readily from the skin into the surrounding air. A dehumidifier makes one more comfortable even when the temperature remains high.

As is the case with so many body functions, temperature regulation is complex and involves several parts of the body, including certain centers in the brain.

Box 7-2

CLINICAL PERSPECTIVES

Medication Patches: No Bitter Pill to Swallow

For most people, pills are a convenient way to take medication, but for others, they have drawbacks. Pills must be taken at regular intervals to ensure consistent dosing, and they must be digested and absorbed into the bloodstream before they can begin to work. For those who have difficulty swallowing or digesting pills, transdermal (TD) patches offer an effective alternative to oral medications.

TD patches deliver a consistent dose of medication that diffuses at a constant rate through the skin into the bloodstream. There is no daily schedule to follow, nothing to swallow, and no stomach upset. TD patches can also deliver medication to unconscious patients, who would otherwise require intravenous drug delivery. TD patches are used in hormone replacement therapy, to treat heart disease, to manage pain, and to suppress motion sickness. Nicotine patches are also used as part of programs to quit smoking.

TD patches must be used carefully. Drug diffusion through the skin takes time, so it is important to know how long the patch must be in place before it is effective. It is also important to know how long the medication's effects take to disappear after the patch is removed. Because the body continues to absorb what has already diffused into the skin, removing the patch does not entirely remove the medicine.

A recent advance in TD drug delivery is iontophoresis. Based on the principle that like charges repel each other, this method uses a mild electrical current to move ionic drugs through the skin. A small electrical device attached to the patch uses positive current to "push" positively charged drug molecules through the skin, and a negative current to push negatively charged ones. Even though very low levels of electricity are used, people with pacemakers should not use iontophoretic patches. Another disadvantage is that they can move only ionic drugs through the skin.

Collection of Sensory Information

Because of its many nerve endings and other special receptors, the skin may be regarded as one of the chief sensory organs of the body. Free nerve endings detect pain and moderate changes in temperature. Other types of sensory receptors in the skin respond to light touch and deep pressure. Figure 7-1 shows some free nerve endings, a touch receptor (Meissner corpuscle), and a deep pressure receptor (Pacinian corpuscle) in a section of skin.

Many of the reflexes that make it possible for humans to adjust themselves to the environment begin as sensory impulses from the skin. As elsewhere in the body, the skin works with the brain and the spinal cord to accomplish these important functions.

Other Activities of the Skin

Substances can be absorbed through the skin in limited amounts. Some drugs, for example, estrogens, other steroids, anesthetics, and medications to control motion sickness, can be absorbed from patches placed on the skin. (See Box 7-2, Medication Patches: No Bitter Pill to Swallow.) Most medicated ointments used on the skin, however, are for the treatment of local conditions only. Even medication injected into the subcutaneous tissues is absorbed very slowly.

There is also a minimal amount of excretion through the skin. Water and electrolytes (salts) are excreted in sweat (perspiration). Some nitrogen-containing wastes are eliminated through the skin, but even in disease, the amount of waste products excreted by the skin is small.

Vitamin D needed for the development and maintenance of bone tissue is manufactured in the skin under the effects of ultraviolet radiation in sunlight.

Note that the human skin does not "breathe." The pores of the epidermis serve only as outlets for perspiration from the sweat glands and sebum (oil) from the sebaceous glands. They are not used for exchange of gases.

Checkpoint Question

7. What two mechanisms are used to regulate temperature through the skin?

THE SKELETON

The skeleton is the strong framework on which the body is constructed. Much like the frame of a building, the skeleton must be strong enough to support and protect all the body structures. Bone tissue is the most dense form of the connective tissues. Bones work with muscles to produce movement at the joints. The bones and joints, together with supporting connective tissue, form the skeletal system.

BONES

Bones have a number of functions, several of which are not evident in looking at the skeleton:

- To serve as a firm framework for the entire body
- To protect such delicate structures as the brain and the spinal cord

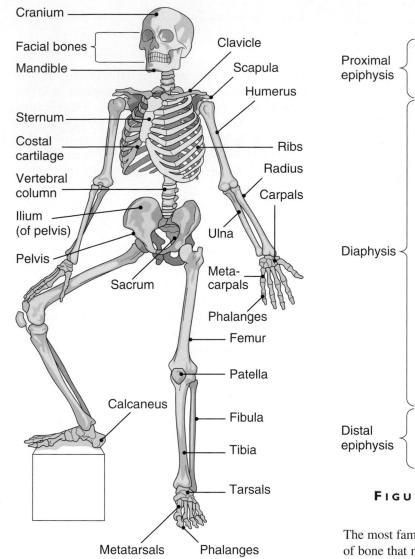

FIGURE 7-6. The skeleton. The axial skeleton is shown in yellow; the appendicular, in blue.

- To serve as levers, working with attached muscles to produce movement
- To serve as a storehouse for calcium salts, which may be resorbed into the blood if there is not enough calcium in the diet
- To produce blood cells (in the red marrow)

Bone Structure

The complete bony framework of the body, known as the **skeleton** (Fig. 7-6), consists of 206 bones. It is divided into a central portion, the axial skeleton, and the extremities, which make up the appendicular skeleton. The individual bones in these two divisions will be described in detail later in this chapter. The bones of the skeleton can be of several different shapes. They may be flat (ribs, cranium), short (carpals of wrist, tarsals of ankle), or irregular (vertebrae, facial bones).

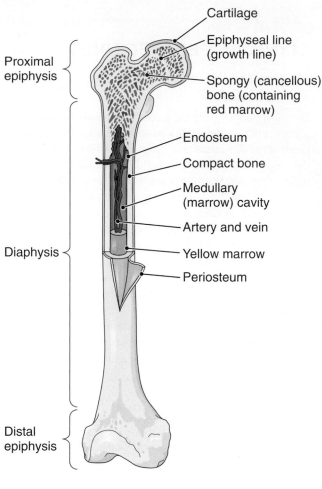

FIGURE 7-7. The structure of a long bone.

The most familiar shape, however, is the long bone, the type of bone that makes up almost all of the skeleton of the arms and legs. The long narrow shaft of this type of bone is called the **diaphysis** (di-AF-ih-sis). At the center of the diaphysis is a **medullary** (MED-u-lar-e) **cavity**, which contains bone marrow. The long bone also has two irregular ends, a proximal and a distal **epiphysis** (eh-PIF-ih-sis) (Fig. 7-7).

Bone Tissue

Bones are not lifeless. Even though the spaces between the cells of bone tissue are permeated with stony deposits of calcium salts, the bone cells themselves are very much alive. Bones are organs, with their own system of blood vessels, lymphatic vessels, and nerves.

There are two types of bone tissue, also known as **osseous** (OS-e-us) tissue. One type is compact bone, which is hard and dense (Fig. 7-8). This tissue makes up the main shaft of a long bone and the outer layer of other bones. The cells in this type of bone are located in rings of bone tissue around a central **haversian** (ha-VER-shan) **canal** containing nerves and blood vessels. The bone cells live in spaces (lacunae) between the rings and extend out into many small radiating channels so

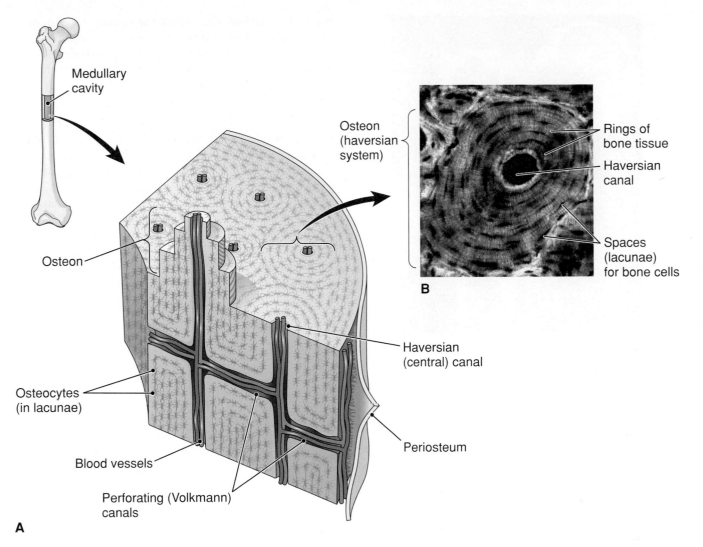

FIGURE 7-8. Compact bone tissue. **(A)** This section shows osteocytes (bone cells) within osteons (haversian systems). It also shows the canals that penetrate the tissue. **(B)** Microscopic view of compact bone in cross section (×300) showing a complete osteon. In living tissue, osteocytes (bone cells) reside in spaces (lacunae) and extend out into channels that radiate from these spaces. (Reprinted with permission from Gartner LP, Hiatt JL. Color Atlas of Histology. 4th ed. Philadelphia: Lippincott Williams & Wilkins, 2005.)

that they can be in contact with nearby cells. Each ringlike unit with its central canal makes up a **haversian system**, also known as an **osteon** (OS-te-on) (see Fig. 7-8B). Forming a channel across the bone, from one side of the shaft to the other, are many **perforating** (Volkmann) **canals**, which also house blood vessels and nerves.

The second type of bone tissue, called spongy, or **cancellous, bone**, has more spaces than compact bone. It is made of a meshwork of small, bony plates filled with red marrow. Spongy bone is found at the epiphyses (ends) of the long bones and at the center of other bones. Figure 7-9 shows a photograph of both compact and spongy tissue in a bone section.

 Checkpoint Questions

8. A long bone has a long, narrow shaft and two irregular ends. What are the scientific names for the shaft and the ends of a long bone?

9. What are the two types of osseous (bone) tissue and where is each type found?

Bone Marrow

Bones contain two kinds of marrow. Red marrow is found at the ends of the long bones and at the center of other bones (see Fig. 7-7). Red bone marrow manufactures blood cells. Yellow marrow is found chiefly in the central cavities of the long bones. Yellow marrow is composed largely of fat.

Bone Membranes

Bones are covered on the outside (except at the joint region) by a membrane called the **periosteum** (per-e-OS-te-um) (see Fig. 7-7). The inner layer of this membrane contains

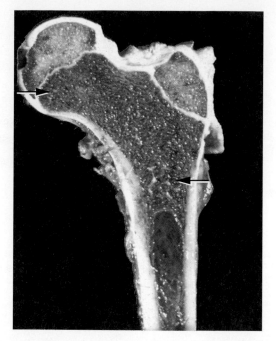

FIGURE 7-9. Bone tissue, longitudinal section. Spongy (cancellous) bone makes up most of the epiphysis (end) of this long bone, shown by the arrows. (Reprinted with permission from Rubin R, Strayer DS. Rubin's Pathology: Clinicopathologic Foundations of Medicine, 5th ed. Philadelphia: Lippincott Williams & Wilkins, 2007.)

cells (osteoblasts) that are essential in bone formation, not only during growth but also in the repair of injuries. Blood vessels and lymphatic vessels in the periosteum play an important role in the nourishment of bone tissue. Nerve fibers in the periosteum make their presence known when one suffers a fracture, or when one receives a blow, such as on the shinbone. A thinner membrane, the **endosteum** (en-DOS-te-um), lines the marrow cavity of a bone; it too contains cells that aid in the growth and repair of bone tissue.

TYPES OF MUSCLE

There are three kinds of muscle tissue: smooth, cardiac, and skeletal muscle. After a brief description of all three types (Table 7-1), this section concentrates on skeletal muscle, which has been studied the most.

Smooth Muscle

Smooth muscle makes up the walls of the hollow body organs as well as those of the blood vessels and respiratory passageways. It moves involuntarily and produces the wavelike motions of **peristalsis** that move substances through a system. Smooth muscle can also regulate the diameter of an opening, such as the central opening of blood vessels, or produce contractions of hollow organs, such as the uterus. Smooth muscle fibers (cells) are tapered at each end and have a single, central nucleus. The cells appear smooth under the microscope because they do not contain the visible

bands, or **striations**, that are seen in the other types of muscle cells. Smooth muscle may contract in response to a nerve impulse, hormonal stimulation, stretching, and other stimuli. The muscle contracts and relaxes slowly and can remain contracted for a long time.

Cardiac Muscle

Cardiac muscle, also involuntary, makes up the wall of the heart and creates the pulsing action of that organ. The cells of cardiac muscle are striated, like those of skeletal muscle. They differ in having one nucleus per cell and branching interconnections. The membranes between the cells are specialized to allow electrical impulses to travel rapidly through them, so that contractions can be better coordinated. These membranes appear as dark lines between the cells (see Table 7-1) and are called intercalated (in-TER-kah-la-ted) disks, because they are "inserted between" the cells. The electrical impulses that produce contractions of cardiac muscle are generated within the muscle itself but can be modified by nervous stimuli and hormones.

Skeletal Muscle

When viewed under the microscope, skeletal muscle cells appear heavily striated. The arrangement of protein threads within the cell that produces these striations is described later. The cells are very long and cylindrical and have multiple nuclei per cell. During development, the nuclei of these cells divide repeatedly by mitosis without division of the cell contents, resulting in a large, multinucleated cell. Such cells can contract as a large unit when stimulated. The nervous system stimulates skeletal muscle to contract, and the tissue usually contracts and relaxes rapidly. Because it is under conscious control, skeletal muscle is described as voluntary.

Skeletal muscle is so named because most of these muscles are attached to bones and produce movement at the joints. There are a few exceptions. The muscles of the abdominal wall, for example, are partly attached to other muscles, and the muscles of facial expression are attached to the skin. Skeletal muscles constitute the largest amount of the body's muscle tissue, making up about 40% of the total body weight. This muscular system is composed of more than 600 individual skeletal muscles. Although each one is a distinct structure, muscles usually act in groups to execute body movements.

 Checkpoint Question

10. What are the three types of muscle?

THE MUSCULAR SYSTEM

The three primary functions of skeletal muscles are:

- Movement of the skeleton. Muscles are attached to bones and contract to change the position of the bones at a joint.

Table 7-1 COMPARISON OF THE DIFFERENT TYPES OF MUSCLE

	Smooth	Cardiac	Skeletal
Location	Wall of hollow organs, vessels, respiratory passageways	Wall of heart	Attached to bones
Cell characteristics	Tapered at each end, branching networks, nonstriated	Branching networks; special membranes (intercalated disks) between cells; single nucleus; lightly striated	Long and cylindrical; multinucleated; heavily striated
Control	Involuntary	Involuntary	Voluntary
Action	Produces peristalsis; contracts and relaxes slowly; may sustain contraction	Pumps blood out of heart; self-excitatory but influenced by nervous system and hormones	Produces movement at joints; stimulated by nervous system; contracts and relaxes rapidly

- Maintenance of posture. A steady partial contraction of muscle, known as muscle tone, keeps the body in position. Some of the muscles involved in maintaining posture are the large muscles of the thighs, back, neck, and shoulders as well as the abdominal muscles.
- Generation of heat. Muscles generate most of the heat needed to keep the body at 37°C (98.6°F). Heat is a natural byproduct of muscle cell metabolism. When we are cold, muscles can boost their heat output by the rapid small contractions we know of as shivering.

Checkpoint Question

11. What are the three main functions of skeletal muscle?

Structure of a Muscle

In forming whole muscles, individual muscle fibers are arranged in bundles, or **fascicles** (FAS-ih-kls), held together by fibrous connective tissue (Fig. 7-10, Table 7-2). The deepest layer of this connective tissue, the **endomysium** (en-do-MIS-e-um) surrounds the individual fibers in the fascicles. Around each fascicle is a connective tissue layer known as the **perimysium** (per-ih-MIS-e-um). The entire muscle is then encased in a tough connective tissue sheath, the **epimysium** (ep-ih-MIS-e-um), which forms the innermost layer of the deep **fascia**, the tough, fibrous sheath that encloses a muscle. (Note that all these layers are named with prefixes that describe their position added to the root *my/o,* meaning "muscle.") All of these supporting tissues merge to form the **tendon**, the band of connective tissue that attaches a muscle to a bone (see Fig. 7-10).

Muscle Cells in Action

Nerve impulses coming from the brain and the spinal cord stimulate skeletal muscle fibers. Because these impulses are traveling away from the central nervous system (CNS), they are described as **motor** impulses (as contrasted to sensory impulses traveling toward the CNS), and the neurons (nerve cells) that carry these impulses are described as motor neurons. As the neuron contacts the muscle, its axon (fiber) branches to supply from a few to hundreds of individual muscle cells, or in some cases more than 1000 (Fig. 7-11).

A single neuron and all the muscle fibers it stimulates comprise a **motor unit**. Small motor units are used in fine coordination, as in movements of the eye. Larger motor units are used for maintaining posture or for broad movements, such as walking or swinging a tennis racquet.

The Neuromuscular Junction

The point at which a nerve fiber contacts a muscle cell is called the **neuromuscular junction** (NMJ) (Fig. 7-12). It is here that a chemical classified as a **neurotransmitter** is released from the neuron to stimulate the muscle fiber. The specific

Table 7-2   CONNECTIVE TISSUE LAYERS IN SKELETAL MUSCLE

Name of Layer	Location
Endomysium	Around each individual muscle fiber.
Perimysium	Around fascicles (bundles) of muscle fibers.
Epimysium	Around entire muscle; forms the innermost layer of the deep fascia.

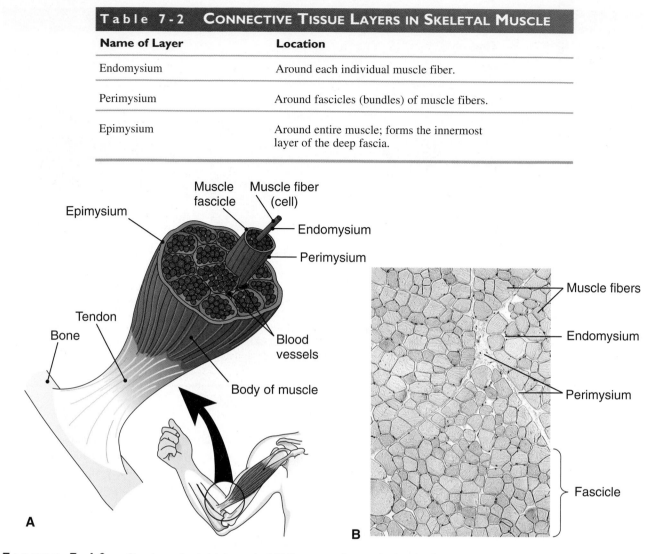

FIGURE 7-10.   Structure of a skeletal muscle. **(A)** Structure of a muscle showing the tendon that attaches it to a bone. **(B)** Muscle tissue seen under a microscope. Portions of several fascicles are shown with connective tissue coverings. (B, Reprinted with permission from Gartner LP, Hiatt JL. Color Atlas of Histology. 3rd ed. Philadelphia: Lippincott Williams & Wilkins, 2000.)   *ZOOMING IN—What is the innermost layer of connective tissue in a muscle? What layer of connective tissue surrounds a fascicle of muscle fibers?*

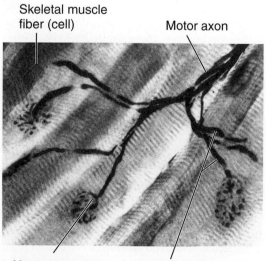

FIGURE 7-11.   Nervous stimulation of skeletal muscle. A motor axon branches to stimulate multiple muscle fibers (cells). The point of contact between the neuron and the muscle cell is the neuromuscular junction. (Reprinted with permission from Cormack DH. Essential Histology. 2nd ed. Philadelphia: Lippincott Williams & Wilkins, 2001.)

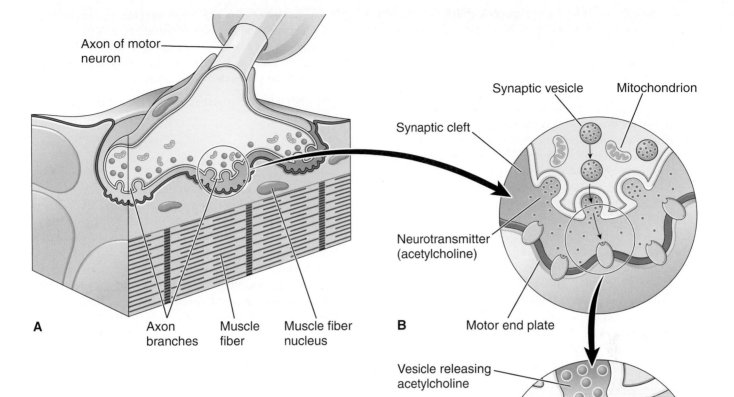

Axon of motor neuron

Axon branches

Muscle fiber

Muscle fiber nucleus

A

Synaptic vesicle

Mitochondrion

Synaptic cleft

Neurotransmitter (acetylcholine)

Motor end plate

B

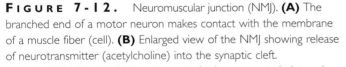

Vesicle releasing acetylcholine

Receptor binds acetylcholine

C

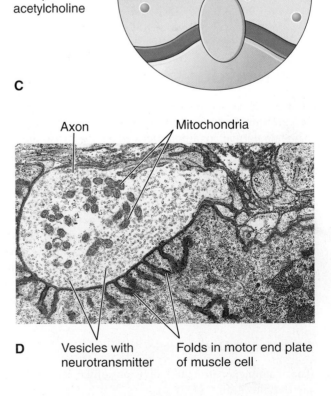

Axon

Mitochondria

Vesicles with neurotransmitter

Folds in motor end plate of muscle cell

D

FIGURE 7-12. Neuromuscular junction (NMJ). **(A)** The branched end of a motor neuron makes contact with the membrane of a muscle fiber (cell). **(B)** Enlarged view of the NMJ showing release of neurotransmitter (acetylcholine) into the synaptic cleft. **(C)** Acetylcholine attaches to receptors in the motor end plate, whose folds increase surface area. **(D)** Electron microscope photograph of the neuromuscular junction. (D, Courtesy of A. Sima.)

neurotransmitter released here is **acetylcholine** (as-e-til-KO-lene), abbreviated ACh, which is found elsewhere in the body as well. A great deal is known about the events that occur at this junction, and this information is important in understanding muscle action.

The neuromuscular junction is an example of a **synapse** (SIN-aps), a point of communication between cells. Between the cells there is a tiny space, the synaptic cleft, across which the neurotransmitter must travel. Until its release, the neurotransmitter is stored in tiny membranous sacs, called vesicles, in the endings of the nerve fiber. Once released, the neurotransmitter crosses the synaptic cleft and attaches to receptors, which are proteins embedded in the muscle cell membrane. The membrane forms multiple folds at this point that increase surface area and hold a maximum number of receptors. The receiving membrane of the muscle cell is known as the **motor end plate**.

Muscle fibers, like nerve cells, show the property of **excitability**; that is, they are able to transmit electrical current along the plasma membrane. When the muscle is stimulated at the neuromuscular junction, an electrical impulse is generated that spreads rapidly along the muscle cell membrane. This spreading wave of electrical current is called the **action potential** because it calls the muscle cell into action.

Checkpoint Questions

12. Muscles are activated by the nervous system. What is the name of the special synapse where a nerve cell makes contact with a muscle cell?
13. What neurotransmitter is involved in the stimulation of skeletal muscle cells?

THE NERVOUS SYSTEM

None of the body systems is capable of functioning alone. All are interdependent and work together as one unit to maintain normal conditions, termed *homeostasis*. The nervous system serves as the chief coordinating agency for all systems. Conditions both within and outside the body are constantly changing. The nervous system must detect and respond to these changes (known as *stimuli*) so that the body can adapt itself to new conditions. The nervous system has been compared with a telephone exchange, in that the brain and the spinal cord act as switching centers and the nerves act as cables for carrying messages to and from these centers.

Although all parts of the nervous system work in coordination, portions may be grouped together on the basis of either structure or function.

Structural Divisions

The anatomic, or structural, divisions of the nervous system are as follows (Fig. 7-13):

- The **central nervous system** (CNS) includes the brain and spinal cord.

- The **peripheral** (per-IF-er-al) **nervous system** (PNS) is made up of all the nerves outside the CNS. It includes all the cranial nerves that carry impulses to and from the brain and all the spinal nerves that carry messages to and from the spinal cord.

The CNS and PNS together include all of the nervous tissue in the body.

Functional Divisions

Functionally, the nervous system is divided according to whether control is voluntary or involuntary and according to what type of tissue is stimulated (Table 7-3). Any tissue or organ that carries out a command from the nervous system is called an **effector**, all of which are muscles or glands.

The **somatic nervous system** is controlled voluntarily (by conscious will), and all its effectors are skeletal muscles. The involuntary division of the nervous system is called the **autonomic nervous system** (ANS), making reference to its automatic activity. It is also called the visceral nervous system because it controls smooth muscle, cardiac muscle, and glands, much of which make up the soft body organs, the viscera.

The ANS is further subdivided into a **sympathetic nervous system** and a **parasympathetic nervous system** based on organization and how each affects specific organs. The ANS is described later in this chapter.

Although these divisions are helpful for study purposes, the lines that divide the nervous system according to function are not as distinct as those that classify the system structurally. For example, the diaphragm, a skeletal muscle, typically functions in breathing without conscious thought. In addition, we have certain rapid reflex responses involving skeletal muscles—drawing the hand away from a hot stove, for example—that do not involve the brain. In contrast, people can be trained to consciously control involuntary functions, such as blood pressure, heart rate, and breathing rate, by techniques known as *biofeedback*.

Checkpoint Questions

14. What are the two divisions of the nervous system based on structure?
15. The nervous system can be divided functionally into two divisions based on type of control and effectors. What division is voluntary and controls skeletal muscle, and what division is involuntary and controls involuntary muscles and glands?

NEURONS AND THEIR FUNCTIONS

The functional cells of the nervous system are highly specialized cells called **neurons** (Fig. 7-14). These cells have a unique structure related to their function.

Table 7-3 FUNCTIONAL DIVISIONS OF THE NERVOUS SYSTEM

| | Characteristics | | |
Division	Control	Effectors	Subdivisions
Somatic nervous system	Voluntary	Skeletal muscle	None
Autonomic nervous system	Involuntary	Smooth muscle, cardiac muscle, and glands	Sympathetic and parasympathetic systems

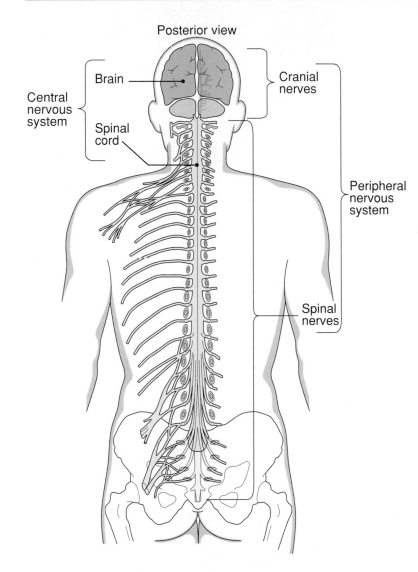

FIGURE 7-13. Anatomic divisions of the nervous system.

Structure of a Neuron

The main portion of each neuron, the cell body, contains the nucleus and other organelles typically found in cells. A distinguishing feature of the neurons, however, are the long, threadlike fibers that extend out from the cell body and carry impulses across the cell (Fig. 7-15). There are two kinds of fibers: dendrites and axons.

• **Dendrites** are neuron fibers that conduct impulses *to* the cell body. Most dendrites have a highly branched, treelike appearance (see Fig. 7-14). In fact, the name comes from a Greek word meaning "tree." Dendrites function as **receptors** in the nervous system. That is, they receive the stimulus that begins a neural pathway.

• **Axons** (AK-sons) are neuron fibers that conduct impulses *away from* the cell body (see Fig. 7-14). These impulses may be delivered to another neuron, to a muscle, or to a gland. An axon is a single fiber, which may be quite long and which branches at its end.

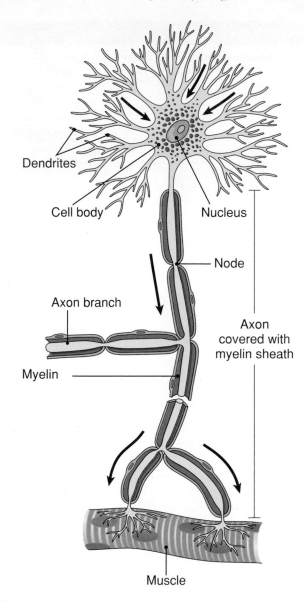

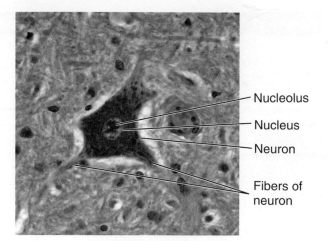

FIGURE 7-15. A typical neuron as seen under the microscope. The nucleus, nucleolus, and multiple fibers of the neuron are visible. (Reprinted with permission from Cormack DH. Essential Histology. 2nd ed. Philadelphia: Lippincott Williams & Wilkins, 2001.)

FIGURE 7-14. Diagram of a motor neuron. The break in the axon denotes length. The arrows show the direction of the nerve impulse. *ZOOMING IN—Is the neuron shown here a sensory or a motor neuron?*

The Myelin Sheath

Some axons are covered with a fatty material called **myelin** that insulates and protects the fiber (see Fig. 7-14). In the PNS, this covering is produced by special connective tissue cells called **Schwann** (shvahn) **cells** that wrap around the axon like a jelly roll, depositing layers of myelin (Fig. 7-16). When the sheath is complete, small spaces remain between the individual cells. These tiny gaps, called **nodes** (originally, nodes of Ranvier), are important in speeding the conduction of nerve impulses.

The outermost membranes of the Schwann cells form a thin coating known as the **neurilemma** (nu-rih-LEM-mah). This covering is a part of the mechanism by which some

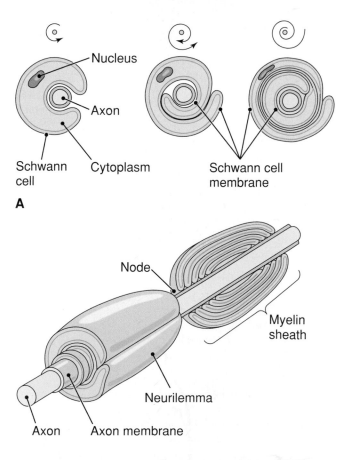

FIGURE 7-16. Formation of a myelin sheath. **(A)** Schwann cells wrap around the axon, creating a myelin coating. **(B)** The outermost layer of the Schwann cell forms the neurilemma. Spaces between the cells are the nodes (of Ranvier).

peripheral nerves repair themselves when injured. Under some circumstances, damaged nerve cell fibers may regenerate by growing into the sleeve formed by the neurilemma. Cells of the brain and the spinal cord are myelinated, not by Schwann cells, but by other types of connective tissue cells. As a result, they have no neurilemma. If they are injured, the damage is permanent. Even in the peripheral nerves, however, repair is a slow and uncertain process.

Myelinated axons, because of myelin's color, are called white fibers and are found in the **white matter** of the brain and spinal cord as well as in the nerve trunks in all parts of the body. The fibers and cell bodies of the **gray matter** are not covered with myelin.

Checkpoint Questions

16. The neuron, the functional unit of the nervous system, has long fibers extending from the cell body. What is the name of the fiber that carries impulses toward the cell body, and what is the name of the fiber that carries impulses away from the cell body?

17. Myelin is a substance that covers and protects some axons. What color describes myelinated fibers, and what color describes unmyelinated tissue of the nervous system?

Types of Neurons

The job of neurons in the PNS is to relay information constantly either to or from the CNS. Neurons that conduct impulses *to* the spinal cord and brain are described as **sensory** neurons, also called **afferent** neurons. Those cells that carry impulses *from* the CNS out to muscles and glands are **motor** neurons, also called **efferent** neurons. Neurons that relay information within the CNS are **interneurons,** also called *central* or *association neurons.*

THE BRAIN

The brain occupies the cranial cavity and is covered by membranes, fluid, and the bones of the skull. Although the brain's various regions communicate and function together, the brain may be divided into distinct areas for ease of study (Fig. 7-17, Table 7-4):

- The **cerebrum** (SER-e-brum) is the largest part of the brain. It is divided into right and left cerebral hemispheres by a deep groove called the longitudinal fissure (Fig. 7-18). Each hemisphere is further subdivided into lobes.
- The **diencephalon** (di-en-SEF-ah-lon) is the area between the cerebral hemispheres and the brain stem. It includes the thalamus and the hypothalamus.
- The **brain stem** connects the cerebrum and diencephalon with the spinal cord. The superior portion of

the brain stem is the **midbrain**. Inferior to the midbrain is the **pons** (ponz), followed by the **medulla oblongata** (meh-DUL-lah ob-long-GAH-tah). The pons connects the midbrain with the medulla, whereas the medulla connects the brain with the spinal cord through a large opening in the base of the skull (foramen magnum).

- The **cerebellum** (ser-eh-BEL-um) is located immediately below the posterior part of the cerebral hemispheres and is connected with the cerebrum, brain stem, and spinal cord by means of the pons. The word *cerebellum* means "little brain."

Each of these divisions is described in greater detail later in this chapter. Damage to any of these brain structures can have severe consequences on brain function (see Box 7-3, Brain Injury: A Heads-Up).

Checkpoint Question

18. What are the main divisions of the brain?

PROTECTIVE STRUCTURES OF THE BRAIN AND SPINAL CORD

The **meninges** (men-IN-jeez) are three layers of connective tissue that surround both the brain and spinal cord to form a complete enclosure (Fig. 7-19). The outermost of these membranes, the **dura mater** (DU-rah MA-ter), is the thickest and toughest of the meninges. (*Mater* is from the Latin meaning "mother," referring to the protective function of the meninges; *dura* means "hard.") Around the brain, the dura mater is in two layers, and the outer layer is fused to the bones of the cranium. In certain places, these two layers separate to provide venous channels, called dural sinuses, for the drainage of blood coming from the brain tissue.

The middle layer of the meninges is the **arachnoid** (ah-RAK-noyd). This membrane is loosely attached to the deepest of the meninges by weblike fibers, allowing a space for the movement of cerebrospinal fluid (CSF) between the two membranes. (The arachnoid is named from the Latin word for spider because of its weblike appearance).

The innermost layer around the brain, the **pia mater** (PI-ah MA-ter), is attached to the nervous tissue of the brain and spinal cord and follows all the contours of these structures (see Fig. 7-19). It is made of a delicate connective tissue (*pia* meaning "tender" or "soft"). The pia mater holds blood vessels that supply nutrients and oxygen to the brain and spinal cord.

Checkpoint Question

19. The meninges are protective membranes around the brain and spinal cord. What are the names of the three layers of the meninges from the outermost to the innermost?

Table 7-4   ORGANIZATION OF THE BRAIN

Division	Description	Functions
Cerebrum	Largest and uppermost portion of the brain Divided into two hemispheres, each subdivided into lobes	Cortex (outer layer) is site for conscious thought, memory, reasoning, and abstract mental functions, all localized within specific lobes
Diencephalon	Between the cerebrum and the brain stem Contains the thalamus and hypothalamus	Thalamus sorts and redirects sensory input; hypothalamus maintains homeostasis, controls autonomic nervous system and pituitary gland
Brain stem Midbrain	Anterior region below the cerebrum Below the center of the cerebrum	Connects cerebrum and diencephalon with spinal cord Has reflex centers concerned with vision and hearing; connects cerebrum with lower portions of the brain
Pons	Anterior to the cerebellum	Connects cerebellum with other portions of the brain; helps to regulate respiration
Medulla oblongata	Between the pons and the spinal cord	Links the brain with the spinal cord; has centers for control of vital functions, such as respiration and the heartbeat
Cerebellum	Below the posterior portion of the cerebellum Divided into two hemispheres	Coordinates voluntary muscles; maintains balance and muscle tone

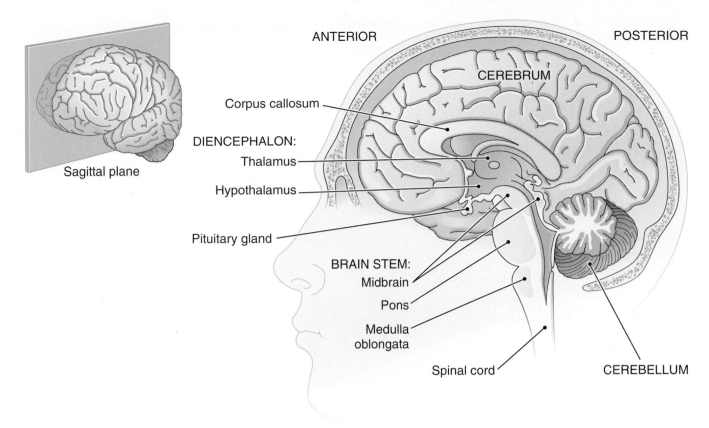

ANTERIOR POSTERIOR

CEREBRUM

Corpus callosum

DIENCEPHALON:

Thalamus

Hypothalamus

Pituitary gland

BRAIN STEM:

Midbrain

Pons

Medulla oblongata

Spinal cord

CEREBELLUM

Sagittal plane

FIGURE 7-17. Brain, sagittal section. Main divisions are shown.

Box 7-3

CLINICAL PERSPECTIVES

Brain Injury: A Heads-Up

Traumatic brain injury is a leading cause of death and disability in the United States. Each year, approximately 1.5 million Americans sustain a brain injury, of whom about 50,000 will die and 80,000 will suffer long-term or permanent disability. The leading causes of traumatic brain injury are motor vehicle accidents, gunshot wounds, and falls. Other causes include shaken baby syndrome (caused by violent shaking of an infant or toddler) and second impact syndrome (when a second head injury occurs before the first has fully healed).

Brain damage occurs either from penetrating head trauma or acceleration-deceleration events where a head in motion suddenly comes to a stop. Nervous tissue, blood vessels, and possibly the meninges may be bruised, torn, lacerated, or ruptured, which may lead to swelling, hemorrhage, and hematoma. The best protection from brain injury is to prevent it. The following is a list of safety tips:

- Always wear a seat belt and secure children in approved car seats.

- Never drive after using alcohol or drugs or ride with an impaired driver.
- Always wear a helmet during activities such as biking, motorcycling, in-line skating, horseback riding, football, ice hockey, and batting and running bases in baseball and softball.
- Inspect playground equipment and supervise children using it. Never swing children around to play "airplane," nor vigorously bounce or shake them.
- Allow adequate time for healing after a head injury before resuming potentially dangerous activities.
- Prevent falls by using a nonslip bathtub or shower mat and using a step stool to reach objects on high shelves. Use a safety gate at the bottom and top of stairs to protect young children (and adults with dementia or other disorienting conditions).
- Keep unloaded firearms in a locked cabinet or safe and store bullets in a separate location.

For more information, contact the Brain Injury Association of America.

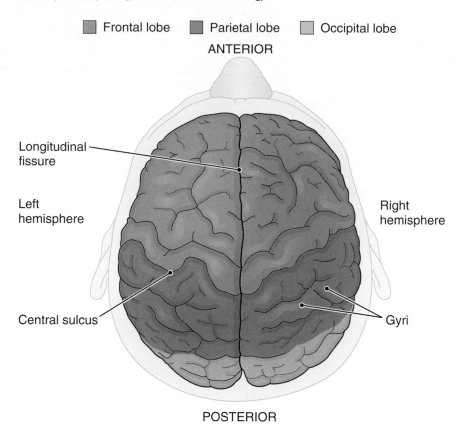

☐ Frontal lobe   ☐ Parietal lobe   ☐ Occipital lobe

ANTERIOR

Longitudinal
fissure

Left
hemisphere

Right
hemisphere

Central sulcus

Gyri

POSTERIOR

FIGURE 7-18. External surface of the brain, superior view. The division into two hemispheres and into lobes is visible.

Cerebrospinal Fluid

Cerebrospinal (ser-e-bro-SPI-nal) **fluid** is a clear liquid that circulates in and around the brain and spinal cord (Fig. 7-20). The function of the CSF is to support nervous tissue and to cushion shocks that would otherwise injure these delicate structures. This fluid also carries nutrients to the cells and transports waste products from the cells.

CSF flows freely through passageways in and around the brain and spinal cord and finally flows out into the subarachnoid space of the meninges. Much of the fluid then returns to the blood through projections called *arachnoid villi* in the dural sinuses (see Figs. 7-19 and 7-20).

Ventricles

CSF forms in four spaces within the brain called **ventricles** (VEN-trih-klz) (Fig. 7-21). A vascular network in each ventricle, the **choroid** (KOR-oyd) **plexus**, forms CSF by filtration of the blood and by cellular secretion.

The four ventricles that produce CSF extend somewhat irregularly into the various parts of the brain. The largest are the lateral ventricles in the two cerebral hemispheres. Their extensions into the lobes of the cerebrum are called horns. These paired ventricles communicate with a midline space, the third ventricle, by means of openings called **foramina** (fo-RAM-in-ah). The third ventricle is surrounded by the diencephalon. Continuing down from the third ventricle, a small

canal, called the cerebral aqueduct, extends through the midbrain into the fourth ventricle, which is located between the brain stem and the cerebellum. This ventricle is continuous with the central canal of the spinal cord. In the roof of the fourth ventricle are three openings that allow the escape of CSF to the area that surrounds the brain and spinal cord.

Box 7-4, The Blood-Brain Barrier: Access Denied, presents information on protecting the brain.

 Checkpoint Question

20. In addition to the meninges, CSF helps to support and protect the brain and spinal cord. Where is CSF produced?

THE SENSORY SYSTEM

The sensory system protects a person by detecting changes in the environment. An environmental change becomes a *stimulus* when it initiates a nerve impulse, which then travels to the central nervous system (CNS) by way of a sensory (afferent) neuron. A stimulus becomes a sensation—something we experience—only when a specialized area of the cerebral cortex interprets the nerve impulse it generates. Many stimuli arrive from the external environment and are detected at or near the body surface. Others, such as stimuli from the viscera, originate internally and help to maintain homeostasis.

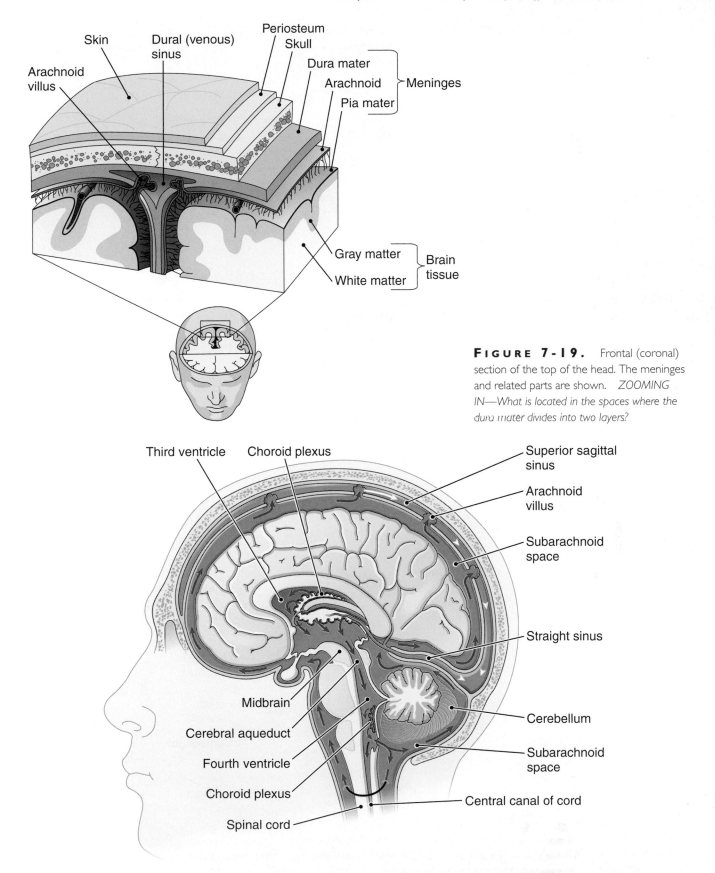

FIGURE 7-19. Frontal (coronal) section of the top of the head. The meninges and related parts are shown. *ZOOMING IN—What is located in the spaces where the dura mater divides into two layers?*

FIGURE 7-20. Flow of cerebrospinal fluid (CSF). Black arrows show the flow of CSF from the choroid plexuses and back to the blood in dural sinuses; white arrows show the flow of blood. (The actual passageways through which the CSF flows are narrower than those shown here, which have been enlarged for visibility.) *ZOOMING IN—Which ventricle is continuous with the central canal of the spinal cord?*

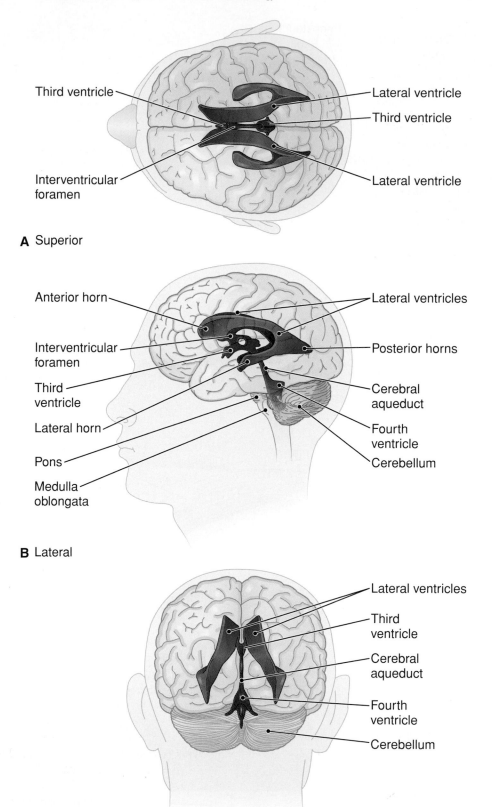

A Superior

B Lateral

C Posterior

FIGURE 7-21.   Ventricles of the brain. Three views are shown.   *ZOOMING IN—Which are the largest ventricles?*

Box 7-4

A CLOSER LOOK

The Blood-Brain Barrier: Access Denied

Neurons in the central nervous system (CNS) function properly only if the composition of the extracellular fluid bathing them is carefully regulated. The semipermeable blood-brain barrier helps maintain this stable environment by allowing some substances to cross it while blocking others. Whereas it allows glucose, amino acids, and some electrolytes to cross, it prevents passage of hormones, drugs, neurotransmitters, and other substances that might adversely affect the brain.

Structural features of CNS capillaries create this barrier. In most parts of the body, capillaries are lined with simple squamous epithelial cells that are loosely attached to each other. The small spaces between cells let materials move between the bloodstream and the tissues. In CNS capillaries, the simple squamous epithelial cells are joined by tight junctions that limit passage of materials between them. Astrocytes—specialized neuroglial cells that wrap around capillaries and limit their permeability—also contribute to this barrier.

The blood-brain barrier excludes pathogens, although some viruses, including poliovirus and herpesvirus, can bypass it by traveling along peripheral nerves into the CNS. Some streptococci also can breach the tight junctions. Disease processes, such as hypertension, ischemia (lack of blood supply), and inflammation, can increase the blood-brain barrier's permeability.

The blood-brain barrier is an obstacle to delivering drugs to the brain. Some antibiotics can cross it, whereas others cannot. Neurotransmitters also pose problems. In Parkinson disease, the neurotransmitter dopamine is deficient in the brain. Dopamine itself will not cross the barrier, but a related compound, L-dopa, will. L-dopa crosses the blood-brain barrier and is then converted to dopamine. Mixing a drug with a concentrated sugar solution and injecting it into the bloodstream is another effective delivery method. The solution's high osmotic pressure causes water to osmose out of capillary cells, shrinking them and opening tight junctions through which the drug can pass.

Sensory Receptors

The part of the nervous system that detects a stimulus is the sensory **receptor.** In structure, a sensory receptor may be one of the following:

- The free dendrite of a sensory neuron, such as the receptors for pain.
- A modified ending, or **end-organ**, on the dendrite of an afferent neuron, such as those for touch and temperature.
- A specialized cell associated with an afferent neuron, such as the rods and cones of the retina of the eye and the receptors in the other special sense organs.

Receptors can be classified according to the type of stimulus to which they respond:

- Chemoreceptors, such as receptors for taste and smell, detect chemicals in solution.
- Photoreceptors, located in the retina of the eye, respond to light.
- Thermoreceptors detect change in temperature. Many of these receptors are located in the skin.
- Mechanoreceptors respond to movement, such as stretch, pressure, or vibration. These include pressure receptors in the skin, receptors that monitor body position, and the receptors of hearing and equilibrium in the ear, which are activated by the movement of cilia on specialized receptor cells.

Any receptor must receive a stimulus of adequate intensity, that is, at least a threshold **stimulus**, in order to respond and generate a nerve impulse.

Special and General Senses

Another way of classifying the senses is according to the distribution of their receptors. A special sense is localized in a special sense organ; a general sense is widely distributed throughout the body.

- **Special senses:**
  - Vision from receptors in the eye.
  - Hearing from receptors in the internal ear.
  - **Equilibrium** from receptors in the internal ear.
  - Taste from the tongue receptors.
  - Smell from receptors in the upper nasal cavities.
- **General senses:**
  - Pressure, temperature, pain, and touch from receptors in the skin and internal organs.
  - Sense of position from receptors in the muscles, tendons, and joints.

THE EYE AND VISION

In the embryo, the eye develops as an outpocketing of the brain. It is a delicate organ, protected by a number of structures:

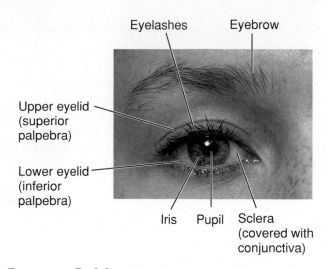

Eyelashes   Eyebrow

Upper eyelid
(superior
palpebra)

Lower eyelid
(inferior
palpebra)

Iris   Pupil   Sclera
(covered with
conjunctiva)

FIGURE 7-22. Protective structures of the eye.
(Reprinted with permission from Bickley LS. Bates' Guide to Physical Examination and History Taking. 8th ed. Philadelphia: Lippincott Williams & Wilkins, 2003.)

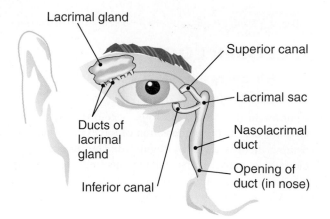

Lacrimal gland

Superior canal

Lacrimal sac

Ducts of
lacrimal
gland

Nasolacrimal
duct

Opening of
duct (in nose)

Inferior canal

FIGURE 7-23. The lacrimal apparatus. The lacrimal (tear) gland and its associated ducts are shown.

- The skull bones form the walls of the eye orbit (cavity) and protect more than half of the posterior part of the eyeball.
- The upper and lower eyelids aid in protecting the eye's anterior portion (Fig. 7-22). The eyelids can be closed to keep harmful materials out of the eye, and blinking helps to lubricate the eye. A muscle, the levator palpebrae, is attached to the upper eyelid. When this muscle contracts, it keeps the eye open. If the muscle becomes weaker with age, the eyelids may droop and interfere with vision, a condition called *ptosis.*
- The eyelashes and eyebrow help to keep foreign matter out of the eye.
- A thin membrane, the **conjunctiva** (kon-junk-TI-vah), lines the inner surface of the eyelids and covers the visible portion of the white of the eye (sclera). Cells within the conjunctiva produce mucus that aids in lubricating the eye. Where the conjunctiva folds back from the eyelid to the anterior of the eye, a sac is formed. The lower portion of the conjunctival sac can be used to instill drops of medication. With age, the conjunctiva often thins and dries, resulting in inflammation and enlarged blood vessels.
- Tears, produced by the **lacrimal** (LAK-rih-mal) glands (Fig. 7-23), lubricate the eye and contain an enzyme that protects against infection. As tears flow across the eye from the lacrimal gland, located in the upper lateral part of the orbit, they carry away small particles that may have entered the eye. The tears then flow into ducts near the nasal corner of the eye where they drain into the nose by way of the nasolacrimal (na-zo-LAK-rih-mal) duct (see Fig. 7-23). An excess of tears causes a "runny nose"; a greater overproduction of them results in the spilling of tears onto the cheeks. With age,

the lacrimal glands produce less secretion, but tears still may overflow onto the cheek if the nasolacrimal ducts become plugged.

 Checkpoint Question

21. What are some structures that protect the eye?

Coats of the Eyeball

The eyeball has three separate coats, or tunics (Fig. 7-24). The outermost tunic, called the **sclera** (SKLE-rah), is made of tough connective tissue. It is commonly referred to as the *white of the eye.* It appears white because of the collagen it contains and because it has no blood vessels to add color. (Reddened or "bloodshot" eyes result from inflammation and swelling of blood vessels in the conjunctiva).

The second tunic of the eyeball is the **choroid** (KO-royd). This coat is composed of a delicate network of connective tissue interlaced with many blood vessels. It also contains much dark brown pigment. The choroid may be compared to the dull black lining of a camera in that it prevents incoming light rays from scattering and reflecting off the inner surface of the eye. The blood vessels at the posterior, or fundus, of the eye can reveal signs of disease, and visualization of these vessels with an **ophthalmoscope** (of-THAL-mo-skope) is an important part of a medical examination.

The innermost tunic, the **retina** (RET-ih-nah), is the actual receptor layer of the eye. It contains light-sensitive cells known as **rods** and **cones**, which generate the nerve impulses associated with vision.

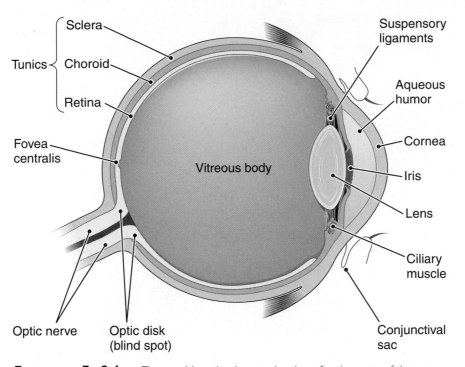

F IGURE 7 - 2 4 .   The eye. Note the three tunics, the refractive parts of the eye (cornea, aqueous humor, lens, vitreous body), and other structures involved in vision.

Checkpoint Question

22. What are the names of the tunics of the eyeball?

THE EAR

The ear is the sense organ for both hearing and equilibrium (Fig. 7-25). It is divided into three main sections:

- The outer ear includes an outer projection and a canal ending at a membrane.
- The middle ear is an air space containing three small bones.
- The inner ear is the most complex and contains the sensory receptors for hearing and equilibrium.

The Outer Ear

The external portion of the ear consists of a visible projecting portion, the **pinna** (PIN-nah), also called the auricle (AW-rih-kl), and the external auditory canal, or **meatus** (me-A-tus), that leads into the deeper parts of the ear. The pinna directs sound waves into the ear, but it is probably of little importance in humans. The external auditory canal extends medially from the pinna for about 2.5 cm or more, depending on which wall of the canal is measured. The skin lining this tube is thin and, in the first part of the canal, contains many wax-producing ceruminous (seh-RU-mih-nus) glands. The wax, or **cerumen** (seh-RU-men), may become dried and im-

pacted in the canal and must then be removed. The same kinds of disorders that involve the skin elsewhere—atopic dermatitis, boils, and other infections—may also affect the skin of the external auditory canal.

The **tympanic** (tim-PAN-ik) **membrane**, or eardrum, is at the end of the external auditory canal. It is a boundary between this canal and the middle ear cavity, and it vibrates freely as sound waves enter the ear.

The Middle Ear and Ossicles

The middle ear cavity is a small, flattened space that contains three small bones, or **ossicles** (OS-ih-klz) (see Fig. 7-25). The three ossicles are joined in such a way that they amplify the sound waves received by the tympanic membrane as they transmit the sounds to the inner ear. The first bone is shaped like a hammer and is called the malleus (MAL-e-us) (Fig. 7-26). The handlelike part of the malleus is attached to the tympanic membrane, whereas the headlike part is connected to the second bone, the incus (ING-kus). The incus is shaped like an anvil, an iron block used in shaping metal, as is used by a blacksmith. The innermost ossicle is shaped somewhat like the stirrup of a saddle and is called the stapes (STA-peze). The base of the stapes is in contact with the inner ear.

Checkpoint Question

23. What are the ossicles of the ear and what do they do?

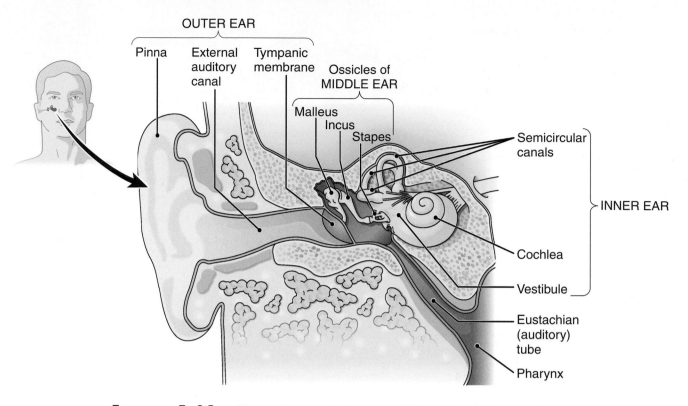

FIGURE 7-25. The ear. Structures in the outer, middle, and inner divisions are shown.

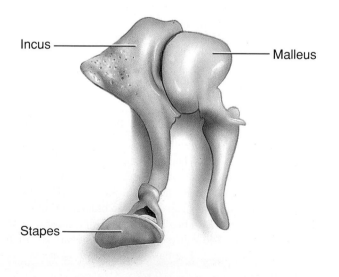

FIGURE 7-26. The ossicles of the middle ear. The handle of the malleus is in contact with the tympanic membrane, and the headlike part with the incus. The base of the stapes is in contact with the inner ear. (Image provided by Anatomical Chart Co.)

The Eustachian Tube

The **eustachian** (u-STA-shun) **tube** (auditory tube) connects the middle ear cavity with the throat, or **pharynx** (FAR-inks) (see Fig. 7-25). This tube opens to allow pressure to equalize on the two sides of the tympanic membrane. A valve that closes the tube can be forced open by swallowing hard, yawning, or blowing with the nose and mouth sealed, as one often does when experiencing pain from pressure changes in an airplane.

The mucous membrane of the pharynx is continuous through the eustachian tube into the middle ear cavity. At the posterior of the middle ear cavity is an opening into the mastoid air cells, which are spaces inside the mastoid process of the temporal bone.

The Inner Ear

The most complicated and important part of the ear is the internal portion, which is described as a *labyrinth* (LAB-ih-rinth) because it has a complex mazelike construction. It consists of three separate areas containing sensory receptors. The skeleton of the inner ear is called the bony labyrinth (Fig. 7-27). It has three divisions:

- The **vestibule** consists of two bony chambers that contain some of the receptors for equilibrium.
- The **semicircular canals** are three projecting bony tubes located toward the posterior. Areas at the bases of the semicircular canals also contain receptors for equilibrium.

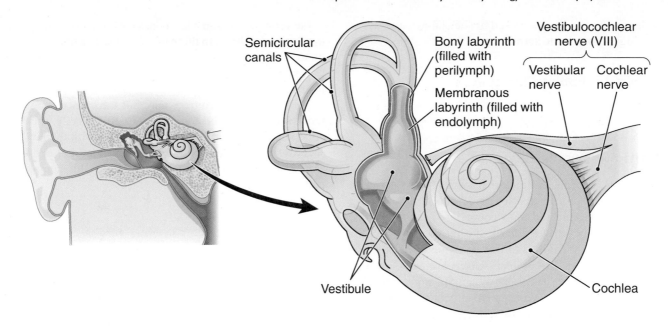

FIGURE 7-27. The inner ear. The vestibule, semicircular canals, and cochlea are made of a bony shell (labyrinth) with an interior membranous labyrinth. Endolymph fills the membranous labyrinth and perilymph is around it in the bony labyrinth.

- The **cochlea** (KOK-le-ah) is coiled like a snail shell and is located toward the anterior. It contains the receptors for hearing.

All three divisions of the bony labyrinth contain a fluid called **perilymph** (PER-e-limf).

Within the bony labyrinth is an exact replica of this bony shell made of membrane, much like an inner tube within a tire. The tubes and chambers of this membranous labyrinth are filled with a fluid called **endolymph** (EN-do-limf) (see Fig. 7-27). The endolymph is within the membranous labyrinth, and the perilymph surrounds it. These fluids are important to the sensory functions of the inner ear.

THE ENDOCRINE SYSTEM

The endocrine system consists of a group of glands that produces regulatory chemicals called **hormones**. The endocrine system and the nervous system work together to control and coordinate all other systems of the body. The nervous system controls such rapid actions as muscle movement and intestinal activity by means of electrical and chemical stimuli. The effects of the endocrine system occur more slowly and over a longer period. They involve chemical stimuli only, and these chemical messengers have widespread effects on the body.

Although the nervous and endocrine systems differ in some respects, the two systems are closely related. For example, the activity of the pituitary gland, which in turn regulates other glands, is controlled by the brain's hypothalamus. The connections between the nervous system and the endocrine system enable endocrine function to adjust to the demands of a changing environment.

HORMONES

Hormones are chemical messengers that have specific regulatory effects on certain cells or organs. Hormones from the endocrine glands are released directly into the bloodstream, which carries them to all parts of the body. They regulate growth, metabolism, reproduction, and behavior. Some hormones affect many tissues, for example, growth hormone, thyroid hormone, and insulin. Others affect only specific tissues. For example, one pituitary hormone, thyroid-stimulating hormone (TSH), acts only on the thyroid gland; another, adrenocorticotropic hormone (ACTH), stimulates only the outer portion of the adrenal gland.

The specific tissue acted on by each hormone is the **target tissue**. The cells that make up these tissues have **receptors** in the plasma membrane or within the cytoplasm to which the hormone attaches. Once a hormone binds to a receptor on or in a target cell, it affects cell activities, regulating the manufacture of proteins, changing the permeability of the membrane, or affecting metabolic reactions.

Hormone Chemistry

Chemically, hormones fall into two main categories:

- **Amino acid** compounds. These hormones are proteins or related compounds also made of amino acids. All hormones except those of the adrenal cortex and the sex glands fall into this category.
- **Steroids**. These hormones are types of lipids derived from the steroid cholesterol. Steroid hormones are produced by the adrenal cortex and the sex glands. Steroid

hormones can be recognized by the ending –*one*, as in progesterone, testosterone.

 Checkpoint Question

24. What are hormones and what are some effects of hormones?

Hormone Regulation

The amount of each hormone that is secreted is normally kept within a specific range. Negative feedback, described in Chapter 5, is the method most commonly used to regulate these levels. In negative feedback, the hormone itself (or the result of its action) controls further hormone secretion. Each endocrine gland tends to oversecrete its hormone, exerting more effect on the target tissue. When the target tissue becomes too active, there is a negative effect on the endocrine gland, which then decreases its secretory action.

We can use as an example the secretion of thyroid hormones (Fig. 7-28). As described in more detail later in the chapter, a pituitary hormone, called *thyroid-stimulating hormone* (TSH), triggers secretion of hormones from the thyroid gland located in the neck. As blood levels of these hormones rise under the effects of TSH, they act as negative feedback messengers to inhibit TSH release from the pituitary. With less TSH, the thyroid releases less hormone and blood levels drop. When hormone levels fall below the normal range, the pituitary can again begin to release TSH. This is a typical example of the kind of self-regulating system that keeps hormone levels within a set normal range.

Less commonly, some hormones are produced in response to positive feedback. In this case, response to a hormone promotes further hormone release. Examples are the action of oxytocin during labor, and the release of some hormones in the menstrual cycle.

The release of hormones may fall into a rhythmic pattern. Hormones of the adrenal cortex follow a 24-hour cycle related to a person's sleeping pattern, with the level of secretion greatest just before arising and least at bedtime. Hormones of the female menstrual cycle follow a monthly pattern.

 Checkpoint Question

25. Hormone levels are normally kept within a specific range. What is the most common method used to regulate secretion of hormones?

THE ENDOCRINE GLANDS AND THEIR HORMONES

Refer to Figure 7-29 to locate each of the endocrine glands as you study them. Table 7-5 summarizes the information on the endocrine glands and their hormones.

Although most of the discussion centers on the endocrine glands, it is important to note that many tissues—other than the endocrine glands—also secrete hormones. That is, they produce substances that act on other tissues, usually at some distance from where they are produced. These tissues include the brain, digestive organs, and kidney.

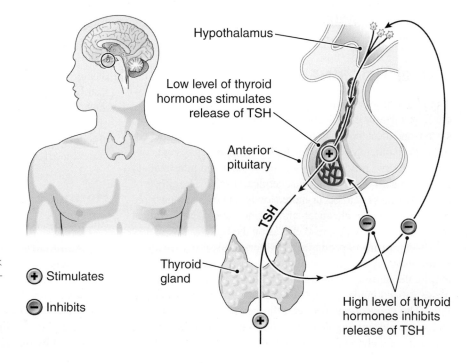

FIGURE 7-28. Negative feedback control of thyroid hormones. The anterior pituitary releases thyroid stimulating hormone (TSH) when the blood level of thyroid hormones is low. A high level of thyroid hormones inhibits release of TSH and thyroid hormone levels fall.

⊕ Stimulates

⊖ Inhibits

Hypothalamus

Low level of thyroid hormones stimulates release of TSH

Anterior pituitary

TSH

Thyroid gland

High level of thyroid hormones inhibits release of TSH

Table 7-5   THE ENDOCRINE GLANDS AND THEIR HORMONES

Gland	Hormone	Principal Functions
Anterior pituitary	GH (growth hormone)	Promotes growth of all body tissues
	TSH (thyroid-stimulating hormone)	Stimulates thyroid gland to produce thyroid hormones
	ACTH (adrenocorticotropic hormone)	Stimulates adrenal cortex to produce cortical hormones; aids in protecting body in stress situations (injury, pain)
	PRL (prolactin)	Stimulates secretion of milk by mammary glands
	FSH (follicle-stimulating hormone)	Stimulates growth and hormone activity of ovarian follicles; stimulates growth of testes; promotes development of sperm cells
	LH (luteinizing hormone); ICSH (interstitial cell-stimulating hormone) in males	Causes development of corpus luteum at site of ruptured ovarian follicle in female; stimulates secretion of testosterone in male
Posterior pituitary	ADH (antidiuretic hormone)	Promotes reabsorption of water in kidney tubules; at high concentration stimulates constriction of blood vessels
	Oxytocin	Causes contraction of uterine muscle; causes ejection of milk from mammary glands
Thyroid	Thyroxine (T_4) and triiodothyronine (T_3)	Increases metabolic rate, influencing both physical and mental activities; required for normal growth
	Calcitonin	Decreases calcium level in blood
Parathyroids	Parathyroid hormone (PTH)	Regulates exchange of calcium between blood and bones; increases calcium level in blood
Adrenal medulla	Epinephrine and norephinephrine	Increases blood pressure and heart rate; activates cells influenced by sympathetic nervous system plus many not affected by sympathetic nerves
Adrenal cortex	Cortisol (95% of glucocorticoids)	Aids in metabolism of carbohydrates, proteins, and fats; active during stress
	Aldosterone (95% of mineralocorticoids)	Aids in regulating electrolytes and water balance
	Sex hormones	May influence secondary sexual characteristics
Pancreatic islets	Insulin	Needed for transport of glucose into cells; required for cellular metabolism of foods, especially glucose; decreases blood sugar levels
	Glucagon	Stimulates liver to release glucose, thereby increasing blood sugar levels
Testes	Testosterone	Stimulates growth and development of sexual organs (testes, penis) plus development of secondary sexual characteristics, such as hair growth on body and face and deepening of voice; stimulates maturation of sperm cells
Ovaries	Estrogens (*e.g.,* estradiol)	Stimulates growth of primary sexual organs (uterus, tubes) and development of secondary sexual organs, such as breasts, plus changes in pelvis to ovoid, broader shape
	Progesterone	Stimulates development of secretory parts of mammary glands; prepares uterine lining for implantation of fertilized ovum; aids in maintaining pregnancy
Thymus	Thymosin	Promotes growth of T cells active in immunity
Pineal	Melatonin	Regulates mood, sexual development, and daily cycles in response to the amount of light in the environment

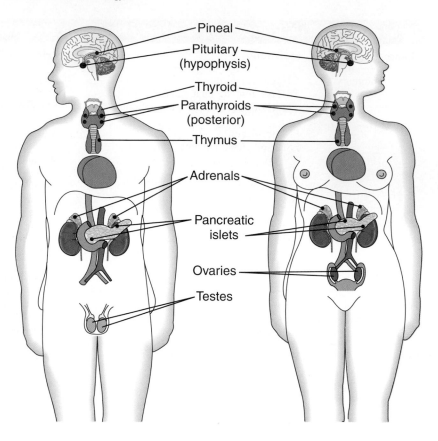

FIGURE 7-29.   The endocrine glands.

THE HEART AND CIRCULATION

The continuous one-way circuit of blood through the body in the blood vessels is known as the circulation. The prime mover that propels blood throughout the body is the **heart**. This chapter examines the structure and function of the heart to lay the foundation for the detailed discussion of blood vessels that follows.

The importance of the heart has been recognized for centuries. Strokes (the contractions) of this pump average about 72 per minute and are carried on unceasingly for the whole of a lifetime. The beating of the heart is affected by the emotions, which may explain the frequent references to it in song and poetry. However, the vital functions of the heart are of more practical concern. Failure of the heart to pump sufficient quantities of blood throughout the body may have life-threatening consequences (see Box 7-5, Artificial Hearts: Saving Lives With Technology).

Location of the Heart

The heart is slightly bigger than a person's fist. This organ is located between the lungs in the center and a bit to the left of the midline of the body (Fig. 7-30). It occupies most of the mediastinum, the central region of the thorax. The heart's **apex**, the pointed, inferior portion, is directed toward the left. The broad, superior base is the area of attachment for the large vessels carrying blood into and out of the heart.

STRUCTURE OF THE HEART

The heart is a hollow organ, with walls formed of three different layers. Just as a warm coat might have a smooth lining, a thick and bulky interlining, and an outer layer of a third fabric, so the heart wall has three tissue layers (Fig. 7-31, Table 7-6). Starting with the innermost layer, these are as follows:

- The **endocardium** (en-do-KAR-de-um) is a thin, smooth layer of epithelial cells that lines the heart's interior. The endocardium provides a smooth surface for easy flow as blood travels through the heart. Extensions of this membrane cover the flaps (cusps) of the heart valves.
- The **myocardium** (mi-o-KAR-de-um), the heart muscle, is the thickest layer and pumps blood through the vessels. Cardiac muscle's unique structure is described in more detail next.
- The **epicardium** (ep-ih-KAR-de-um) is a serous membrane that forms the thin, outermost layer of the heart wall.

The Pericardium

The **pericardium** (per-ih-KAR-de-um) is the sac that encloses the heart (Fig. 7-31, Table 7-7). The outermost and heaviest layer of this sac is the fibrous pericardium. Connective tissue anchors this pericardial layer to the

Box 7-5

HOT TOPICS

Artificial Hearts: Saving Lives With Technology

More than 2000 Americans receive a heart transplant each year. Because, unfortunately, the number of individuals waiting to receive a transplant far exceeds the number of donor hearts available, researchers are inventing alternate technologies.

The ventricular assist device (VAD) is a mechanical pump that helps a patient's damaged heart to pump blood. The device is surgically implanted into a patient's chest or abdomen and connected to either the left or right ventricle. Powered by an external battery connected to it by a thin wire, the VAD pulls blood from the ventricle and pumps it to the aorta (in the case of a left VAD) or the pulmonary artery (in the case of a right VAD). These devices were first designed to help a patient survive until a suitable donor heart could be found, but a permanent model has recently been approved for use in the United States.

More than thirty years ago, researchers began experimenting with total artificial hearts, which are designed to completely replace a patient's damaged heart. The best known of these pumps is the Jarvik-7, an air-driven pump that required tubes and wires to remain connected through the skin to a large external unit. Unfortunately, all of the patients who received this device died of complications shortly after surgery and testing was discontinued. Today, researchers are experimenting with a new completely self-contained artificial heart that uses a wireless rechargeable external battery. A computer implanted in the abdomen closely monitors and controls the heart's pumping speed. If the experiments are successful, total artificial hearts may become a real alternative for patients who would otherwise die waiting for a heart transplant.

Table 7-6 LAYERS OF THE HEART WALL

Layer	Location	Description	Function
Endocardium	Innermost layer of the heart wall	Thin, smooth layer of epithelial cells	Lines the interior of the chambers and covers the heart valves
Myocardium	Middle layer of the heart wall	Thick layer of cardiac muscle	Contracts to pump blood into the arteries
Epicardium	Outermost layer of the heart wall	Thin serous membrane	Covers the heart and forms the visceral layer of the serous pericardium

diaphragm, located inferiorly; the sternum, located anteriorly; and to other structures surrounding the heart, thus holding the heart in place. A serous membrane lines this fibrous sac and folds back at the base to cover the heart's surface. Anatomically, the outer layer of this serous membrane is called the parietal layer, and the inner layer is the visceral layer, also known as the epicardium, as previously noted. A thin film of fluid between these two layers reduces friction as the heart moves within the pericardium. Normally the visceral and parietal layers are very close together, but fluid may accumulate in the region between them, the pericardial cavity, under certain disease conditions.

Checkpoint Questions

26. What are the names of the innermost, middle, and outermost layers of the heart?
27. What is the name of the sac that encloses the heart?

Special Features of the Myocardium

Cardiac muscle cells are lightly striated (striped) based on alternating actin and myosin filaments, as seen in skeletal muscle cells. Unlike skeletal muscle cells, however, cardiac muscle cells have a single nucleus instead of multiple nuclei. Also, cardiac muscle tissue is involuntarily controlled. There are specialized partitions between cardiac muscle cells that show faintly under a microscope (Fig. 7-32). These **intercalated** (in-TER-cah-la-ted) **disks** are actually modified plasma membranes that firmly attach adjacent cells to each other but allow for rapid transfer of electrical impulses between them. The adjective *intercalated* is from Latin and means "inserted between."

Another feature of cardiac muscle tissue is the branching of the muscle fibers (cells). These fibers are interwoven so that the stimulation that causes the contraction of one fiber results in the contraction of a whole group. The intercalated disks and the branching cellular networks allow cardiac muscle cells to contract in a coordinated manner.

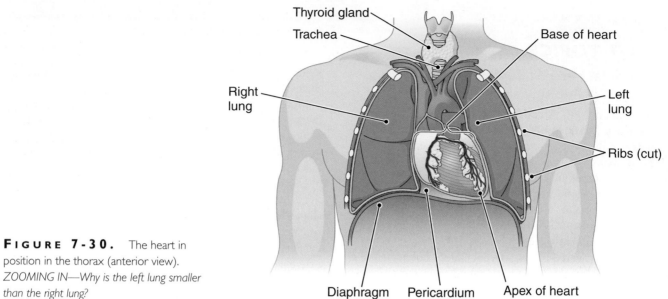

FIGURE 7-30. The heart in position in the thorax (anterior view). *ZOOMING IN—Why is the left lung smaller than the right lung?*

Labels: Thyroid gland, Trachea, Right lung, Base of heart, Left lung, Ribs (cut), Diaphragm, Pericardium, Apex of heart

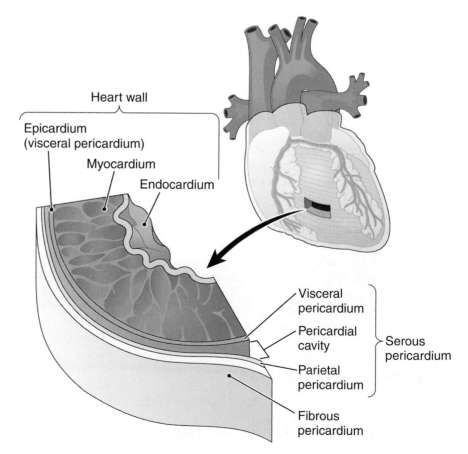

FIGURE 7-31. Layers of the heart wall and pericardium. The serous pericardium covers the heart and lines the fibrous pericardium. *ZOOMING IN—Which layer of the heart wall is the thickest?*

Labels: Heart wall, Epicardium (visceral pericardium), Myocardium, Endocardium, Visceral pericardium, Pericardial cavity, Parietal pericardium, Serous pericardium, Fibrous pericardium

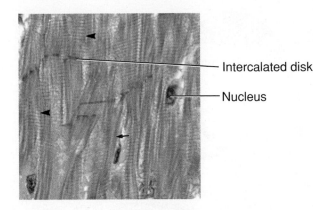

FIGURE 7-32. Cardiac muscle tissue viewed under the microscope (×540). The sample shows light striations (arrowheads), intercalated disks, and branching fibers (arrow). (Reprinted with permission from Gartner LP, Hiatt JL. Color Atlas of Histology. 3rd ed. Philadelphia: Lippincott Williams & Wilkins, 2000.)

Divisions of the Heart

Healthcare professionals often refer to the *right heart* and the *left heart,* because the human heart is really a double pump (Fig. 7-33). The right side pumps blood low in oxygen to the lungs through the **pulmonary circuit**. The left side pumps oxygenated blood to the remainder of the body through the **systemic circuit**. Each side of the heart is divided into two chambers.

Four Chambers

The upper chambers on the right and left sides, the **atria** (A-tre-ah), are mainly blood-receiving chambers (Fig. 7-34, Table 7-8). The lower chambers on the right and left side, the **ventricles** (VEN-trih-klz), are forceful pumps. The chambers, listed in the order in which blood flows through them, are as follows:

1. The right atrium (A-tre-um) is a thin-walled chamber that receives the blood returning from the body tissues. This blood, which is low in oxygen, is carried in **veins**, the blood vessels leading back to the heart from the body tissues. The superior vena cava brings blood from the head, chest, and arms; the inferior vena cava delivers blood from the trunk and legs. A third vessel that opens into the right atrium brings blood from the heart muscle itself, as described later in this chapter.

2. The right ventricle pumps the venous blood received from the right atrium to the lungs. It pumps into a large pulmonary trunk, which then divides into right and left pulmonary arteries, which branch to the lungs. An **artery** is a vessel that takes blood from the heart to the tissues. Note that the pulmonary arteries in Figure 7-34 are colored blue because they are carrying deoxygenated blood, unlike other arteries, which carry oxygenated blood.

3. The left atrium receives blood high in oxygen content as it returns from the lungs in pulmonary veins. Note that the pulmonary veins in Figure 7-34 are colored red because they are carrying oxygenated blood, unlike other veins, which carry deoxygenated blood.

4. The left ventricle, which is the chamber with the thickest wall, pumps oxygenated blood to all parts of the body. This blood goes first into the **aorta** (a-OR-tah), the largest artery, and then into the branching systemic arteries that take blood to the tissues. The heart's apex, the lower pointed region, is formed by the wall of the left ventricle (see Fig. 7-31).

The heart's chambers are completely separated from each other by partitions, each of which is called a **septum**. The interatrial (in-ter-A-tre-al) septum separates the two atria, and the interventricular (in-ter-ven-TRIK-u-lar) septum separates the two ventricles. The septa, like the heart wall, consist largely of myocardium.

 Checkpoint Question

28. The heart is divided into four chambers. What is the upper receiving chamber on each side called? What is the lower pumping chamber called?

Table 7-7 LAYERS OF THE PERICARDIUM

Layer	Location	Description	Function
Fibrous pericardium	Outermost layer	Fibrous sac	Encloses and protects the heart; anchors heart to surrounding structures
Serous pericardium	Between the fibrous pericardium and the myocardium	Doubled membranous sac with fluid between layers	Fluid reduces friction within the pericardium as the heart functions
Parietal layer	Lines the fibrous pericardium	Serous membrane	Forms the outer layer of the serous pericardium
Visceral layer	Surface of the heart	Serous membrane	Forms the inner layer of the serous pericardium; also called the epicardium

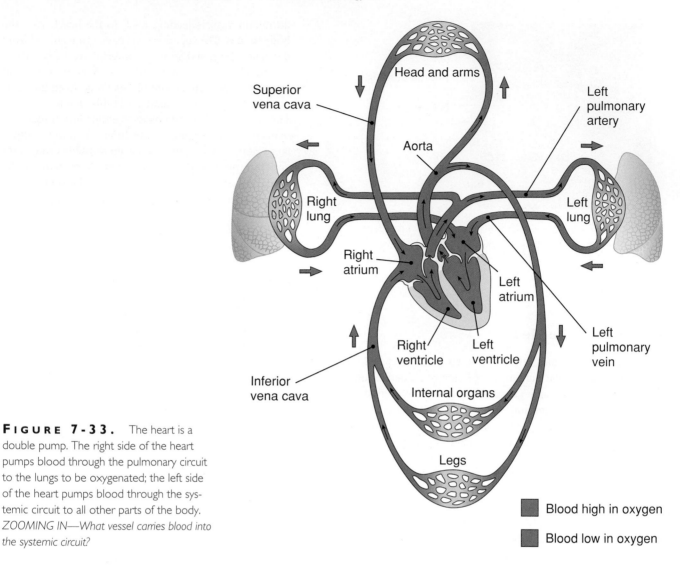

FIGURE 7-33. The heart is a double pump. The right side of the heart pumps blood through the pulmonary circuit to the lungs to be oxygenated; the left side of the heart pumps blood through the systemic circuit to all other parts of the body. *ZOOMING IN—What vessel carries blood into the systemic circuit?*

THE LYMPHATIC SYSTEM

The lymphatic system is a widespread system of tissues and vessels. Its organs are not in continuous order, but are scattered throughout the body, and it services almost all regions. Only bone tissue, cartilage, epithelium, and the central nervous system are not in direct communication with this system.

Functions of the Lymphatic System

The functions of the lymphatic system are just as varied as its locations. These functions fall into three categories:

- **Fluid balance**. As blood circulates through the capillaries in the tissues, water and dissolved substances are constantly exchanged between the bloodstream and the interstitial (in-ter-STISH-al) fluids that bathe the cells. Ideally, the volume of fluid that leaves the blood should be matched by the amount that returns to the blood. However, there is always a slight excess of fluid left behind in the tissues. In addition, some proteins escape

from the blood capillaries and are left behind. This fluid and protein would accumulate in the tissues if not for a second drainage pathway through lymphatic vessels (Fig. 7-35).

In addition to the blood-carrying capillaries, the tissues also contain microscopic lymphatic capillaries. These small vessels pick up excess fluid and protein left behind in the tissues (Fig. 7-36). The capillaries then drain into larger vessels, which eventually return these materials to the venous system near the heart.

The fluid that circulates in the lymphatic system is called **lymph** (limf), a clear fluid similar in composition to interstitial fluid. Although lymph is formed from the components of blood plasma, it differs from the plasma in that it has much less protein.

- **Protection from infection**. The lymphatic system is an important component of the immune system, which fights infection. One group of white blood cells, the lymphocytes, can live and multiply in the lymphatic system, where they attack and destroy foreign organisms. Lymphoid tissue scattered throughout the body

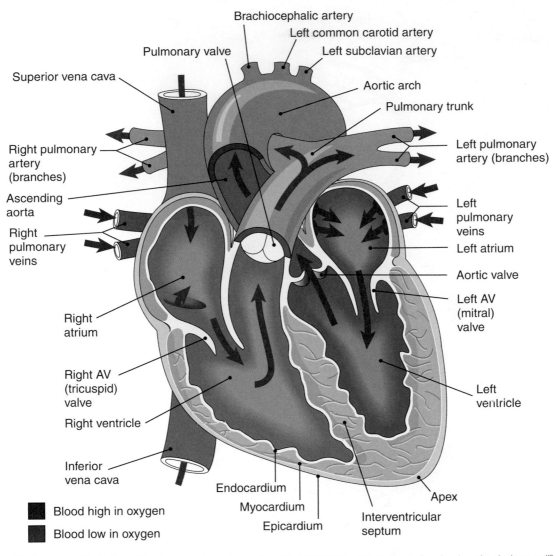

FIGURE 7-34. The heart and great vessels. *ZOOMING IN—Which heart chamber has the thickest wall?*

Table 7-8	CHAMBERS OF THE HEART	
Chamber	**Location**	**Function**
Right atrium	Upper right chamber	Receives blood from the vena cavae and the coronary sinus; pumps blood into the right ventricle
Right ventricle	Lower right chamber	Receives blood from the right atrium and pumps blood into the pulmonary artery, which carries blood to the lungs to be oxygenated
Left atrium	Upper left chamber	Receives oxygenated blood coming back to the heart from the lungs in the pulmonary veins; pumps blood into the left ventricle
Left ventricle	Lower left chamber	Receives blood from the left atrium and pumps blood into the aorta to be carried to tissues in the systemic circuit

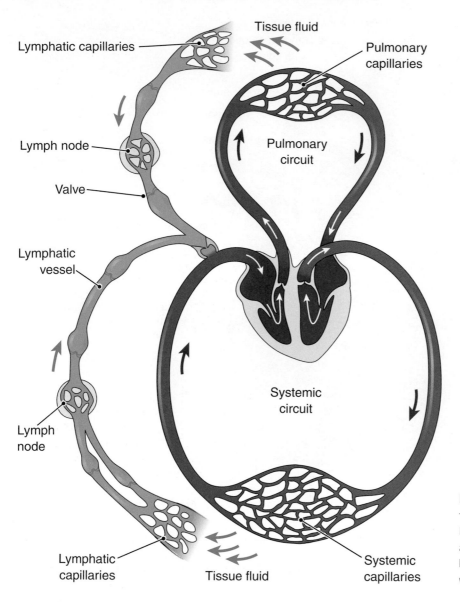

Tissue fluid

Lymphatic capillaries

Pulmonary capillaries

Lymph node

Valve

Pulmonary circuit

Lymphatic vessel

Systemic circuit

Lymph node

Lymphatic capillaries

Tissue fluid

Systemic capillaries

FIGURE 7-35. The lymphatic system in relation to the cardiovascular system. Lymphatic vessels pick up fluid in the tissues and return it to the blood in vessels near the heart. *ZOOMING IN—What type of blood vessel receives lymph collected from the body?*

filters out pathogens, other foreign matter, and cellular debris in body fluids.

- **Absorption of fats**. Following the chemical and mechanical breakdown of food in the digestive tract, most nutrients are absorbed into the blood through intestinal capillaries. Many digested fats, however, are too large to enter the blood capillaries and are instead absorbed into lymphatic capillaries. These fats are added to the blood when lymph joins the bloodstream.

Checkpoint Question

29. What are three functions of the lymphatic system?

LYMPHATIC CIRCULATION

Lymph travels through a network of small and large channels that are in some ways similar to the blood vessels.

However, the system is not a complete circuit. It is a one-way system that begins in the tissues and ends when the lymph joins the blood (see Fig. 7-35).

Lymphatic Capillaries

The walls of the lymphatic capillaries resemble those of the blood capillaries in that they are made of one layer of flattened (squamous) epithelial cells. This thin layer, also called *endothelium*, allows for easy passage of soluble materials and water (Fig. 7-37). The gaps between the endothelial cells in the lymphatic capillaries are larger than those of the blood capillaries. The lymphatic capillaries are thus more permeable, allowing for easier entrance of relatively large protein particles. The proteins do not move back out of the vessels because the endothelial cells overlap slightly, forming one-way valves to block their return.

Unlike the blood capillaries, the lymphatic capillaries arise blindly; that is, they are closed at one end and do not

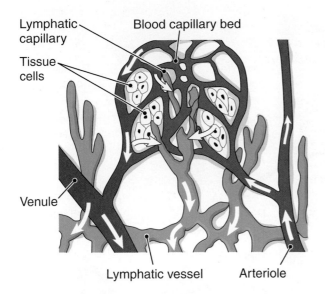

FIGURE 7-36. Pathway of lymphatic drainage in the tissues. Lymphatic capillaries are more permeable than blood capillaries and can pick up fluid and proteins left in the tissues as blood leaves the capillary bed to travel back toward the heart.

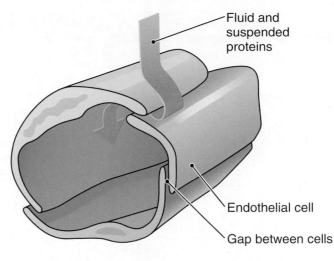

FIGURE 7-37. Structure of a lymphatic capillary. Fluid and proteins can enter the capillary with ease through gaps between the endothelial cells. Overlapping cells act as valves to prevent the material from leaving.

form a bridge between two larger vessels. Instead, one end simply lies within a lake of tissue fluid, and the other communicates with a larger lymphatic vessel that transports the lymph toward the heart (see Figs. 7-35 and 7-36).

Some specialized lymphatic capillaries located in the lining of the small intestine absorb digested fats. Fats taken into these **lacteals** (LAK-te-als) are transported in the lymphatic vessels until the lymph is added to the blood.

 Checkpoint Question

30. What are two differences between blood capillaries and lymphatic capillaries?

Lymphatic Vessels

The lymphatic vessels are thin walled and delicate and have a beaded appearance because of indentations where valves are located (see Fig. 7-35). These valves prevent back flow in the same way as do those found in some veins.

Lymphatic vessels (Fig. 7-38) include superficial and deep sets. The surface lymphatics are immediately below the skin, often lying near the superficial veins. The deep vessels are usually larger and accompany the deep veins.

Lymphatic vessels are named according to location. For example, those in the breast are called mammary lymphatic vessels, those in the thigh are called femoral lymphatic vessels, and those in the leg are called tibial lymphatic vessels. At certain points, the vessels drain through lymph nodes, small masses of lymphatic tissue that filter the lymph. The nodes are in groups that serve a particular region. For example, nearly all the lymph from the upper extremity and the breast passes through the axillary lymph nodes, whereas lymph from the lower extremity passes through the inguinal nodes. Lymphatic vessels carrying lymph away from the regional nodes eventually drain into one of two terminal vessels, the right lymphatic duct or the thoracic duct, both of which empty into the bloodstream.

The Right Lymphatic Duct

The right lymphatic duct is a short vessel, about 1.25 cm (½ inch) long, that receives only the lymph that comes from the superior right quadrant of the body: the right side of the head, neck, and thorax, as well as the right upper extremity. It empties into the right subclavian vein near the heart (see Fig. 7-38B). Its opening into this vein is guarded by two pocket-like semilunar valves to prevent blood from entering the duct. The rest of the body is drained by the thoracic duct.

The Thoracic Duct

The thoracic duct, or left lymphatic duct, is the larger of the two terminal vessels, measuring about 40 cm (16 inches) in length. As shown in Figure 7-38, the thoracic duct receives lymph from all parts of the body except those above the diaphragm on the right side. This duct begins in the posterior part of the abdominal cavity, below the attachment of the diaphragm. The first part of the duct is enlarged to form a cistern, or temporary storage pouch, called the **cisterna chyli** (sis-TER-nah KI-li). **Chyle** (kile) is the milky fluid that drains from the intestinal lacteals, and is formed by the combination of fat globules and lymph. Chyle passes through the intestinal lymphatic vessels and the lymph nodes of the mesentery, finally entering the cisterna chyli. In addition to

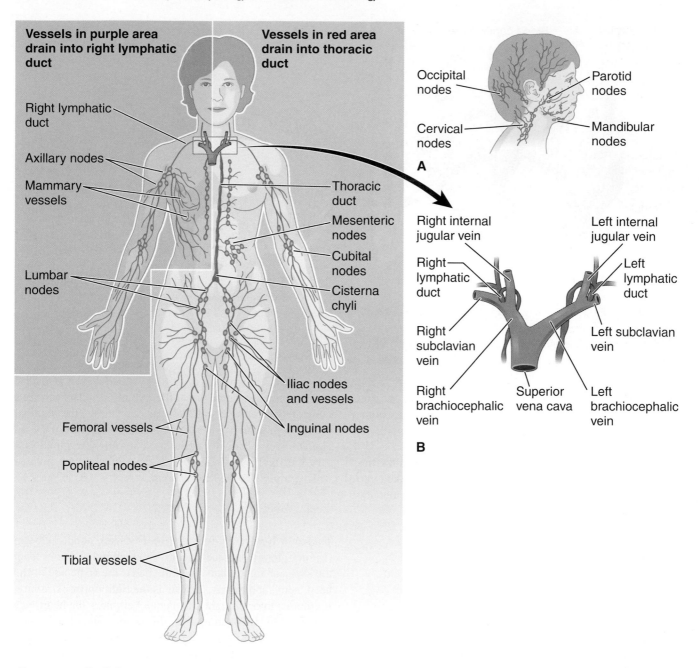

F I G U R E   7 - 3 8 .   Vessels and nodes of the lymphatic system. **(A)** Lymph nodes and vessels of the head. **(B)** Drainage of right lymphatic duct and thoracic duct into subclavian veins.

chyle, all the lymph from below the diaphragm empties into the cisterna chyli, passing through the various clusters of lymph nodes. The thoracic duct then carries this lymph into the bloodstream.

The thoracic duct extends upward through the diaphragm and along the posterior wall of the thorax into the base of the neck on the left side. Here, it receives the left jugular lymphatic vessels from the head and neck, the left subclavian vessels from the left upper extremity, and other lymphatic vessels from the thorax and its parts. In addition to the valves along the duct, there are two valves at its opening into the left subclavian vein to prevent the passage of blood into the duct.

Checkpoint Question

31. What are the two main lymphatic vessels?

Movement of Lymph

The segments of lymphatic vessels located between the valves contract rhythmically, propelling the lymph along. The contraction rate is related to the volume of fluid in the vessel—the more fluid, the more rapid the contractions.

Lymph is also moved by the same mechanisms that promote venous return of blood to the heart. As skeletal muscles contract during movement, they compress the lymphatic vessels and drive lymph forward. Changes in pressures within the abdominal and thoracic cavities caused by breathing aid the movement of lymph during passage through these body cavities.

LYMPHOID TISSUE

Lymphoid (LIM-foyd) tissue is distributed throughout the body and makes up the specialized organs of the lymphatic system. The lymph nodes have already been described relative to describing lymphatic circulation, but these tissues and other components of the lymphatic system are discussed in greater detail in the next section.

Lymph Nodes

The lymph nodes, as noted, are designed to filter the lymph once it is drained from the tissues (Fig. 7-39). They are also sites where lymphocytes of the immune system multiply and work to combat foreign organisms. The lymph nodes are small, rounded masses varying from pinhead size to as long as 2.5 cm (1 inch). Each has a fibrous connective tissue capsule from which partitions (trabeculae) extend into the substance of the node. At various points in the node's surface, afferent lymphatic vessels pierce the capsule to carry lymph into the node. An indented area called the **hilum** (HI-lum) is the exit point for efferent lymphatic vessels carrying lymph out of the node. At this region, other structures, including blood vessels and nerves, connect with the node.

Each node is subdivided into lymph-filled spaces (sinuses) and cords of lymphatic tissue. Pulplike nodules in the outer region, or cortex, have germinal centers where certain immune lymphocytes multiply. The inner region, the medulla, has populations of immune cells, including lymphocytes and macrophages (phagocytes) along open channels that lead into the efferent vessels.

Lymph nodes are seldom isolated. As a rule, they are massed together in groups, varying in number from 2 or 3 to well over 100. Some of these groups are placed deeply, whereas others are superficial. The main groups include the following:

- **Cervical nodes**, located in the neck in deep and superficial groups, drain various parts of the head and neck. They often become enlarged during upper respiratory infections.
- **Axillary nodes**, located in the axillae (armpits), may become enlarged after infections of the upper extremities and the breasts. Cancer cells from the breasts often metastasize (spread) to the axillary nodes.
- **Tracheobronchial** (tra-ke-o-BRONG-ke-al) **nodes** are found near the trachea and around the larger bronchial tubes. In people living in highly polluted areas, these nodes become so filled with carbon particles that they are solid black masses resembling pieces of coal.

- **Mesenteric** (mes-en-TER-ik) nodes are found between the two layers of peritoneum that form the mesentery (membrane around the intestines). There are some 100 to 150 of these nodes.
- **Inguinal nodes**, located in the groin region, receive lymph drainage from the lower extremities and from the external genital organs. When they become enlarged, they are often referred to as buboes (BU-bose), from which bubonic plague got its name.

Box 7-6 explains the role of lymph node biopsy in the treatment of cancer.

Checkpoint Question

32. What is the function of the lymph nodes?

PHASES OF RESPIRATION

Most people think of respiration simply as the process by which air moves into and out of the lungs, that is, *breathing.* By scientific definition, respiration is the process by which oxygen is obtained from the environment and delivered to the cells. Carbon dioxide is transported to the outside in a reverse pathway (Fig. 7-40).

Respiration includes three phases:

- **Pulmonary ventilation,** which is the exchange of air between the atmosphere and the air sacs (alveoli) of the lungs. This is normally accomplished by the inhalation and exhalation of breathing.
- **External exchange of gases**, which occurs in the lungs as oxygen (O_2) diffuses from the air sacs into the blood and carbon dioxide (CO_2) diffuses out of the blood to be eliminated.
- **Internal exchange of gases**, which occurs in the tissues as oxygen diffuses from the blood to the cells, whereas carbon dioxide passes from the cells into the blood.

Gas exchange requires close association of the respiratory system with the circulatory system, as the circulating blood is needed to transport oxygen to the cells and transport carbon dioxide back to the lungs.

The term *respiration* is also used to describe a related process that occurs at the cellular level. In **cellular respiration**, oxygen is taken into a cell and used in the breakdown of nutrients with the release of energy. Carbon dioxide is the waste product of cellular respiration.

Checkpoint Question

33. What are the three phases of respiration?

THE RESPIRATORY SYSTEM

The respiratory system is an intricate arrangement of spaces and passageways that conduct air into the lungs (Fig. 7-41).

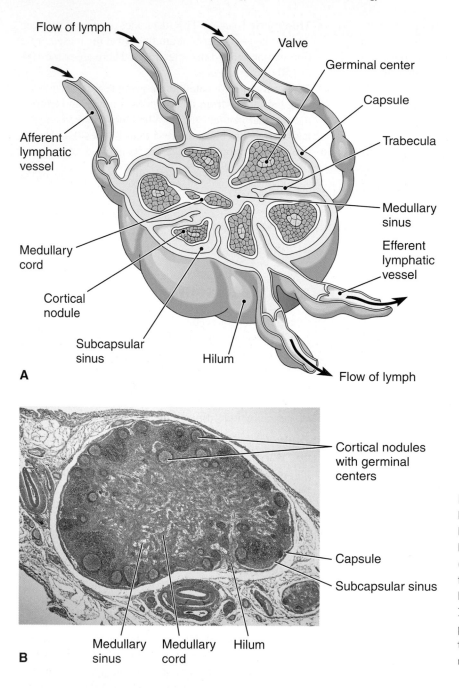

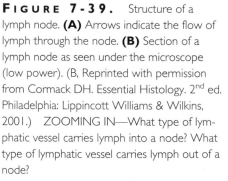

FIGURE 7-39. Structure of a lymph node. **(A)** Arrows indicate the flow of lymph through the node. **(B)** Section of a lymph node as seen under the microscope (low power). (B, Reprinted with permission from Cormack DH. Essential Histology. 2ⁿᵈ ed. Philadelphia: Lippincott Williams & Wilkins, 2001.)   ZOOMING IN—What type of lymphatic vessel carries lymph into a node? What type of lymphatic vessel carries lymph out of a node?

These spaces include the nasal cavities; the **pharynx** (FAR-inks), which is common to the digestive and respiratory systems; the voice box, or **larynx** (LAR-inks); the windpipe, or **trachea** (TRA-ke-ah); and the **lungs** themselves, with their conducting tubes and air sacs. The entire system might be thought of as a pathway for air between the atmosphere and the blood.

The Nasal Cavities

Air enters the body through the openings in the nose called the nostrils, or nares *(NA-reze)* (sing., naris). Immediately inside the nostrils, located between the roof of the mouth and the cranium, are the two spaces known as the **nasal cavities**.

These two spaces are separated from each other by a partition, the nasal septum. The superior portion of the septum is formed by a thin plate of the ethmoid bone that extends downward, and the inferior portion is formed by the vomer. An anterior extension of the septum is made of hyaline cartilage. The septum and the walls of the nasal cavity are covered with mucous membrane. On the lateral walls of each nasal cavity are three projections called the **conchae** (KONG-ke). The shell-like conchae greatly increase the surface area of the mucous membrane over which air travels on its way through the nasal cavities.

The mucous membrane lining the nasal cavities contains many blood vessels that deliver heat and moisture. The cells of this membrane secrete a large amount of fluid—up to 1

Box 7-6

HOT TOPICS

Sentinel Node Biopsy: Finding Cancer Before it Spreads

Ordinarily, the lymphatic system is one of the body's primary defenses against disease. In cancer, though, it can be a vehicle for the spread (metastasis) of disease. When cancer cells enter the lymphatic vessels, they travel to other parts of the body, where they may establish new tumors. Along the way, some cancer cells become lodged in the lymph nodes.

In breast cancer, the degree of invasion of nearby lymph nodes helps determine what treatments are required after surgical removal of the tumor. Until recently, a mastectomy often included the removal of nearby lymphatic vessels and nodes (a procedure called axillary lymph node dissection). Biopsy of the nodes determined whether or not they contained cancerous cells, and if they did, radiation treatment or chemotherapy was required. In many women with early-stage breast cancer, however, the axillary bodies do not contain cancerous cells. In addition, about 20 percent of the women whose lymphatic vessels and nodes have been removed suffer impaired lymph flow. The results are lymphedema, pain, disability, and an increased risk of infection.

Sentinel node biopsy is a new diagnostic procedure that may minimize the need to perform axillary lymph node dissection, while still detecting metastasis. Surgeons use radioactive tracers to identify the first nodes that receive lymph from the area of a tumor. Biopsy of only these "sentinel nodes" reveals whether tumor cells are present, providing the earliest indication of metastasis. Research shows that sentinel lymph node biopsy is associated with less pain, fewer complications, and faster recovery than axillary lymph node dissection. However, because the procedure is relatively new, more clinical trials are required to determine whether sentinel node biopsy is as successful as axillary dissection in finding cancer before it spreads.

---

quart each day. The following changes are produced in the air as it comes in contact with the lining of the nose:

- Foreign bodies, such as dust particles and pathogens, are filtered out by the hairs of the nostrils or caught in the surface mucus.
- Air is warmed by blood in the well-vascularized mucous membrane.
- Air is moistened by the liquid secretion.

To allow for these protective changes to occur, it is preferable to breathe through the nose rather than through the mouth.

The **sinuses** are small cavities lined with mucous membrane in the skull bones. They are resonating chambers for the voice and lessen the weight of the skull. The sinuses communicate with the nasal cavities, and they are highly susceptible to infection.

 Checkpoint Question

34. What happens to air as it passes over the nasal mucosa?

The Pharynx

The muscular pharynx, or throat, carries air into the respiratory tract and carries foods and liquids into the digestive system (see Fig. 7-41). The superior portion, located immediately behind the nasal cavity, is called the **nasopharynx** (na-zo-FAR-inks); the middle section, located posterior to the mouth, is called the **oropharynx** (o-ro-FAR-inks); and the most inferior portion is called the **laryngeal** (lah-RIN-je-al) **pharynx.** This last section opens into the larynx toward the anterior and into the esophagus toward the posterior.

The Larynx

The larynx, commonly called the *voice box* (Fig. 7-42), is located between the pharynx and the trachea. It has a framework of cartilage, part of which is the thyroid cartilage that protrudes in the front of the neck. The projection formed by the thyroid cartilage is commonly called the *Adam's apple* because it is considerably larger in the male than in the female.

Folds of mucous membrane used in producing speech are located on both sides at the superior portion of the larynx. These are the vocal folds, or **vocal cords** (Fig. 7-43), which vibrate as air flows over them from the lungs. Variations in the length and tension of the vocal cords and the distance between them regulate the pitch of sound. The amount of air forced over them regulates volume. A difference in the size of the larynx and the vocal cords is what accounts for the difference between adult male and female voices. In general, a man's larynx is larger than a woman's. His vocal cords are thicker and longer, so they vibrate more slowly, resulting in a lower range of pitch. Muscles of the pharynx, tongue, lips, and face also are used to form clear pronunciations. The mouth, nasal cavities, paranasal sinuses, and the pharynx all serve as resonating chambers for speech, just as does the cabinet for an audio speaker.

The space between the vocal cords is called the **glottis** (GLOT-is). This is somewhat open during normal breathing but widely open during forced breathing (see Fig. 7-43). The

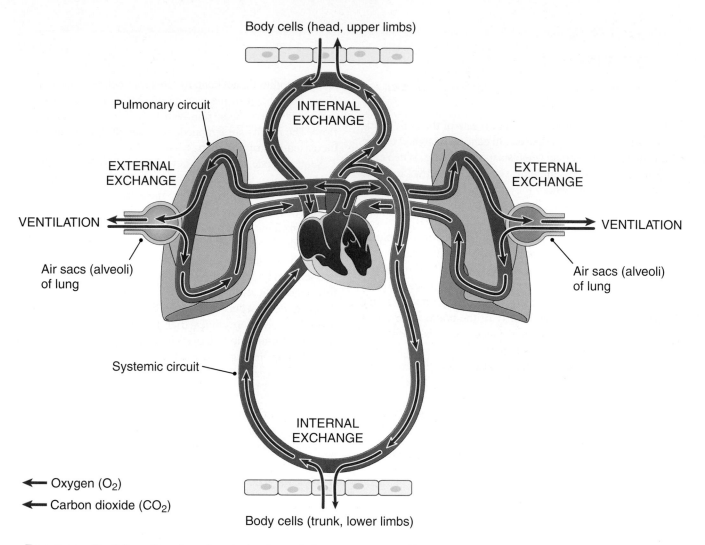

Body cells (head, upper limbs)

Pulmonary circuit

INTERNAL EXCHANGE

EXTERNAL EXCHANGE

EXTERNAL EXCHANGE

VENTILATION

VENTILATION

Air sacs (alveoli) of lung

Air sacs (alveoli) of lung

Systemic circuit

INTERNAL EXCHANGE

← Oxygen (O_2)

← Carbon dioxide (CO_2)

Body cells (trunk, lower limbs)

FIGURE 7-40.   *Overview of respiration. In ventilation, gases are moved into and out of the lungs. In external exchange, gases move between the air sacs (alveoli) of the lungs and the blood. In internal exchange, gases move between the blood and body cells. The circulation transports gases in the blood.*

little leaf-shaped cartilage that covers the larynx during swallowing is called the **epiglottis** (ep-ih-GLOT-is). The glottis and epiglottis help keep food and liquids out of the remainder of the respiratory tract. As the larynx moves upward and forward during swallowing, the epiglottis moves downward, covering the opening into the larynx. You can feel the larynx move upward toward the epiglottis during this process by placing the flat ends of your fingers on your larynx as you swallow. Muscles in the larynx assist in keeping foreign materials out of the respiratory tract by closing the glottis during swallowing. Muscles also close the glottis when one holds his or her breath and strains, as to defecate or lift a heavy weight.

The Trachea

The trachea, commonly called the *windpipe,* is a tube that extends from the inferior edge of the larynx to the upper part of

the chest superior to the heart. The trachea's purpose is to conduct air between the larynx and the lungs.

A framework of separate cartilages reinforces the trachea and keeps it open. These cartilages, each shaped somewhat like a tiny horseshoe or the letter C, are found along the trachea's entire length. The open sections in the cartilages are lined up at their posterior so that the esophagus can expand into this region during swallowing.

Checkpoint Questions

35. What are the scientific names for the throat, voice box, and windpipe?

36. What are the three regions of the pharynx?

The Bronchi

At its inferior end, the trachea divides into two primary, or main-stem, **bronchi** (BRONG-ki), which enter the lungs (see

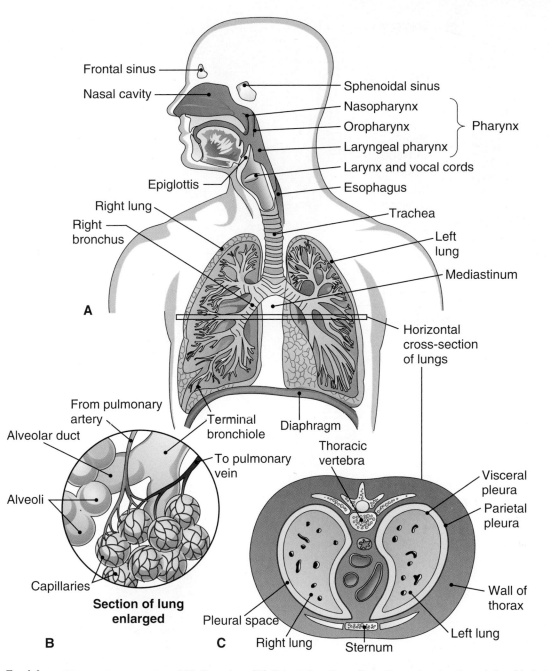

Frontal sinus
Nasal cavity
Sphenoidal sinus
Nasopharynx
Oropharynx
Laryngeal pharynx
} Pharynx
Larynx and vocal cords
Epiglottis
Esophagus
Right lung
Trachea
Right bronchus
Left lung
Mediastinum

A

Horizontal cross-section of lungs

From pulmonary artery
Alveolar duct
Terminal bronchiole
Diaphragm
Thoracic vertebra
To pulmonary vein
Alveoli
Visceral pleura
Parietal pleura
Capillaries
Section of lung enlarged
Pleural space
Wall of thorax
Left lung
B
C
Right lung
Sternum

F I G U R E 7 - 4 1 . The respiratory system. **(A)** Overview. **(B)** Enlarged section of lung tissue showing the relationship between the alveoli (air sacs) of the lungs and the blood capillaries. **(C)** A transverse section through the lungs. *ZOOMING IN—What organ is located in the medial depression of the left lung?*

Fig. 7-42). The right bronchus is considerably larger in diameter than the left and extends downward in a more vertical direction. Therefore, if a foreign body is inhaled, it is likely to enter the right lung. Each bronchus enters the lung at a notch or depression called the **hilum** (HI-lum). Blood vessels and nerves also connect with the lung in this region.

The Lining of the Air Passageways

The trachea, bronchi, and other conducting passageways of the respiratory tract are lined with a special type of epithelium (Fig. 7-44). Basically, it is simple columnar epithelium, but the cells are arranged in such a way that they

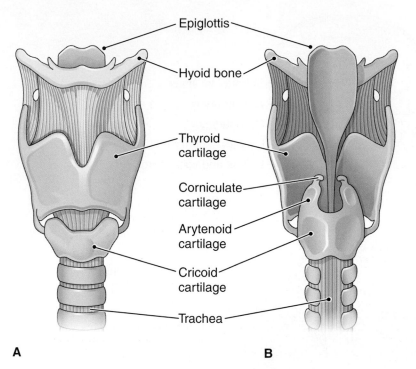

F I G U R E   7 - 4 2 .   The larynx. **(A)** Anterior view. **(B)** Posterior view.

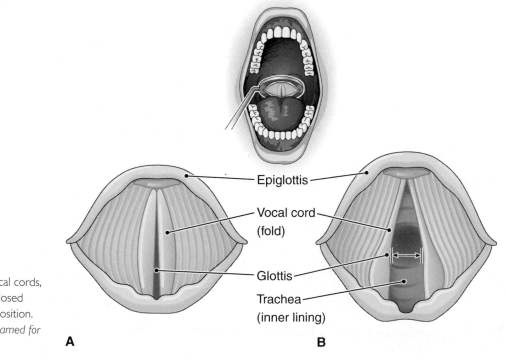

F I G U R E   7 - 4 3 .   The vocal cords, superior view. **(A)** The glottis in closed position. **(B)** The glottis in open position. *ZOOMING IN—What cartilage is named for its position above the glottis?*

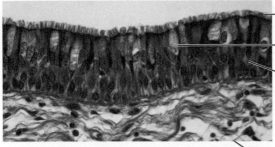

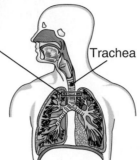

— Cilia

— Goblet cell
(secretes mucus)

— Columnar
epithelium
(pseudostratified)

Trachea

FIGURE 7-44. Microscopic view of ciliated epithelium. Ciliated epithelium lines the respiratory passageways, as shown here in the trachea. (Micrograph reprinted with permission from Cormack DH. Essential Histology. 2nd ed. Philadelphia: Lippincott Williams & Wilkins, 2001.)

appear stratified. The tissue is thus described as *pseudostratified*, meaning "falsely stratified." These epithelial cells have cilia to filter out impurities and to create fluid movement within the conducting tubes. The cilia beat to drive impurities toward the throat, where they can be swallowed or eliminated by coughing, sneezing, or blowing the nose.

 Checkpoint Question

37. The cells that line the respiratory passageways help to keep impurities out of the lungs. What feature of these cells enables them to filter impurities and move fluids?

The Lungs

The lungs are the organs in which gas diffusion takes place through the extremely thin and delicate lung tissues (see Fig. 7-42). The two lungs are set side by side in the thoracic (chest) cavity. Between them are the heart, the great blood vessels, and other organs of the **mediastinum** (me-de-as-TI-num), the space between the lungs, including the esophagus, trachea, and lymph nodes.

On its medial side, the left lung has an indentation that accommodates the heart. The right lung is subdivided by fissures into three lobes; the left lung is divided into two lobes. Each lobe is then further subdivided into segments and then lobules. These subdivisions correspond to subdivisions of the bronchi as they branch throughout the lungs.

Each primary bronchus enters the lung at the hilum and immediately subdivides. The right bronchus divides into three secondary bronchi, each of which enters one of the three lobes of the right lung. The left bronchus gives rise to two secondary bronchi, which enter the two lobes of the left lung. Because the bronchial subdivisions resemble the branches of a tree, they have been given the common name *bronchial tree*. The bronchi subdivide again and again, be-

coming progressively smaller as they branch through lung tissue.

The smallest of these conducting tubes are called **bronchioles** (BRONG-ke-oles). The bronchi contain small bits of cartilage, which give firmness to their walls and hold the passageways open so that air can pass in and out easily. As the bronchi become smaller, however, the cartilage decreases in amount. In the bronchioles, there is no cartilage at all; what remains is mostly smooth muscle, which is under the control of the autonomic (involuntary) nervous system.

The Alveoli

At the end of the terminal bronchioles, the smallest subdivisions of the bronchial tree, there are clusters of tiny air sacs in which most gas exchange takes place. These sacs are known as **alveoli** (al-VE-o-li) (sing., alveolus) (see Fig. 7-42). The wall of each alveolus is made of a single-cell layer of squamous (flat) epithelium. This thin wall provides easy passage for the gases entering and leaving the blood as the blood circulates through the millions of tiny capillaries covering the alveoli.

Certain cells in the alveolar wall produce **surfactant** (sur-FAK-tant), a substance that reduces the surface tension ("pull") of the fluids that line the alveoli. This surface action prevents collapse of the alveoli and eases expansion of the lungs.

There are about 300 million alveoli in the human lungs. The resulting surface area in contact with gases approximates 60 square meters (some books say even more). This area is equivalent, as an example, to the floor surface of a classroom that measures about 24 by 24 feet. As with many other systems in the body, there is great functional reserve; we have about three times as much lung tissue as is minimally necessary to sustain life. Because of the many air spaces, the lung is light in weight; normally, a piece of lung tissue dropped into a glass of water will float. Figure 7-45 shows a microscopic view of lung tissue.

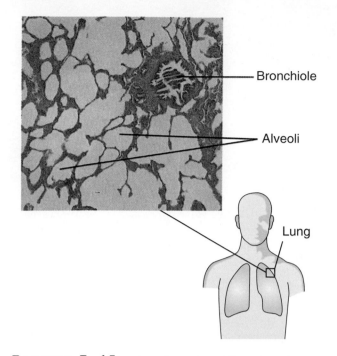

F IGURE 7 - 4 5 .   Lung tissue viewed through a micro-scope. (Micrograph courtesy of Dana Morse Bittus and BJ Cohen.)

The pulmonary circuit brings blood to and from the lungs. In the lungs, blood passes through the capillaries around the alveoli, where gas exchange takes place.

The Lung Cavities and Pleura

The lungs occupy a considerable portion of the thoracic cavity, which is separated from the abdominal cavity by the muscular partition known as the **diaphragm.** A continuous doubled sac, the **pleura,** covers each lung. The two layers of the pleura are named according to location. The portion of the pleura that is attached to the chest wall is the parietal pleura, and the portion that is attached to the surface of the lung is called the visceral pleura. Each closed sac completely surrounds the lung, except in the place where the bronchus and blood vessels enter the lung, a region known as the *root* of the lung.

Between the two layers of the pleura is the pleural space containing a thin film of fluid that lubricates the membranes. The effect of this fluid is the same as between two flat pieces of glass joined by a film of water; that is, the surfaces slide easily on each other but strongly resist separation. Thus, the lungs are able to move and enlarge effortlessly in response to changes in the thoracic volume that occur during breathing.

Checkpoint Questions

38. In what structures does gas exchange occur in the lung?

39. What is the name of the membrane that encloses the lung?

THE DIGESTIVE SYSTEM

Every body cell needs a constant supply of nutrients. The energy contained in these nutrients is used to do cell work. In addition, the cell rearranges the chemical building blocks of the nutrients to manufacture cellular materials for metabolism, growth, and repair. Food as we take it in, however, is too large to enter the cells. It must first be broken down into particles small enough to pass through the cells' plasma membrane. This breakdown process is known as **digestion**.

After digestion, the circulation must carry nutrients to the cells in every part of the body. The transfer of nutrients into the circulation is called **absorption**. Finally, undigested waste material must be eliminated from the body. Digestion, absorption, and elimination are the three chief functions of the digestive system.

For our purposes, the digestive system may be divided into two groups of organs:

- the digestive tract, a continuous passageway beginning at the mouth, where food is taken in, and terminating at the anus, where the solid waste products of digestion are expelled from the body
- the accessory organs, which are necessary for the digestive process but are not a direct part of the digestive tract. They release substances into the digestive tract through ducts. These organs are the salivary glands, liver, gallbladder, and pancreas.

Checkpoint Question

40. Why does food have to be digested before cells can use it?

Before describing the individual organs of the digestive tract, we will pause to discuss the general structure of these organs. We will also describe the large membrane (peritoneum) that lines the abdominopelvic cavity, which contains most of the digestive organs.

The Wall of the Digestive Tract

Although modified for specific tasks in different organs, the wall of the digestive tract, from the esophagus to the anus, is similar in structure throughout. The general pattern consists of four layers:

- mucous membrane
- submucosa
- smooth muscle
- serous membrane

Refer to the diagram of the small intestine in Figure 7-46 as we describe the layers of this wall from the innermost to the outermost surface.

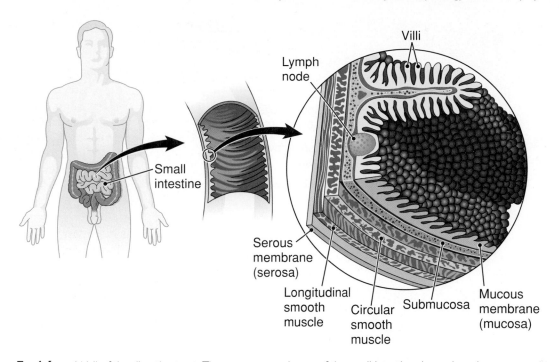

F IGURE 7 - 4 6 . Wall of the digestive tract. The mucous membrane of the small intestine shown here has numerous projections called villi. *ZOOMING IN—What type of tissue is between the submucosa and the serous membrane in the digestive tract wall?*

First is the mucous membrane, or **mucosa**, so called because its epithelial layer contains many mucus-secreting cells. From the mouth through the esophagus, and also in the anus, the epithelium consists of multiple layers of squamous (flat) cells, which help to protect deeper tissues. Throughout the remainder of the digestive tract, the type of epithelium in the mucosa is simple columnar. Many of the cells that secrete digestive juices are located in the mucosa. Figure 7-47 is a microscopic view of a representative section of the digestive tract taken from the small intestine. Mucus-secreting cells (goblet cells) appear as clear areas between epithelial cells. Note that the small intestine's lining has fingerlike extensions (villi) that aid in the absorption of nutrients, as will be described later.

The layer of connective tissue beneath the mucosa is the **submucosa**, which contains blood vessels and some of the nerves that help regulate digestive activity. In the small intestine, the submucosa has many glands that produce mucus to protect that organ from the highly acidic material it receives from the stomach.

The next layer is composed of smooth muscle. Most of the digestive organs have two layers of smooth muscle: an inner layer of circular fibers, and an outer layer of longitudinal fibers. When a section of the circular muscle contracts, the lumen of the organ narrows; when the longitudinal muscle contracts, a section of the wall shortens and the lumen becomes wider. These alternating muscular contractions create the wavelike movement, called **peristalsis** (per-ih-STAL-sis), that propels food through the digestive tract and mixes it with digestive juices.

The esophagus differs slightly from this pattern in having striated muscle in its upper portion, and the stomach has an additional third layer of smooth muscle in its wall to add strength for churning food.

The digestive organs in the abdominopelvic cavity have an outermost layer of serous membrane, or **serosa**, a thin, moist tissue composed of simple squamous epithelium and loose connective tissue. This membrane forms part of the **peritoneum** (per-ih-to-NE-um). The esophagus above the diaphragm has instead an outer layer composed of fibrous connective tissue.

 Checkpoint Question

41. The digestive tract has a wall that is basically similar throughout its length and is composed of four layers. What are the typical four layers of this wall?

The Peritoneum

The abdominopelvic cavity (Fig. 7-48) is lined with a thin, shiny serous membrane that also folds back to cover most of the organs contained within the cavity. The outer portion of this membrane, the layer that lines the cavity, is called the parietal peritoneum; that covering the organs is called the visceral peritoneum. This slippery membrane allows the organs to slide over each other as they function. The peritoneum also carries blood vessels, lymphatic vessels, and

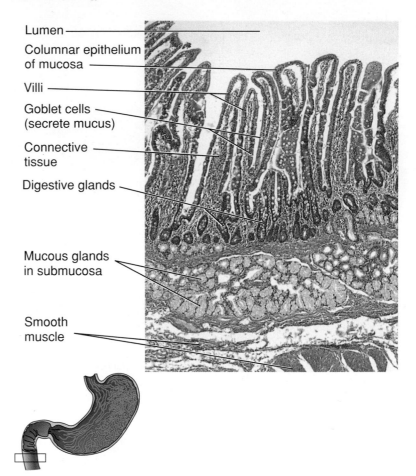

Lumen
Columnar epithelium of mucosa
Villi
Goblet cells (secrete mucus)
Connective tissue
Digestive glands
Mucous glands in submucosa
Smooth muscle

FIGURE 7-47. Microscopic view of small intestine. The layers of the intestinal wall are visible (except for the serous membrane). (Micrograph reprinted with permission from Cormack DH. Essential Histology. 2nd ed. Philadelphia: Lippincott Williams & Wilkins, 2001.)

nerves. In some places, it supports the organs and binds them to each other. Subdivisions of the peritoneum around the various organs have special names.

Subdivisions of the Peritoneum

The **mesentery** (MES-en-ter-e) is a double-layered portion of the peritoneum shaped somewhat like a fan. The handle portion is attached to the posterior abdominal wall, and the expanded long edge is attached to the small intestine. Between the two membranous layers of the mesentery are the vessels and nerves that supply the intestine. The section of the peritoneum that extends from the colon to the posterior abdominal wall is the **mesocolon** (mes-o-KO-lon).

A large double layer of the peritoneum containing much fat hangs like an apron over the front of the intestine. This greater **omentum** (o-MEN-tum) extends from the lower border of the stomach into the pelvic part of the abdomen and then loops back up to the transverse colon. A smaller membrane, called the lesser **omentum**, extends between the stomach and the liver.

Checkpoint Question

42. What is the name of the large serous membrane that lines the abdominopelvic cavity and covers the organs it contains?

ORGANS OF THE DIGESTIVE TRACT

The digestive tract is a muscular tube extending through the body. It is composed of several parts: the **mouth, pharynx, esophagus, stomach, small intestine**, and **large intestine**. The digestive tract is sometimes called the alimentary tract, from the word *aliment*, meaning "food." It is more commonly referred to as the **gastrointestinal (GI) tract** because of the major importance of the stomach and intestine in the process of digestion.

Figure 7-49 provides a diagram of all digestive organs.

THE URINARY SYSTEM

The urinary system is also called the *excretory system* because one of its main functions is **excretion**, removal and

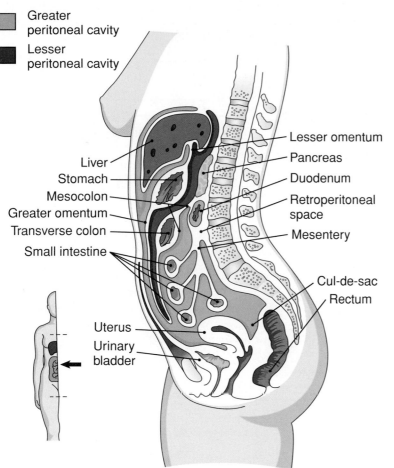

Greater peritoneal cavity

Lesser peritoneal cavity

Liver
Stomach
Mesocolon
Greater omentum
Transverse colon
Small intestine

Lesser omentum
Pancreas
Duodenum
Retroperitoneal space
Mesentery

Cul-de-sac
Rectum

Uterus
Urinary bladder

FIGURE 7-48. The abdominopelvic cavity. Subdivisions of the peritoneum fold over, supporting and separating individual organs. *ZOOMING IN— What part of the peritoneum is around the small intestine?*

elimination of metabolic waste products from the blood. It has many other functions as well, including regulation of the volume, acid–base balance (pH), and electrolyte composition of body fluids.

Although the focus of this section is the urinary system, certain aspects of other systems are also discussed, because body systems work interdependently to maintain homeostasis (internal balance). The systems active in excretion and some of the substances they eliminate are the following:

- The **urinary system** excretes water, nitrogen-containing waste products, and salts. These are all constituents of the urine.
- The **digestive system** elimiinates water, some salts, and bile in addition to digestive residue, all of which are contained in the feces. The liver is important in eliminating the products of red blood cell destruction and in breaking down certain drugs and toxins.
- The **respiratory system** eliminates carbon dioxide and water. The latter appears as vapor, as can be demonstrated by breathing on a windowpane.
- The skin, or **integumentary system**, excretes water, salts, and very small quantities of nitrogenous wastes.

These all appear in perspiration, although water also evaporates continuously from the skin without our being conscious of it.

Checkpoint Question

43. The main function of the urinary system is to eliminate waste. What are some other systems that eliminate waste?

ORGANS OF THE URINARY SYSTEM

The main parts of the urinary system, shown in Figure 7-50, are as follows:

- two **kidneys**. These organs extract wastes from the blood, balance body fluids, and form urine
- two **ureters** (U-re-ters). These tubes conduct urine from the kidneys to the urinary bladder
- a single **urinary bladder**. This reservoir receives and stores the urine brought to it by the two ureters
- a single **urethra** (u-RE-thrah). This tube conducts urine from the bladder to the outside of the body for elimination.

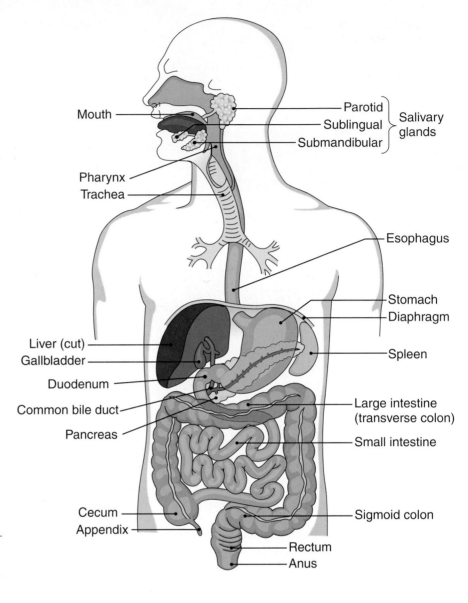

FIGURE 7-49. The digestive system. *ZOOMING IN—What accessory organs of digestion secrete into the mouth?*

Checkpoint Question

44. What are the organs of the urinary system?

Checkpoint Question

45. The kidneys are located in the retroperitoneal space. Where is this space?

THE KIDNEYS

The kidneys lie against the back muscles in the upper abdomen at about the level of the last thoracic and first three lumbar vertebrae. The right kidney is slightly lower than the left to accommodate the liver. Each kidney is firmly enclosed in a membranous renal capsule made of fibrous connective tissue. In addition, there is a protective layer of fat called the adipose capsule around the organ. An outermost layer of fascia (connective tissue) anchors the kidney to the peritoneum and abdominal wall. The kidneys, as well as the ureters, lie posterior to the peritoneum. Thus, they are not in the peritoneal cavity but rather in an area known as the **retroperitoneal** (ret-ro-per-ih-to-NE-al) space.

Functions of the Kidney

The kidneys are involved in the following processes:

- Excretion of unwanted substances, such as cellular metabolic waste, excess salts, and toxins. One product of amino acid metabolism is nitrogen-containing waste material, a chief form of which is **urea** (u-RE-ah). After synthesis in the liver, urea is transported in the blood to the kidneys for elimination. The kidneys have a specialized mechanism for the elimination of urea and other nitrogenous (ni-TROJ-en-us) wastes.
- Maintenance of water balance. Although the amount of water gained and lost in a day can vary tremendously, the kidneys can adapt to these variations, so that the

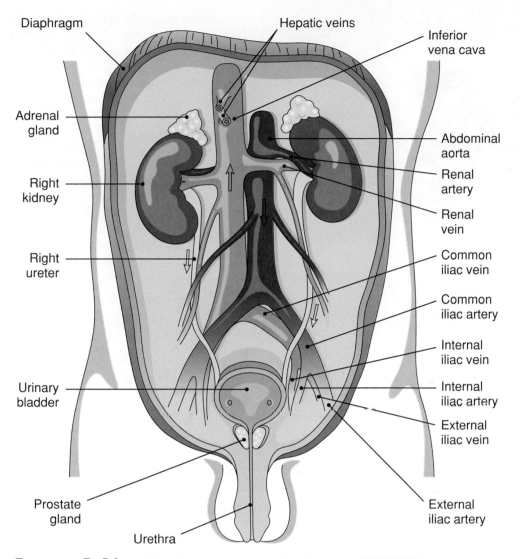

Diaphragm

Hepatic veins

Inferior vena cava

Adrenal gland

Right kidney

Right ureter

Urinary bladder

Prostate gland

Urethra

Abdominal aorta

Renal artery

Renal vein

Common iliac vein

Common iliac artery

Internal iliac vein

Internal iliac artery

External iliac vein

External iliac artery

FIGURE 7-50. Male urinary system, showing blood vessels. *ZOOMING IN—What vessel supplies blood to the kidney? What vessel drains the kidney?*

volume of body water remains remarkably stable from day to day.

- Regulation of the acid–base balance of body fluids. Acids are constantly being produced by cellular metabolism. Certain foods can yield acids or bases, and people may also ingest antacids, such as bicarbonate. However, if the body is to function normally, the pH of body fluids must remain in the range of 7.35 to 7.45.

- Regulation of blood pressure. The kidneys depend on blood pressure to filter the blood. If blood pressure falls too low for effective filtration, the cells of the JG apparatus release renin. This enzyme activates **angiotensin** (an-je-o-TEN-sin), a blood protein that causes blood vessels to constrict, thus raising blood pressure. Angiotensin also stimulates the adrenal cortex to produce the hormone aldosterone, which promotes retention of sodium and water, also raising blood pressure.

- Regulation of red blood cell production. When the kidneys do not get enough oxygen, they produce the hormone **erythropoietin** (eh-rith-ro-POY-eh-tin) (**EPO**), which stimulates the red cell production in the bone marrow. EPO made by genetic engineering is now available to treat severe anemia, such as occurs in the end stage of kidney failure.

 Checkpoint Question

46. What substance is produced by the JG apparatus and under what conditions is it produced?

THE URETERS

Each of the two ureters is a long, slender, muscular tube that extends from the kidney down to and through the inferior portion of the urinary bladder (see Fig. 7-50). The ureters, which

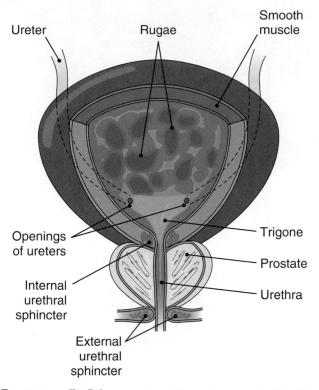

Ureter   Rugae   Smooth muscle

Openings of ureters

Internal urethral sphincter

External urethral sphincter

Trigone

Prostate

Urethra

FIGURE 7-51.   Interior of the male urinary bladder. The trigone is a triangular region in the floor of the bladder marked by the openings of the ureters and the urethra.   *ZOOMING IN—What gland does the urethra pass through in the male?*

are located posterior to the peritoneum and, at the distal portion, below the peritoneum, are entirely extraperitoneal. Their length naturally varies with the size of the individual, and they may be anywhere from 25 to 32 cm (10–13 inches) long. Nearly 2.5 cm (1 inch) of the ureter's distal portion enters the bladder by passing obliquely (at an angle) through the inferior bladder wall. Because of the oblique direction the ureter takes through the wall, a full bladder compresses the ureter and prevents the backflow of urine.

THE URINARY BLADDER

When it is empty, the urinary bladder (Fig. 7-51) is located below the parietal peritoneum and posterior to the pubic joint. When filled, it pushes the peritoneum upward and may extend well into the abdominal cavity proper. The urinary bladder is a temporary reservoir for urine, just as the gallbladder is a storage sac for bile.

The bladder wall has many layers. It is lined with mucous membrane containing transitional epithelium. The bladder's lining, like that of the stomach, is thrown into folds called *rugae* when the organ is empty. Beneath the mucosa is a layer of connective tissue, followed by a three-layered coat of involuntary muscle tissue that can stretch considerably. Finally, there is an incomplete coat of peritoneum that covers only the superior portion of the bladder.

When the bladder is empty, the muscular wall becomes thick, and the entire organ feels firm. As the bladder fills, the muscular wall becomes thinner, and the organ may increase from a length of 5 cm (2 inches) up to as much as 12.5 cm (5 inches) or even more. A moderately full bladder holds about 470 mL (1 pint) of urine.

THE URETHRA

The urethra is the tube that extends from the bladder to the outside (see Fig. 7-51) and is the means by which the bladder is emptied. The urethra differs in men and women; in the male, it is part of both the reproductive system and the urinary system, and it is much longer than is the female urethra.

The male urethra is about 20 cm (8 inches) in length. Proximally, it passes through the prostate gland, where it is joined by two ducts carrying male germ cells (spermatozoa) from the testes and glandular secretions. From here, it leads to the outside through the **penis** (PE-nis), the male organ of copulation. The male urethra serves the dual purpose of conveying semen with the germ cells and draining the bladder.

The urethra in the female is a thin-walled tube about 4 cm (1.5 inches) long. It is located posterior to the pubic joint and is embedded in the muscle of the vagina's anterior wall. The external opening, called the urinary meatus (me-A-tus), is located just anterior to the vaginal opening between the labia minora. The female urethra drains the bladder only and is entirely separate from the reproductive system.

REPRODUCTION

The simplest forms of life, one-celled organisms, usually need no partner to reproduce; they simply divide by themselves. This form of reproduction is known as **asexual** (nonsexual) reproduction.

In most animals, however, reproduction is **sexual**, meaning that there are two kinds of individuals, males and females, each of which has specialized cells designed specifically for the perpetuation of the species. These specialized sex cells are known as **germ cells**, or **gametes** (GAM-etes). In the male, they are called **spermatozoa** (sper-mah-to-ZO-ah) (sing., spermatozoon), or simply sperm cells, and in the female, they are called **ova** (O-vah) (sing., ovum) or egg cells.

Gametes are characterized by having half as many chromosomes as are found in any other body cell. During their formation, they go through a special process of cell division, called **meiosis** (mi-O-sis), which halves the number of chromosomes. In humans, meiosis reduces the chromosome number in a cell from 46 to 23.

 Checkpoint Question

47. What is the process of cell division that halves the chromosome number in a cell to produce a gamete?

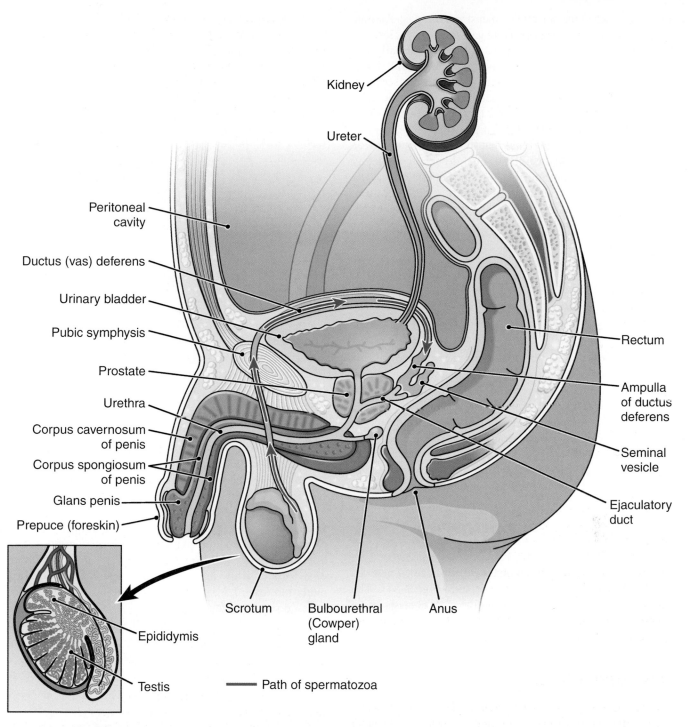

FIGURE 7-52. Male reproductive system. Organs of the urinary system are also shown. *ZOOMING IN—What four glands empty secretions into the urethra?*

THE MALE REPRODUCTIVE SYSTEM

The male reproductive system, like that of the female, may be divided into two groups of organs: primary and accessory (see Fig. 7-52).

- The primary organs are the **gonads** (GO-nads), or sex glands; they produce the germ cells and manufacture hormones. The male gonad is the testis. (In comparison, the female gonad is the ovary, as explained below.)

- The **accessory organs** include a series of ducts that transport the germ cells as well as various exocrine glands.

The Testes

The male gonads, the **testes** (TES-teze) (sing., testis) are located outside the body proper, suspended between the thighs in a sac called the **scrotum** (SKRO-tum). The testes are oval organs measuring about 4.0 cm (1.5 inches) in length and about 2.5 cm

(1 inch) in each of the other two dimensions. During embryonic life, each testis develops from tissue near the kidney.

A month or two before birth, the testis normally descends (moves downward) through the **inguinal** (ING-gwih-nal) **canal** in the abdominal wall into the scrotum. Each testis then remains suspended by a **spermatic cord** (Fig. 7-53) that extends through the inguinal canal. This cord contains blood vessels, lymphatic vessels, nerves, and the tube (ductus deferens) that transports spermatozoa away from the testis. The gland must descend completely if it is to function normally; to produce spermatozoa, the testis must be kept at the temperature of the scrotum, which is several degrees lower than that of the abdominal cavity.

   Checkpoint Question

48. What is the male gonad?

The Urethra and Penis

The male urethra serves the dual purpose of conveying urine from the bladder and carrying the reproductive cells with their accompanying secretions to the outside. The ejection of semen into the receiving canal (vagina) of the female is made possible by the erection, or stiffening and enlargement, of the penis, through which the longest part of the urethra extends. The penis is made of spongy tissue containing many blood spaces that are relatively empty when the organ is flaccid but fill with blood and distend when the penis is erect.

THE FEMALE REPRODUCTIVE SYSTEM

The female gonads are the **ovaries** (O-vah-reze), where the female sex cells, or ova, are formed (Fig. 7-54). The remainder of the female reproductive tract consists of an organ (uterus) to hold and nourish a developing infant, various passageways, and the external genital organs.

The Ovaries

The ovary is a small, somewhat flattened oval body measuring about 4 cm (1.6 inches) in length, 2 cm (0.8 inch) in width, and 1 cm (0.4 inch) in depth. Like the testes, the ovaries descend, but only as far as the pelvic portion of the abdomen. Here, they are held in place by ligaments, including the broad ligament, the ovarian ligament, and others, that attach them to the uterus and the body wall.

The Ova and Ovulation

The outer layer of the ovary is made of a single layer of epithelium. Beneath this layer, the female gametes, the ova, are produced. The ovaries of a newborn female contain a large

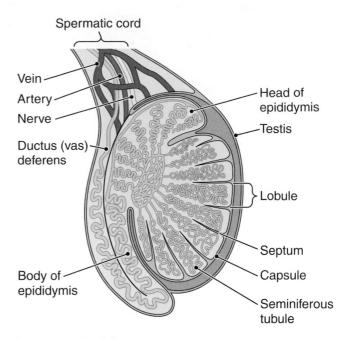

F I G U R E   7 - 5 3 .   Structure of the testis. The epididymis and spermatic cord are also shown.   *ZOOMING IN—What duct receives secretions from the epididymis?*

number of potential ova. Each month during the reproductive years, several ripen, but usually only one is released.

The complicated process of maturation, or "ripening," of an ovum takes place in a small fluid-filled cluster of cells called the **ovarian follicle** (o-VA-re-an FOL-ih-kl) or **Graafian** (GRAF-e-an) **follicle** (Fig. 7-55). As the follicle develops, cells in its wall secrete the hormone estrogen, which stimulates growth of the uterine lining. When an ovum has ripened, the ovarian follicle may rupture and discharge the egg cell from the ovary's surface. The rupture of a follicle allowing the escape of an ovum is called **ovulation** (ov-u-LA-shun). Any developing ova that are not released simply degenerate.

After it is released, the egg cell makes its way to the nearest **oviduct** (O-vih-dukt), a tube that arches over the ovary and leads to the uterus (see Fig. 7-54).

   Checkpoint Questions

49. What is the female gonad called?
50. What is the female gamete called?
51. What is the structure that surrounds the egg as it ripens?
52. What is the process of releasing an egg cell from the ovary called?

The Uterus

The oviducts lead to the **uterus** (U-ter-us), an organ in which a fetus can develop to maturity. The uterus is a pear-shaped, muscular organ about 7.5 cm (3 inches) long, 5 cm (2 inches)

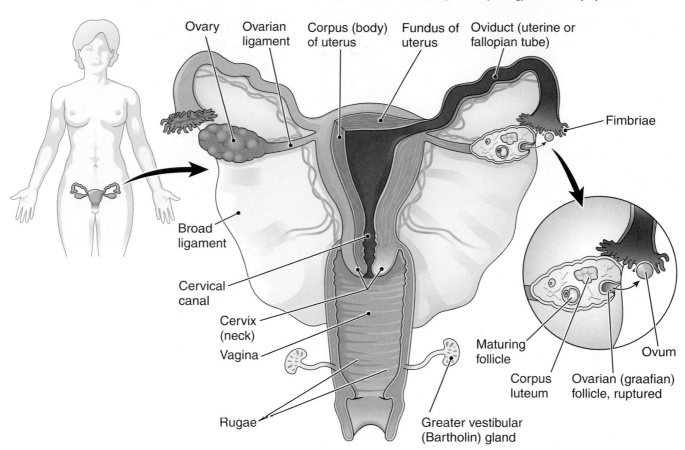

FIGURE 7-54. Female reproductive system. The enlargement (*right*) shows ovulation. *ZOOMING IN—What is the deepest part of the uterus called?*

wide, and 2.5 cm (1 inch) deep. (The organ is typically larger in women who have borne children and smaller in postmenopausal women.) The superior portion rests on the upper surface of the urinary bladder; the inferior portion is embedded in the pelvic floor between the bladder and the rectum. The wider upper region of the uterus is called the **corpus**, or body; the lower, narrower region is the **cervix** (SER-viks), or neck. The small, rounded region above the level of the tubal entrances is known as the **fundus** (FUN-dus) (see Fig. 7-54).

Checkpoint Question

53. In what organ does a fetus develop?

The Vagina

The cervix leads to the **vagina** (vah-JI-nah), the distal part of the birth canal, which opens to the outside of the body. The vagina is a muscular tube about 7.5 cm (3 inches) long connecting the uterine cavity with the outside. The cervix dips into the superior portion of the vagina forming a circular recess known as the **fornix** (FOR-niks). The deepest area of the fornix, located behind the cervix, is the posterior fornix (Fig. 7-56). This recess in the posterior vagina lies adjacent to the

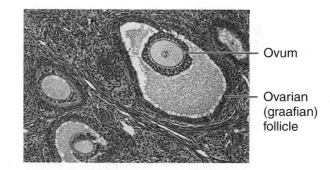

FIGURE 7-55. Microscopic view of the ovary. The photomicrograph shows egg cells (ova) developing within ovarian (graafian) follicles. (Courtesy of Dana Morse Bittus and BJ Cohen.)

most inferior portion of the peritoneal cavity, a narrow passage between the uterus and the rectum named the cul-de-sac (from the French meaning "bottom of the sack"). This area is also known as the rectouterine pouch or the pouch of Douglas. A rather thin layer of tissue separates the posterior fornix from this region, so that abscesses or tumors in the peritoneal cavity can sometimes be detected by vaginal examination.

The lining of the vagina is a wrinkled mucous membrane similar to that found in the stomach. The folds (rugae) permit enlargement so that childbirth usually does not tear the lin-

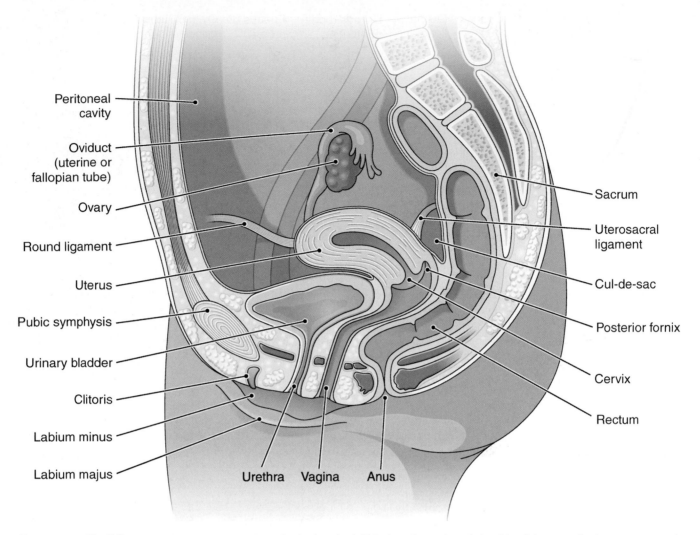

Peritoneal cavity

Oviduct (uterine or fallopian tube)

Ovary

Round ligament

Uterus

Pubic symphysis

Urinary bladder

Clitoris

Labium minus

Labium majus

Sacrum

Uterosacral ligament

Cul-de-sac

Posterior fornix

Cervix

Rectum

Urethra   Vagina   Anus

FIGURE 7-56.   Female reproductive system (sagittal section). This view shows the relationship of the reproductive organs to each other and to other structures in the pelvic cavity.   *ZOOMING IN—Which has the more anterior opening, the vagina or the urethra?*

ing. In addition to being a part of the birth canal, the vagina is the organ that receives the penis during sexual intercourse. A fold of membrane called the **hymen** (HI-men) may sometimes be found at or near the vaginal (VAJ-ih-nal) canal opening.

The Vulva and the Perineum

The external parts of the female reproductive system form the vulva (VUL-vah), which includes two pairs of lips, or **labia** (LA-be-ah); the **clitoris** (KLIT-o-ris), which is a small

organ of great sensitivity; and related structures. Although the entire pelvic floor in both the male and female is properly called the **perineum** (per-ih-NE-um), those who care for pregnant women usually refer to the limited area between the vaginal opening and the anus as the perineum or obstetrical perineum.

Word Anatomy

Medical terms are built from standardized word parts (prefixes, roots, and suffixes). Learning the meanings of these parts can help you remember words and interpret unfamiliar terms.

Word part	Meaning	Example
Structure of the Skin		
derm/o	skin	The *epidermis* is the outermost layer of the skin.
corne/o	horny	The stratum *corneum* is the outermost thickened, horny layer of the skin.
melan/o	dark, black	A *melanocyte* is a cell that produces the dark pigment melanin.
sub-	under, below	The *subcutaneous* layer is under the skin.
Accessory Structures of the Skin		
ap/o-	separation from, derivation from	The *apocrine* sweat glands release some cellular material in their secretions.
pil/o	hair	The arrector *pili* muscle raises the hair to produce "goose bumps."
Skin Color		
alb/i	white	*Albinism* is a condition associated with a lack of pigment, so the skin appears white.
Bones		
dia-	through, between	The *diaphysis*, or shaft, of a long bone is between the two ends, or epiphyses.
oss, osse/o	bone, bone tissue	*Osseous* tissue is another name for bone tissue.
oste/o	bone, bone tissue	The *periosteum* is the fibrous membrane around a bone.
-clast	break	An *osteoclast* breaks down bone in the process of resorption.
Divisions of the Skeleton		
para-	near	The *paranasal* sinuses are near the nose.
pariet/o	wall	The *parietal* bones form the side walls of the skull.
cost/o	rib	*Intercostal* spaces are located between the ribs.
supra-	above, superior	The *supraspinous* fossa is a depression superior to the spine of the scapula.
infra-	below, inferior	The *infraspinous* fossa is a depression inferior to the spine of the scapula.
meta-	near, beyond	The *metacarpal* bones of the palm are near and distal to the carpal bones of the wrist.
The Joints		
arthr/o	joint, articulation	A *synarthrosis* is an immovable joint, such as a suture.
amphi-	on both sides, around, double	An *amphiarthrosis* is a slightly movable joint.
ab-	away from	*Abduction* is movement away from the midline of the body.
ad-	toward, added to	*Adduction* is movement toward the midline of the body.
circum-	around	*Circumduction* is movement around a joint in a circle.
The Muscular System		
my/o	muscle	The *endomysium* is the deepest layer of connective tissue around muscle cells.
sarc/o	flesh	A *sarcomere* is a contracting subunit of skeletal muscle.
troph/o	nutrition, nurture	Muscles undergo *hypertrophy*, an increase in size, under the effects of resistance training.

(continued)

Word part	Meaning	Example
vas/o	vessel	*Vasodilation* (widening) of the blood vessels in muscle tissue during exercise brings more blood into the tissue.
iso-	same, equal	In an *isotonic* contraction, muscle tone remains the same, but the muscle shortens.
ton/o	tone, tension	See preceding example.
metr/o	measure	In an *isometric* contraction, muscle length remains the same, but muscle tension increases.

The Mechanics of Muscle Movement

brachi/o	arm	The biceps *brachii* and triceps *brachii* are in the arm.
erg/o	work	*Synergists* are muscles that work together.

Skeletal Muscle Groups

quadr/i	four	The *quadriceps* muscle group consists of four muscles.

The Nervous System as a Whole

soma-	body	The *somatic* nervous system controls skeletal muscles that move the body.
aut/o	self	The *autonomic* nervous system is automatically controlled and is involuntary.
neur/i	nerve, nervous tissue	The *neurilemma* is the outer membrane of the myelin sheath around an axon.
-lemma	sheath	See preceding example.

The Nervous System at Work

de-	remove	*Depolarization* removes the charge on the plasma membrane of a cell.
re-	again, back	*Repolarization* restores the charge on the plasma membrane of a cell.
post-	after	The *postsynaptic* cell is located after the synapse and receives neurotransmitters from the presynaptic cell.

The Brain and its Protective Structures

cerebr/o	brain	*Cerebrospinal* fluid circulates around the brain and spinal cord.
chori/o	membrane	The *choroid* plexus is the vascular membrane in the ventricle that produces CSF.
gyr/o	circle	A *gyrus* is a circular raised area on the surface of the brain.
encephal/o	brain	The *diencephalon* is the part of the brain located between the cerebral hemispheres and the brain stem.
contra-	opposed, against	The cerebral cortex has *contralateral* control of motor function.
later/o	lateral, side	See preceding example.

Imaging the Brain

tom/o	cut	*Tomography* is a method for viewing sections as if cut through the body.

Cranial Nerves

gloss/o	tongue	The *hypoglossal* nerve controls muscles of the tongue.

The Eye and Vision

ophthalm/o	eye	An *ophthalmologist* is a physician who specializes in treatment of the eye.
-scope	instrument for examination	An *ophthalmoscope* is an instrument used to examine the posterior of the eye.

(continued)

Word part	Meaning	Example
lute/o	yellow	The macula *lutea* is a yellowish spot in the retina that contains the fovea centralis.
presby-	old	*Presbyopia* is farsightedness that occurs with age.

The Ear

Word part	Meaning	Example
tympan/o	drum	The *tympanic* membrane is the eardrum.
equi-	equal	*Equilibrium* is balance (*equi-* combined with the Latin word *libra* meaning "balance").
ot/o	ear	*Otology* is the study of the ear.
lith	stone	*Otoliths* are small crystals in the inner ear that aid in static equilibrium.
-cusis	hearing	*Presbycusis* is hearing loss associated with age.

The Endocrine Glands and Their Hormones

Word part	Meaning	Example
trop/o	acting on, influencing	*Somatotropin* stimulates growth in most body tissues.
cortic/o	cortex	*Adrenocorticotropic* hormone acts on the adrenal cortex.
lact/o	milk	*Prolactin* stimulates production of milk in the breasts.
ur/o	urine	*Antidiuretic* hormone promotes reabsorption of water in the kidneys and decreases excretion of urine.
oxy	sharp, acute	*Oxytocin* stimulates uterine contractions during labor.
toc/o	labor	See preceding example.
ren/o	kidney	The *adrenal* glands are near (ad-) the kidneys.
nephr/o	kidney	*Epinephrine* is another name for adrenaline.
insul/o	pancreatic islet, island	*Insulin* is a hormone produced by the pancreatic islets.
andr/o	male	An *androgen* is any male sex hormone.

Other Hormone-Producing Tissues

Word part	Meaning	Example
–poiesis	making, forming	*Erythropoietin* is a hormone from the kidneys that stimulates production of red blood cells.
natri	sodium (*L. natrium*)	Atrial *natriuretic* peptide stimulates release of sodium in the urine.

Structure of the Heart

Word part	Meaning	Example
cardi/o	heart	The *myocardium* is the heart muscle.
pulmon/o	lung	The *pulmonary* circuit carries blood to the lungs.

Function of the Heart

Word part	Meaning	Example
sin/o	sinus	The *sinoatrial* node is in a space (sinus) in the wall of the right atrium.
brady-	slow	*Bradycardia* is a slow heart rate.
tachy-	rapid	*Tachycardia* is a rapid heart rate.

Heart Studies

Word part	Meaning	Example
steth/o	chest	A *stethoscope* is used to listen to body sounds, such as those heard through the wall of the chest.

Systemic Arteries

Word part	Meaning	Example
brachi/o	arm	The *brachiocephalic* artery supplies blood to the arm and head on the right side.
cephal/o	head	See preceding example.
clav/o	clavicle	The *subclavian* artery extends under the clavicle on each side.
cost/o	rib	The *intercostal* arteries are between the ribs.
celi/o	abdomen	The *celiac* trunk branches to supply blood to the abdominal organs.

(continued)

Word part	Meaning	Example
gastr/o	stomach	The *gastric* artery goes to the stomach.
splen/o	spleen	The *splenic* artery goes to the spleen.
hepat/o	liver	The *hepatic* artery supplies blood to the liver.
enter/o	intestine	The *mesenteric* arteries supply blood to the intestines.
phren/o	diaphragm	The *phrenic* artery supplies blood to the diaphragm.
ped/o	foot	The dorsalis *pedis* artery supplies blood to the foot.
stoma	mouth	An *anastomosis* is a communication between two vessels.

The Physiology of Circulation

sphygm/o	pulse	A *sphygmomanometer* is used to measure blood pressure.
man/o	pressure	See preceding example.

Lymphoid Tissue

-oid	like, resembling	*Lymphoid* tissue makes up the specialized organs of the lymphatic system.
aden/o	gland	The *adenoids* are gland-like tonsils.
lingu/o	tongue	The *lingual* tonsils are at the back of the tongue.

The Respiratory System

nas/o	nose	The *nasopharynx* is behind the nasal cavity.
or/o	mouth	The *oropharynx* is behind the mouth.
laryng/o	larynx	The *laryngeal* pharynx opens into the pharynx.
pleur/o	side, rib	The *pleura* covers the lung and lines the chest wall (rib cage).

The Process of Respiration

spir/o	breathing	A *spirometer* is an instrument used to record breathing volumes.
capn/o	carbon dioxide	*Hypercapnia* is a rise in the blood level of carbon dioxide.
-pnea	breathing	*Hypopnea* is a decrease in the rate and depth of breathing.
orth/o-	straight	*Orthopnea* can be relieved by sitting in an upright position.

Function and Design of the Digestive System

ab-	away from	In *absorption*, digested materials are taken from the digestive tract into the circulation.
enter/o	intestine	The *mesentery* is the portion of the peritoneum around the intestine.
mes/o-	middle	The *mesocolon*, like the mesentery, comes from the middle layer of cells in the embryo, the mesoderm.

Organs of the Digestive Tract

gastr/o	stomach	The *gastrointestinal* tract consists mainly of the stomach and intestine.

The Kidneys

retro-	backward, behind	The *retroperitoneal* space is posterior to the peritoneal cavity.
ren/o	kidney	The *renal* artery carries blood to the kidney.
nephr/o	kidney	The *nephron* is the functional unit of the kidney.
juxta-	next to	The *juxtaglomerular* apparatus is next to the glomerulus.

The Ureters

extra-	beyond, outside of	The ureters are *extraperitoneal*.

The Effects of Aging

noct/i	night	*Nocturia* is excessive urination at night.

Fluid Compartments

intra-	within	*Intracellular* fluid is within a cell.
extra-	outside of, beyond	*Extracellular* fluid is outside the cells.
semi-	partial, half	A *semipermeable* membrane is partially permeable.

(continued)

Word part	Meaning	Example
Water Balance		
poly-	many	*Polydipsia* is excessive thirst.
osmo-	osmosis	*Osmoreceptors* detect changes in osmotic concentration of fluids.
The Male Reproductive System		
semin/o	semen, seed	Sperm cells are produced in the *seminiferous* tubules.
test/o	testis	The hormone *testosterone* is produced in the testis.
acr/o	extreme end	The *acrosome* covers the head of a sperm cell.
fer	to carry	The ductus *deferens* carries spermatozoa away from (de-) the testis.
circum-	around	A cut is made around the glans to remove part of the foreskin in a *circumcision*.
The Female Reproductive System		
ov/o, ov/i	egg	An *ovum* is an egg cell.
ovar, ovari/o	ovary	The *ovarian* follicle encloses a maturing ovum.
metr/o	uterus	The *myometrium* is the muscular (my/o) layer of the uterus.
rect/o	rectum	The *rectouterine* pouch is between the uterus and rectum.

8

Metabolism, Nutrition, and Body Temperature

CHAPTER OBJECTIVES

In this chapter, you'll learn:

1. To differentiate between catabolism and anabolism.
2. To differentiate between the anaerobic and aerobic phases of cellular respiration and give the end products and the relative amount of energy released by each.
3. To define *metabolic rate* and name several factors that affect the metabolic rate.
4. To explain the roles of glucose and glycogen in metabolism.
5. To compare the energy contents of fats, proteins, and carbohydrates.
6. To define *essential amino acid.*
7. To explain the roles of minerals and vitamins in nutrition and give examples of each.

8. To list the recommended percentages of carbohydrate, fat, and protein in the diet.
9. To distinguish between simple and complex carbohydrates, giving examples of each.
10. To compare saturated and unsaturated fats.
11. To list some adverse effects of alcohol consumption.
12. To explain how heat is produced and lost in the body.
13. To describe the role of the hypothalamus in regulating body temperature.
14. To show how word parts are used to build words related to metabolism, nutrition, and body temperature (see Word Anatomy at the end of the chapter).

KEY TERMS

anabolism
catabolism
glucose

glycogen
hypothalamus
kilocalorie

malnutrition
metabolic rate
mineral

oxidation
vitamin

METABOLISM

Nutrients absorbed from the digestive tract are used for all the cellular activities of the body, which together make up **metabolism**. These activities fall into two categories:

- **Catabolism**, which is the breakdown of complex compounds into simpler compounds. Catabolism includes the digestion of food into small molecules and the release of energy from these molecules within the cell.
- **Anabolism**, which is the building of simple compounds into substances needed for cellular activities and for the growth and repair of tissues.

Through the steps of catabolism and anabolism, there is a constant turnover of body materials as energy is consumed, cells function and grow, and waste products are generated.

? Checkpoint Question

1. What are the two phases of metabolism?

Cellular Respiration

Energy is released from nutrients in a series of reactions called **cellular respiration** (see Table 8-1 and Fig. 8-1). Early studies on cellular respiration were done with **glucose** as the starting compound. Glucose is a simple sugar that is the main energy source for the body.

The Anaerobic Phase

The first steps in the breakdown of glucose do not require oxygen; that is, they are **anaerobic**. This phase of catabolism, known as **glycolysis** (gli-KOL-ih-sis), occurs in the cytoplasm of the cell. It yields a small amount of energy, which is used to make ATP (adenosine triphosphate), the cells' energy compound. Each glucose molecule yields enough energy by this process to produce 2 molecules of ATP.

The anaerobic breakdown of glucose is incomplete and ends with formation of an organic product called **pyruvic** (pi-RU-vik) **acid**. This organic acid is further metabolized in the next phase of cellular respiration, which requires oxygen. In muscle cells operating briefly under anaerobic conditions, pyruvic acid is converted to lactic acid, which accumulates as the cells build up an oxygen debt. Lactic acid induces muscle fatigue, so the body is forced to rest and recover. During the recovery phase immediately after exercise, breathing restores the oxygen needed to convert lactic acid back to pyruvic acid, which is then metabolized further. During this recovery phase, reserves stored in muscles are also replenished.

ANAEROBIC

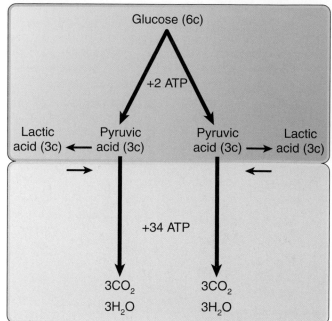

AEROBIC

FIGURE 8-1. Cellular respiration. This diagram shows the catabolism of glucose without oxygen (anaerobic) and with oxygen (aerobic). (C = carbon atoms in one molecule of a substance.) In cellular respiration, glucose first yields two molecules of pyruvic acid, which will convert to lactic acid under anaerobic conditions, as during intense exercise. (Lactic acid must eventually be converted back to pyruvic acid.) Typically, however, pyruvic acid is broken down aerobically (using oxygen) to CO_2 and H_2O (aerobically). *ZOOMING IN—What does pyruvic acid produce in cellular respiration under anaerobic conditions? Under aerobic conditions?*

These compounds are myoglobin, which stores oxygen; glycogen, which can be broken down for glucose; and creatine phosphate, which stores energy.

The Aerobic Phase

To generate enough energy for survival, the body's cells must break pyruvic acid down more completely in the second phase of cellular respiration, which requires oxygen. These **aerobic** reactions occur within the mitochondria of the cell. They result in the transfer of most of the energy remaining in the nutrients to ATP. On average, about 34 to 36 molecules of ATP can be formed aerobically per glucose molecule — quite an increase over anaerobic metabolism.

Table 8-1	SUMMARY OF CELLULAR RESPIRATION OF GLUCOSE		
Phase	**Location in Cell**	**End Product(s)**	**Energy Yield/Glucose**
Anaerobic (glycolysis)	Cytoplasm	Pyruvic acid	2 ATP
Aerobic	Mitochondria	Carbon dioxide and water	34–36 ATP

During the aerobic steps of cellular respiration, the cells form carbon dioxide, which then must be transported to the lungs for elimination. In addition, water is formed by the combination of oxygen with the hydrogen that is removed from nutrient molecules. Because of the type of chemical reactions involved, and because oxygen is used in the final steps, cellular respiration is described as an **oxidation** of nutrients. Note that enzymes are required as catalysts in all the reactions of cellular respiration. Many of the vitamins and minerals described later in this chapter are parts of these enzymes.

Although the oxidation of food is often compared to the burning of fuel, this comparison is inaccurate. Burning fuel results in a sudden and often wasteful release of energy in the form of heat and light. In contrast, metabolic oxidation occurs in small steps, and much of the energy released is stored as ATP for later use by the cells; some of the energy is released as heat, which is used to maintain body temperature, as discussed later in this chapter.

For those who know how to read chemical equations, the net balanced equation for cellular respiration, starting with glucose, is as follows:

$$\underset{\text{glucose}}{C_6H_{12}O_6} + \underset{\text{oxygen}}{6O_2} \rightarrow \underset{\substack{\text{carbon}\\\text{dioxide}}}{6CO_2} + \underset{\text{water}}{6H_2O}$$

Checkpoint Question

2. What name is given to the series of cellular reactions that releases energy from nutrients?

Metabolic Rate

Metabolic rate refers to the rate at which energy is released from nutrients in the cells. It is affected by a person's size, body fat, sex, age, activity, and hormones, especially thyroid hormone (thyroxine). Metabolic rate is high in children and adolescents and decreases with age. **Basal metabolism** is the amount of energy needed to maintain life functions while the body is at rest.

The unit used to measure energy is the **kilocalorie** (kcal), which is the amount of heat needed to raise 1 kilogram of water 1°C. To estimate the daily calories needed taking activity level into account, see Box 8-1.

The Use of Nutrients for Energy

As noted, glucose is the main source of energy in the body. Most of the carbohydrates in the diet are converted to glucose

---

Box 8-1

A CLOSER LOOK
Calorie Counting: Estimating Daily Energy Needs

Basal energy requirements for a day can be estimated with a simple formula. An average woman requires 0.9 kcal/kg/hour, and a man, 1.0 kcal/kg/hour. Multiplying 0.9 by body weight in kilograms* by 24 for a woman, or 1.0 by body weight in kilograms by 24 for a man, yields the daily basal energy requirement. For example, if a woman weighed 132 pounds, the equation would be as follows:

132 pounds ÷ 2.2 pounds/kg = 60 kg

0.9 kcal/kg/hour × 60 kg = 54 kcal/hour

54 kcal/hour × 24 hours/day = 1,296 kcal/day

To estimate total energy needs for a day, a percentage based on activity level ("couch potato" to serious athlete) must also be added to the basal requirement. These percentages are shown in the table below.

The equation to calculate total energy needs for a day is:

Basal energy requirement + (basal energy requirement × activity level)

Using our previous example, and assuming light activity levels, the following equations apply:
At 40% activity:

1,296 kcal/day + (1,296 kcal/day × 40%) = 1,814.4 kcal/day

At 60% activity:

1,296 kcal/day + (1,296 kcal/day × 60%) = 2,073.6 kcal/day

Therefore, the woman in our example would require between 1,814 and 2,073 kcal/day.

Activity Level	Male	Female
Little activity ("couch potato")	25–40%	25–35%
Light activity (*e.g.*, walking to and from class, but little or no intentional exercise)	50–75%	40–60%
Moderate activity (*e.g.*, aerobics several times a week)	65–80%	50–70%
Heavy activity (serious athlete)	90–120%	80–100%

*To convert pounds to kilograms, divide weight in pounds by 2.2.

in the course of metabolism. Reserves of glucose are stored in liver and muscle cells as **glycogen** (GLI-ko-jen), a compound built from glucose molecules. When glucose is needed for energy, glycogen is broken down to yield glucose. Glycerol and fatty acids (from fat digestion) and amino acids (from protein digestion) can also be used for energy, but they enter the breakdown process at different points.

Fat in the diet yields more than twice as much energy as do protein and carbohydrate (*e.g.*, it is more "fattening"); fat yields 9 kcal of energy per gram, whereas protein and carbohydrate each yield 4 kcal per gram. Calories that are ingested in excess of need are converted to fat and stored in adipose tissue.

Before they are oxidized for energy, amino acids must have their nitrogen (amine) groups removed. This removal, called **deamination** (de-am-ih-NA-shun), occurs in the liver, where the nitrogen groups are then formed into urea by combination with carbon dioxide. The blood transports urea to the kidneys to be eliminated.

There are no specialized storage forms of proteins, as there are for carbohydrates (glycogen) and fats (adipose tissue). Therefore, when one needs more proteins than are supplied in the diet, they must be obtained from body substance, such as muscle tissue or plasma proteins. Drawing on these resources becomes dangerous when needs are extreme. Fats and carbohydrates are described as "protein sparing," because they are used for energy before proteins are and thus spare proteins for the synthesis of necessary body components.

Checkpoint Question

3. What is the main energy source for the cells?

Anabolism

Nutrient molecules are built into body materials by anabolic steps, all of which are catalyzed by enzymes.

Essential Amino Acids

Eleven of the 20 amino acids needed to build proteins can be synthesized internally by metabolic reactions. These 11 amino acids are described as *nonessential* because they need not be taken in as food (Table 8-2). The remaining 9 amino acids cannot be made by the body and therefore must be taken in as part of the diet; these are the essential amino acids. Note that some nonessential amino acids may become essential under certain conditions, as during extreme physical stress, or in certain hereditary metabolic diseases.

Essential Fatty Acids

There are also two essential fatty acids (linoleic acid and linolenic acid) that must be taken in as food. These are easily obtained through a healthful, balanced diet.

Checkpoint Question

4. What is meant when an amino acid or a fatty acid is described as essential?

Table 8-2   AMINO ACIDS

Nonessential Amino Acids[a]		Essential Amino Acids[b]	
Name	**Pronunciation**	**Name[c]**	**Pronunciation**
Alanine	AL-ah-nene	Histidine	HIS-tih-dene
Arginine	AR-jih-nene	Isoleucine	i-so-LU-sene
Asparagine	ah-SPAR-ah-jene	Leucine	LU-sene
Aspartic acid	ah-SPAR-tik AH-sid	Lysine	LI-sene
Cysteine	SIS-teh-ene	Methionine	meh-THI-o-nene
Glutamic acid	glu-TAM-ik AH-sid	Phenylalanine	fen-il-AL-ah-nene
Glutamine	GLU-tah-mene	Threonine	THRE-o-nene
Glycine	GLY-sene	Tryptophan	TRIP-to-fane
Proline	PRO-lene	Valine	VA-lene
Serine	SERE-ene		
Tyrosine	TI-ro-sene		

[a]*Nonessential amino acids can be synthesized by the body.*
[b]*Essential amino acids cannot be synthesized by the body; they must be taken in as part of the diet.*
[c]*If you are ever called upon to memorize the essential amino acids, the mnemonic (memory) device Pvt. T. M. Hill gives the first letter of each name.*

Table 8-3 MINERALS

Mineral	Functions	Sources	Results of Deficiency
Calcium (Ca)	Formation of bones and teeth, blood clotting, nerve conduction, muscle contraction	Dairy products, eggs, green vegetables, legumes (peas and beans)	Rickets, tetany, osteoporosis
Phosphorus (P)	Formation of bones and teeth; found in ATP, nucleic acids	Meat, fish, poultry, egg yolk, dairy products	Osteoporosis, abnormal metabolism
Sodium (Na)	Fluid balance; nerve impulse conduction, muscle contraction	Most foods, especially processed foods, table salt	Weakness, cramps, diarrhea, dehydration
Potassium (K)	Fluid balance, nerve and muscle activity	Fruits, meats, seafood, milk, vegetables, grains	Muscular and neurologic disorders
Chloride (Cl)	Fluid balance, hydrochloric acid in stomach	Meat, milk, eggs, processed foods, table salt	Rarely occurs
Iron (Fe)	Oxygen carrier (hemoglobin, myoglobin)	Meat, eggs, fortified cereals, legumes, dried fruit	Anemia, dry skin, indigestion
Iodine (I)	Thyroid hormones	Seafood, iodized salt	Hypothyroidism, goiter
Magnesium (Mg)	Catalyst for enzyme reactions, carbohydrate metabolism	Green vegetables, grains, nuts, legumes	Spasticity, arrhythmia, vasodilation
Manganese (Mn)	Catalyst in actions of calcium and phosphorus; facilitator of many cell processes	Many foods	Possible reproductive disorders
Copper (Cu)	Necessary for absorption and use of iron in formation of hemoglobin; part of some enzymes	Meat, water	Anemia
Chromium (Cr)	Works with insulin to regulate blood glucose levels	Meat, unrefined food, fats and oils	Inability to use glucose
Cobalt (Co)	Part of vitamin B12	Animal products	Pernicious anemia
Zinc (Zn)	Promotes carbon dioxide transport and energy metabolism; found in enzymes	Meat, fish, poultry, grains, vegetables	Alopecia (baldness); possibly related to diabetes
Fluoride (F)	Prevents tooth decay	Fluoridated water, tea, seafood	Dental caries

Minerals and Vitamins

In addition to needing fats, proteins, and carbohydrates, the body requires minerals and vitamins.

Minerals are chemical elements needed for body structure, fluid balance, and such activities as muscle contraction, nerve impulse conduction, and blood clotting. Some minerals are components of vitamins. A list of the main minerals needed in a proper diet is given in Table 8-3. Some additional minerals not listed are also required for good health. Minerals needed in extremely small amounts are referred to as **trace elements**.

Vitamins are complex organic substances needed in very small quantities. Vitamins are parts of enzymes or other substances essential for metabolism, and vitamin deficiencies lead to a variety of nutritional diseases.

The water-soluble vitamins are the B vitamins and vitamin C. These are not stored and must be taken in regularly with food. The fat-soluble vitamins are A, D, E, and K. These vitamins are kept in reserve in fatty tissue. Excess intake of the fat-soluble vitamins can lead to toxicity. A list of vitamins is given in Table 8-4.

Certain substances are valuable in the diet as **antioxidants**. They defend against the harmful effects of **free radicals**, highly reactive and unstable molecules produced from oxygen in the normal course of metabolism (and also from UV radiation, air pollution, and tobacco smoke). Free radicals contribute to aging and disease. Antioxidants react with free radicals to stabilize them and minimize their harmful effects on cells. Vitamins C and E and beta carotene, an orange pigment found in plants that is

Table 8-4   VITAMINS

Vitamins	Functions	Sources	Results of Deficiency
A (retinol)	Required for healthy epithelial tissue and for eye pigments; involved in reproduction and immunity	Orange fruits and vegetables, liver, eggs, dairy products, dark green vegetables	Night blindness; dry, scaly skin; decreased immunity
B1 (thiamin)	Required for enzymes involved in oxidation of nutrients; nerve function	Pork, cereal, grains, meats, legumes, nuts	Beriberi, a disease of nerves
B2 (riboflavin)	In enzymes required for oxidation of nutrients	Milk, eggs, liver, green leafy vegetables, grains	Skin and tongue disorders
B3 (niacin, nicotinic acid)	Involved in oxidation of nutrients	Yeast, meat, liver, grains, legumes, nuts	Pellagra with dermatitis, diarrhea, mental disorders
B6 (pyridoxine)	Amino acid and fatty acid metabolism; formation of niacin; manufacture of red blood cells	Meat, fish, poultry, fruit, grains, legumes, vegetables	Anemia, irritability, convulsions, muscle twitching, skin disorders
Pantothenic acid	Essential for normal growth; energy metabolism	Yeast, liver, eggs, and many other foods	Sleep disturbances, digestive upset
B12 (cyanocobalamin)	Production of cells; maintenance of nerve cells; fatty acid and amino acid metabolism	Animal products	Pernicious anemia
Biotin	Involved in fat and glycogen formation, amino acid metabolism	Peanuts, liver, tomatoes, eggs, and many other foods	Lack of coordination, dermatitis, fatigue
Folate (folic acid)	Required for amino acid metabolism, DNA synthesis, maturation of red blood cells	Vegetables, liver, legumes, seeds	Anemia, digestive disorders, neural tube defects in the embryo
C (ascorbic acid)	Maintains healthy skin and mucous membranes; involved in synthesis of collagen; antioxidant	Citrus fruits, green vegetables, potatoes, orange fruits	Scurvy, poor wound healing, anemia, weak bones
D (calciferol)	Aids in absorption of calcium and phosphorus from intestinal tract	Fatty fish, liver, eggs, fortified milk	Rickets, bone deformities
E (tocopherol)	Protects cell membranes; antioxidant	Seeds, green vegetables, nuts, grains, oils	Anemia, muscle and liver degeneration, pain
K	Synthesis of blood clotting factors, bone formation	Bacteria in digestive tract, liver, cabbage, and leafy green vegetables	Hemorrhage

converted to vitamin A, are antioxidants. There are also many compounds found in plants (*e.g.*, soybeans and tomatoes) that are antioxidants.

 Checkpoint Question

5. Both vitamins and minerals are needed in metabolism. What is the difference between vitamins and minerals?

NUTRITIONAL GUIDELINES

The relative amounts of carbohydrates, fats, and proteins that should be in the daily diet vary somewhat with the individual. Typical recommendations for the number of

calories derived each day from the three types of food are as follows:

- Carbohydrate: 55%–60%.
- Fat: 30% or less.
- Protein: 15%–20%.

It is important to realize that the type as well as the amount of each is a factor in good health. A weight loss diet should follow the same proportions as given above, but with a decrease in portion sizes.

Carbohydrates

Carbohydrates in the diet should be mainly complex, naturally occurring carbohydrates, and simple sugars should be kept to a minimum. Simple sugars are monosaccharides, such as glucose and fructose (fruit sugar), and disaccharides, such as sucrose (table sugar), and lactose (milk sugar). Simple sugars are a source of fast energy because they are metabolized rapidly. However, they boost pancreatic insulin output, and as a result, they cause blood glucose levels to rise and fall rapidly. It is healthier to maintain steady glucose levels, which normally range from approximately 85 to 125 mg/dL throughout the day.

The **glycemic effect** is a measure of how rapidly a particular food raises the blood glucose level and stimulates the release of insulin. The effect is generally low for whole grains, fruit, and dairy products and high for sweets and refined ("white") grains. Note, however, that the glycemic effect of a food also depends on when it is eaten during the day, and if or how it is combined with other foods.

Complex carbohydrates are polysaccharides. Examples are:

- starches, found in grains, legumes, and potatoes
- fibers, such as cellulose, pectins, and gums, which are the structural materials of plants.

Fiber adds bulk to the stool and promotes elimination of toxins and waste. It also slows the digestion and absorption of carbohydrates, thus regulating the release of glucose. It helps in weight control by providing a sense of fullness and limiting caloric intake. Adequate fiber in the diet lowers cholesterol and helps to prevent diabetes, colon cancer, hemorrhoids, appendicitis, and diverticulitis. Foods high in fiber, such as whole grains, fruits, and vegetables, are also rich in vitamins and minerals (see Box 8-2).

Checkpoint Question

6. What is the normal range of blood glucose?

Fats

Fats are subdivided into saturated and unsaturated forms based on their chemical structure. The fatty acids in saturated fats have more hydrogen atoms in their molecules and fewer double bonds between carbons atoms than do those of unsaturated fats (Fig. 8-2). Most saturated fats are from animal sources and are solid at room temperature, such as butter and lard. Also included in this group are the so-called tropical oils: coconut oil and palm oil. **Unsaturated** fats are derived from plants. They are liquid at room temperature and are generally referred to as oils, such as corn, peanut, olive, and canola oils.

Saturated fats should make up less than one third of the fat in the diet (less than 10% of total calories). Diets high in saturated fats are associated with a higher than normal incidence of cancer, heart disease, and cardiovascular problems, although the relation between these factors is not fully understood.

Many commercial products contain fats that are artificially saturated to prevent rancidity and provide a more solid consistency. These are listed on food labels as partially hydrogenated (HI-dro-jen-a-ted) vegetable oils and are found in baked goods, processed peanut butter, vegetable shortening, and solid margarine. Evidence shows that components of hydrogenated fats, known as *trans-fatty acids*, may be just as harmful, if not more so, than natural saturated fats and should be avoided.

Proteins

Because proteins, unlike carbohydrates and fats, are not stored in special reserves, protein foods should be taken in on a regular basis, with attention to obtaining the essential amino acids. Most animal proteins supply all of the essential

---

B o x   8 - 2

HEALTH MAINTENANCE
Dietary Fiber: Bulking Up

Dietary fiber is best known for its ability to improve bowel habits and ease weight loss. But fiber may also help to prevent diabetes, heart disease, and certain digestive disorders such as diverticulitis and gallstones.

Dietary fiber is an indigestible type of carbohydrate found in fruit, vegetables, and whole grains. The amount of fiber recommended for a 2,000-calorie diet is 25 grams per day, but most people in the United States tend to get only half this amount. One should eat fiber-rich foods throughout the day to meet the requirement. It is best to increase fiber in the diet gradually to avoid unpleasant symptoms, such as intestinal bloating and flatulence. If your diet lacks fiber, try adding the following foods over

a period of several weeks:

- Whole grain breads, cereals, pasta, and brown rice. These add 1 to 3 more grams of fiber per serving than the "white" product.
- Legumes, which include beans, peas, and lentils. These add 4 to 12 grams of fiber per serving.
- Fruits and vegetables. Whole, raw, unpeeled versions contain the most fiber, and juices, the least. Apple juice has no fiber, whereas a whole apple has 3 grams.
- Unprocessed bran. This can be sprinkled over almost any food: cereal, soups, and casseroles. One tablespoon adds 2 grams of fiber. Be sure to take adequate fluids with bran.

Saturated
fatty acid
(stearic acid)

Unsaturated
fatty acid
(linoleic acid)

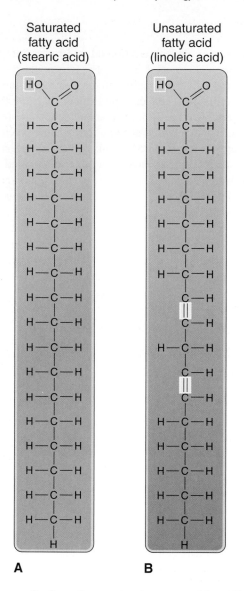

A   B

FIGURE 8-2. Saturated and unsaturated fats. **(A)** Saturated fatty acids contain the maximum numbers of hydrogen atoms attached to carbons and no double bonds between carbon atoms. **(B)** Unsaturated fatty acids have less than the maximum number of hydrogen atoms attached to carbons and one or more double bonds between carbon atoms (highlighted).

amino acids and are described as complete proteins. Most vegetables are lacking in one or more of the essential amino acids. People on strict vegetarian diets must learn to combine foods such as legumes (e.g., beans and peas) with grains (*e.g.*, rice, corn, or wheat), to obtain all the essential amino acids each day. Table 8-5 demonstrates the principles of combining two foods, legumes and grains, to supply essential amino acids that might be missing in one food or the other. Legumes are rich in isoleucine and lysine but poor in methonine and tryptophan, while grains are just the opposite. For illustration purposes, the table includes only the 4 missing essential amino acids (there are 9 total). Traditional ethnic diets reflect these healthy combinations, for example, beans with corn or rice in Mexican dishes or chickpeas and lentils with wheat in Middle Eastern fare.

Vitamin and Mineral Supplements

The need for mineral and vitamin supplements to the diet is a subject of controversy. Some researchers maintain that adequate amounts of these substances can be obtained from a varied, healthful diet. Many commercial foods, including milk, cereal, and bread, are already fortified with minerals and vitamins. Others hold that pollution, depletion of the soils, and the storage, refining, and processing of foods make additional supplementation beneficial. Most agree, however, that children, elderly people, pregnant and lactating women, and teenagers, who often do not get enough of the proper foods, would profit from additional minerals and vitamins.

When required, supplements should be selected by a physician or nutritionist to fit an individual's particular needs. Megavitamin dosages may cause unpleasant reactions and in some cases are hazardous. Vitamins A and D have both been found to cause serious toxic effects when taken in excess.

The Food Guide Pyramid

In 1992, the USDA (United States Department of Agriculture) developed a pyramid to represent the quantities of foods in the different food groups recommended each day

Table 8-5 COMBINING FOODS FOR ESSENTIAL AMINO ACIDS				
	Essential Amino Acids[a]			
	Isoleucine	**Lysine**	**Methionine**	**Tryptophan**
Legumes	x	x		
Grains			x	x
Legumes and grains combined	x	x	x	x

[a] *There are 9 essential amino acids; the table includes 4 for the purposes of illustration.*

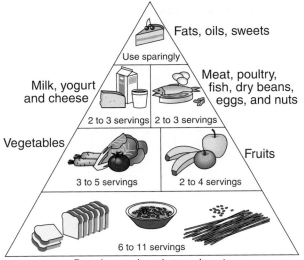

Fats, oils, sweets
Use sparingly

Milk, yogurt and cheese

Meat, poultry, fish, dry beans, eggs, and nuts

2 to 3 servings   2 to 3 servings

Vegetables

Fruits

3 to 5 servings   2 to 4 servings

6 to 11 servings

Bread, cereal, grains, and pasta

FIGURE 8-3. The Food Guide Pyramid. (From U.S. Department of Agriculture/U.S. Department of Health and Human Services.)

for good health (Fig. 8-3). This symbol is under revision, and some suggested improvements include:

- distinguish between unrefined and refined carbohydrates
- distinguish between healthful unsaturated fats, which can be eaten in moderation, and less healthful saturated and processed (trans-) fats, which should be restricted
- accommodate vegetarians, who may avoid not only meats, but dairy products and eggs as well
- specify portion sizes, which are smaller than most people think
- include the need for water
- indicate possible need for vitamin supplements.

Governments in the United States and other countries will continue to study this topic with input from nutritionists and other scientists. The best nutrition guidelines, however, will be of no benefit unless people are educated and motivated to follow them.

Alcohol

Alcohol yields energy in the amount of 7 kcal per gram, but it is not considered a nutrient because it does not yield useful end products. In fact, alcohol interferes with metabolism and contributes to a variety of disorders.

The body can metabolize about .5 ounce of pure alcohol (ethanol) per hour. This amount translates into one glass of wine, one can of beer, or one shot of hard liquor. Consumed at a more rapid rate, alcohol enters the bloodstream and affects many cells, notably in the brain.

Alcohol is rapidly absorbed through the stomach and small intestine and is detoxified by the liver. When delivered in excess to the liver, alcohol can lead to the accumulation of fat as well as inflammation and scarring of liver tissue. It can

eventually cause cirrhosis (sih-RO-sis), which involves irreversible changes in liver structure. Alcohol metabolism ties up enzymes needed for oxidation of nutrients and also results in byproducts that acidify body fluids. Other effects of alcoholism include obesity, **malnutrition**, cancer, ulcers, and fetal alcohol syndrome. Pregnant women are advised not to drink any alcohol. In addition, alcohol impairs judgment and leads to increased involvement in accidents.

Although alcohol consumption is compatible with good health and may even have a beneficial effect on the cardiovascular system, alcohol should be consumed only in moderation.

 Checkpoint Question

7. What are typical recommendations for the relative amounts of carbohydrates, fats, and proteins in the diet?

NUTRITION AND AGING

With age, a person may find it difficult to maintain a balanced diet. Often, the elderly lose interest in buying and preparing food or are unable to do so. Because metabolism generally slows, and less food is required to meet energy needs, nutritional deficiencies may develop. Medications may interfere with appetite and with the absorption and use of specific nutrients.

It is important for older people to seek out foods that are "nutrient dense," that is, foods that have a high proportion of nutrients in comparison with the number of calories they provide. Exercise helps to boost appetite and maintains muscle tissue, which is more active metabolically. Box 8-3 describes how dietitians and nutritionists can help in planning a healthful diet for people of all ages.

BODY TEMPERATURE

Heat is an important byproduct of the many chemical activities constantly occurring in body tissues. At the same time, heat is always being lost through a variety of outlets. Under normal conditions, a number of regulatory devices keep body temperature constant within quite narrow limits. Maintenance of a constant temperature despite both internal and external influences is one phase of homeostasis, the tendency of all body processes to maintain a normal state despite forces that tend to alter them.

Heat Production

Heat is a byproduct of the cellular oxidations that generate energy. The amount of heat produced by a given organ varies with the kind of tissue and its activity. While at rest, muscles may produce as little as 25% of total body heat, but when muscles contract, heat production is greatly multiplied, owing to the increase in metabolic rate. Under basal conditions (at rest), the liver and other abdominal organs produce about 50% of total body heat. The brain produces only 15%

Box 8-3

HEALTH PROFESSIONS

Dietitians and Nutritionists

Dietitians and nutritionists specialize in planning and supervising food programs for institutions such as hospitals, schools, and nursing care facilities. They assess their clients' nutritional needs and design individualized meal plans. Dietitians and nutritionists also work in community settings, educating the public about disease prevention through healthy eating. Increased public awareness about food and nutrition has also led to new opportunities in the food manufacturing industry. To perform their duties, dietitians and nutritionists need a thorough understanding of anatomy and physiology. Most dietitians and nutritionists in the United States receive their training from a college or university and take a licensing exam.

Job prospects for dietitians and nutritionists are good. As the American population continues to age, the need for nutritional planning in hospital and nursing care settings is expected to rise. In addition, many people now place an emphasis on healthy eating and may consult nutritionists privately. For more information about this career, contact the American Dietetic Association.

---

of body heat at rest, and an increase in nervous tissue activity produces little increase in heat production.

Although it would seem from this description that some parts of the body would tend to become much warmer than others, the circulating blood distributes the heat fairly evenly.

Factors Affecting Heat Production

The rate at which heat is produced is affected by a number of factors, including exercise, hormone production, food intake, and age. Hormones, such as thyroxine from the thyroid gland and epinephrine (adrenaline) from the adrenal medulla, increase the rate of heat production.

The intake of food is also accompanied by increased heat production. The nutrients that enter the blood after digestion are available for increased cellular metabolism. In addition, the glands and muscles of the digestive system generate heat as they set to work. These responses do not account for all the increase, however, nor do they account for the much greater increase in metabolism after a meal containing a large amount of protein. Although the reasons are not entirely clear, the intake of food definitely increases metabolism and thus adds to heat production.

 Checkpoint Question

8. What are some factors that affect heat production in the body?

Heat Loss

More than 80% of heat loss occurs through the skin. The remaining 15% to 20% is dissipated by the respiratory system and with the urine and feces. Networks of blood vessels in the skin's dermis (deeper part) can bring considerable quantities of blood near the surface, so that heat can be dissipated to the outside. This release can occur in several ways.

- Heat can be transferred directly to the surrounding air by means **conduction**.

- Heat also travels from its source as heat waves or rays, a process termed **radiation**.
- If the air is moving, so that the layer of heated air next to the body is constantly being carried away and replaced with cooler air (as by an electric fan), the process is known as **convection**.
- Finally, heat may be lost by **evaporation**, the process by which liquid changes to the vapor state.

To illustrate evaporation, rub some alcohol on your skin; it evaporates rapidly, using so much heat from the skin that your arm feels cold. Perspiration does the same thing, although not as quickly. The rate of heat loss through evaporation depends on the humidity of the surrounding air. When it exceeds 60% or so, perspiration does not evaporate so readily, making one feel generally miserable unless some other means of heat loss is available, such as convection caused by a fan.

Prevention of Heat Loss

Factors that play a part in heat loss through the skin include the volume of tissue compared with the amount of skin surface. A child loses heat more rapidly than does an adult. Such parts as fingers and toes are affected most by exposure to cold because they have a great amount of skin compared with total tissue volume.

If the temperature of the surrounding air is lower than that of the body, excessive heat loss is prevented by both natural and artificial means. Clothing checks heat loss by trapping "dead air" in both its material and its layers. This noncirculating air is a good insulator. An effective natural insulation against cold is the layer of fat under the skin. Even when skin temperature is low, this fatty tissue prevents the deeper tissues from losing much heat. On the average, this layer is slightly thicker in females than in males. Naturally, there are individual variations, but as a rule, the degree of insulation depends on the thickness of this subcutaneous fat layer.

Temperature Regulation

Given that body temperature remains almost constant despite wide variations in the rate of heat production or loss, there must be internal mechanisms for regulating temperature.

The Role of the Hypothalamus

Many areas of the body take part in heat regulation, but the most important center is the **hypothalamus**, the area of the brain located just above the pituitary gland. Some of the cells in the hypothalamus control heat production in body tissues, whereas another group of cells controls heat loss. Regulation is based on the temperature of the blood circulating through the brain and also on input from temperature receptors in the skin.

If these two factors indicate that too much heat is being lost, impulses are sent quickly from the hypothalamus to the autonomic (involuntary) nervous system, which in turn causes constriction of the skin blood vessels to reduce heat loss. Other impulses are sent to the muscles to cause shivering, a rhythmic contraction of many muscles, which results in increased heat production. Furthermore, the output of epinephrine may be increased if necessary. Epinephrine increases cell metabolism for a short period, and this in turn increases heat production.

If there is danger of overheating, the hypothalamus stimulates the sweat glands to increase their activity. Impulses from the hypothalamus also cause blood vessels in the skin to dilate, so that increased blood flow to the skin will result in greater heat loss. The hypothalamus may also promote muscle relaxation to minimize heat production.

Muscles are especially important in temperature regulation because variations in the activity of these large tissue masses can readily increase or decrease heat generation. Because muscles form roughly one-third of the body, either an involuntary or an intentional increase in their activity can form enough heat to offset a considerable decrease in the temperature of the environment.

Checkpoint Question

9. What part of the brain is responsible for regulating body temperature?

Age Factors

Very young and very old people are limited in their ability to regulate body temperature when exposed to environmental extremes. A newborn infant's body temperature decreases if the infant is exposed to a cool environment for a long period. Elderly people also are not able to produce enough heat to maintain body temperature in a cool environment.

With regard to overheating in these age groups, heat loss mechanisms are not fully developed in the newborn. The elderly do not lose as much heat from their skin as do younger people. Both groups should be protected from extreme temperatures.

Normal Body Temperature

The normal temperature range obtained by either a mercury or an electronic thermometer may extend from 36.28°C to 37.6°C (97°F to 100°F). Body temperature varies with the time of day. Usually, it is lowest in the early morning because the muscles have been relaxed and no food has been taken in for several hours. Temperature tends to be higher in the late afternoon and evening because of physical activity and consumption of food.

Normal temperature also varies in different parts of the body. Skin temperature obtained in the axilla (armpit) is lower than mouth temperature, and mouth temperature is a degree or so lower than rectal temperature. It is believed that, if it were possible to place a thermometer inside the liver, it would register a degree or more higher than rectal temperature. The temperature within a muscle might be even higher during activity.

Although the Fahrenheit scale is used in the United States, in most parts of the world, temperature is measured with the **Celsius** (SEL-se-us) thermometer. On this scale, the ice point is at 0° and the normal boiling point of water is at 100°, the interval between these two points being divided into 100 equal units. The Celsius scale is also called the **centigrade scale** (think of 100 cents in a dollar).

Checkpoint Question

10. What is normal body temperature?

Word Anatomy

Medical terms are built from standardized word parts (prefixes, roots, and suffixes). Learning the meanings of these parts can help you remember words and interpret unfamiliar terms.

Word part	Meaning	Example
Metabolism		
glyc/o	sugar, sweet	*Glycogen* yields glucose molecules when it breaks down.
-lysis	separating, dissolving	*Glycolysis* is the breakdown of glucose for energy.

Summary

I. Metabolism—life-sustaining reactions that occur in the living cell
1. Catabolism—breakdown of complex compounds into simpler compounds
2. Anabolism—building of simple compounds into substances needed for cellular activities, growth, and repair
   A. Cellular respiration—a series of reactions in which food is oxidized for energy
      1. Anaerobic phase—does not require oxygen
         a. Location—cytoplasm
         b. Yield—2 ATP per glucose
         c. End product—organic (*i.e.*, pyruvic acid)
      2. Aerobic phase—requires oxygen
         a. Location—mitochondria
         b. Yield—34–36 ATP per glucose
         c. End products—carbon dioxide and water
      3. Metabolic rate—rate at which energy is released from food in the cells
         a. Basal metabolism—amount of energy needed to maintain life functions while at rest
   B. Use of nutrients for energy
      1. Glucose—main energy source
      2. Fats—highest energy yield
      3. Proteins—can be used for energy after removal of nitrogen (deamination)
   C. Anabolism
      1. Essential amino acids and fatty acids must be taken in as part of diet
   D. Minerals and vitamins
      1. Minerals—elements needed for body structure and cell activities
         a. Trace elements—elements needed in extremely small amounts
      2. Vitamins—organic substances needed in small amounts
         a. Antioxidants (*e.g.*, vitamins C and E) protect against free radicals

II. Nutritional guidelines
   A. Carbohydrates
      1. 55%–60% of calories
      2. Should be complex (unrefined) not simple (sugars)
      a. Glycemic effect—how quickly a food raises blood glucose and insulin
      b. Plant fiber important
   B. Fats
      1. 30% or less of calories
      2. Unsaturated healthier than saturated
         a. Hydrogenated fats artificially saturated
   C. Proteins
      1. 15%–20% of calories
      2. Complete—all essential amino acids
         a. Need to combine plant foods
   D. Vitamin and mineral supplements
   E. Food Guide Pyramid (USDA)—under revision
   F. Alcohol—metabolized in liver

III. Nutrition and aging

IV. Body temperature
   A. Heat production
      1. Most heat produced in muscles and glands
      2. Distributed by the circulation
      3. Affected by exercise, hormones, food, age
   B. Heat loss
      1. Avenues—skin, urine, feces, respiratory system
      2. Mechanisms—conduction, radiation, convection, evaporation
      3. Prevention of heat loss—clothing, subcutaneous fat
   C. Temperature regulation
      1. Hypothalamus—main temperature-regulating center
         a. Responds to temperature of blood in brain and temperature receptors in skin
      2. Conservation of heat
         a. Constriction of blood vessels in skin
         b. Shivering
         c. Increased release of epinephrine
      3. Release of heat
         a. Dilation of skin vessels
         b. Sweating
         c. Relaxation of muscles
      4. Age factors
      5. Normal body temperature—ranges from 36.2°C to 37.6°C; varies with time of day and location measured

Questions for Study and Review

Building Understanding

Fill in the blanks
1. Building glycogen from glucose is an example of
   _____.
2. The amount of energy needed to maintain life functions while at rest is _____.

3. Reserves of glucose are stored in liver and muscle as
   _____.
4. The most important area of the brain for temperature regulation is the _____.
5. Minerals needed in extremely small amounts are referred to as _____.

Matching
Match each numbered item with the most closely related lettered item.

_____ 6. Main energy source for the body

a. saturated fat

_____ 7. Chemical element required for normal body function

b. vitamin

_____ 8. Complex organic substance required for normal body function

c. mineral

_____ 9. Energy storage molecule with only single bonds between carbon atoms

d. unsaturated fat

_____ 10. Energy storage molecule with one or more double bonds between carbon atoms

e. glucose

Multiple choice

_____ 11. During amino acid catabolism, nitrogen is removed by
a. oxidation
b. the glycemic effect
c. lysis
d. deamination

_____ 12. Which of the following would have the lowest glycemic effect?
a. glucose
b. sucrose
c. lactose
d. starch

_____ 13. Alcohol is catabolized by the
a. small intestine
b. liver
c. pancreas
d. spleen

_____ 14. Amino acids that cannot be made by metabolism are said to be
a. essential
b. nonessential
c. antioxidants
d. free radicals

Understanding Concepts

15. In what part of the cell does anaerobic respiration occur and what are its end products? In what part of the cell does aerobic respiration occur? What are its end products?
16. About how many kilocalories are released from a tablespoon of butter (14 grams)? a tablespoon of sugar (12 grams)? a tablespoon of egg white (15 grams)?
17. If you eat 2000 kcal a day, how many kilocalories should come from carbohydrates? from fats? from protein?
18. How is heat produced in the body? What structures produce the most heat during increased activity?
19. Emily's body temperature increased from 36.2°C to 36.5°C and then decreased to 36.2°C Describe the feedback mechanism regulating Emily's body temperature.
20. Differentiate between the terms in the following pairs:
a. conduction and convection
b. radiation and evaporation
c. antioxidants and free radicals
e. catabolism and anabolism

Conceptual Thinking

21. The oxidation of glucose to form ATP is often compared to the burning of fuel. Why is this analogy inaccurate?
22. It is a hot summer's day and you are trying to keep cool by sitting in front of a fan, but you are still sweating profusely. Describe the two mechanisms of heat loss that you are employing.

9

Development and Birth

CHAPTER OBJECTIVES

In this chapter, you'll learn:

1. To describe fertilization and the early development of the fertilized egg.
2. To describe the structure and function of the placenta.
3. To briefly describe changes that occur in the fetus and the mother during pregnancy.
4. To briefly describe the four stages of labor.
5. To compare fraternal and identical twins.
6. To cite the advantages of breastfeeding.
7. To briefly describe the mechanism of gene function.
8. To explain the difference between dominant and recessive genes.
9. To compare *phenotype* and *genotype* and give examples of each.
10. To describe what is meant by a *carrier* of a genetic trait.
11. To define *meiosis* and explain its function in reproduction.
12. To explain how sex is determined in humans.
13. To describe what is meant by the term *sex-linked* and list several sex-linked traits.
14. To list several factors that may influence the expression of a gene.
15. To define *mutation*.
16. To show how word parts are used to build words related to development and heredity (see Word Anatomy near the end of the chapter).

KEY TERMS

abortion	embryo	heterozygous	phenotype
allele	fertilization	homozygous	placenta
amniotic sac	fetus	implantation	recessive
autosome	gene	lactation	sex-linked trait
chromosome	genotype	meiosis	umbilical cord
dominant	gestation	parturition	zygote

PREGNANCY

Pregnancy begins with **fertilization** of an ovum and ends with delivery of the fetus and afterbirth. During this approximately 38-week period of development, known as **gestation** (jes-TA-shun), all fetal tissues differentiate from a single fertilized egg. Along the way, many changes occur in both the mother and the developing infant.

Fertilization and the Start of Pregnancy

When semen is deposited in the vagina, the many spermatozoa immediately wriggle about in all directions, some traveling into the uterus and oviducts (Fig. 9-1). If an egg cell is present in the oviduct, many spermatozoa cluster around it. Using enzymes, they dissolve the coating around the ovum, so that eventually one sperm cell can penetrate its plasma membrane. The nuclei of the sperm and egg then combine. (See Box 9-1 on artificial methods to assist conception.)

The result of this union is a single cell, called a **zygote** (ZI-gote), with the full human chromosome number of 46. The zygote divides rapidly into two cells and then four cells and soon forms a ball of cells. During this time, the cell cluster is traveling toward the uterine cavity, pushed along by cilia lining the oviduct and by peristalsis (contractions) of the tube. After reaching the uterus, the little ball of cells burrows into the greatly thickened uterine lining and is soon implanted and completely covered. After **implantation** in the uterus, a group of cells within the dividing cluster becomes an **embryo** (EM-bre-o), the term used for the growing offspring in the early stage of gestation. The other cells within the cluster will differentiate into tissue that will support the developing offspring throughout gestation.

 Checkpoint Question

1. What structure is formed by the union of an ovum and a spermatozoon?

The Placenta

For a few days after implantation, the embryo gets nourishment from the endometrium. By the end of the second week, however, the outer cells of the embryonic cluster form villi (projections) that invade the uterine wall and maternal blood channels (venous sinuses). Gradually, tissue in the outer

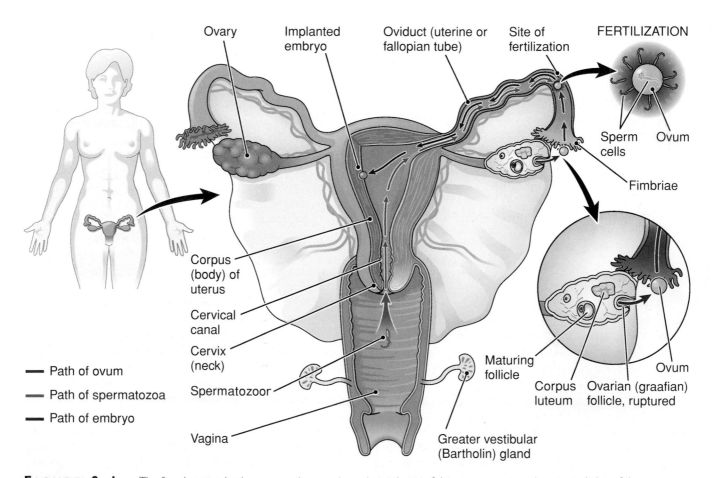

— Path of ovum
— Path of spermatozoa
— Path of embryo

Ovary · Implanted embryo · Oviduct (uterine or fallopian tube) · Site of fertilization · FERTILIZATION · Sperm cells · Ovum · Fimbriae · Corpus (body) of uterus · Cervical canal · Cervix (neck) · Spermatozoor · Vagina · Maturing follicle · Corpus luteum · Ovarian (graafian) follicle, ruptured · Ovum · Greater vestibular (Bartholin) gland

FIGURE 9-1. The female reproductive system. Arrows show the pathway of the spermatozoa and ovum and also of the fertilization and implantation of the fertilized ovum. *ZOOMING IN—Where is the ovum fertilized?*

embryonic layer and in the uterine lining together form the **placenta** (*plah-SEN-tah*), a flat, circular organ that consists of a spongy network of blood-filled channels and capillary-containing villi (Fig. 9-2). (Placenta is from a Latin word meaning "pancake.") The placenta is the organ of nutrition, respiration, and excretion for the developing offspring throughout gestation. Although the blood of the mother and her offspring do not mix — each has its own blood and cardiovascular system — exchanges take place through the capillaries of the placental villi. In this manner, gases (CO_2 and O_2) are exchanged, nutrients are provided to the developing infant, and waste products are released into the maternal blood to be eliminated.

The Umbilical Cord

The embryo is connected to the developing placenta by a stalk of tissue that eventually becomes the **umbilical** (um-BIL-ih-kal) **cord**. This structure carries blood to and from the embryo, later called the **fetus** (FE-tus). The cord encloses two arteries that carry deoxygenated blood from the fetus to the placenta, and one vein that carries oxygenated blood from the placenta to the fetus (see Fig. 9-2). (Note that, like the pulmonary vessels, these arteries carry blood low in oxygen and this vein carries blood high in oxygen.) The fetus has special circulatory features used to carry blood to and from the umbilical cord. Several adaptations in the fetal heart allow blood to bypass the lungs, which are not functional in the fetus (see Box 9-2).

Placental Hormones

In addition to maintaining the fetus, the placenta is an endocrine organ. Beginning soon after implantation, some embryonic cells produce the hormone **human chorionic gonadotropin** (ko-re-ON-ik gon-ah-do-TRO-pin) **(hCG).** This hormone stimulates the ovarian corpus luteum, prolonging its life-span to 11 or 12 weeks and causing it to secrete increasing amounts of progesterone and estrogen. It is hCG that is used in tests as an indicator of pregnancy.

Progesterone is essential for the maintenance of pregnancy. It promotes endometrial secretion to nourish the embryo, maintains the endometrium and decreases the ability of the uterine muscle to contract, thus preventing the embryo from being expelled from the body. During pregnancy, progesterone also helps prepare the breasts for milk secretion.

Estrogen promotes enlargement of the uterus and breasts. By the 11th or 12th week of pregnancy, the corpus luteum is no longer needed; by this time, the placenta itself can secrete adequate amounts of progesterone and estrogen, and the corpus luteum disintegrates. Miscarriages (loss of an embryo or fetus) frequently occur during this critical time when hormone secretion is shifting from the corpus luteum to the placenta.

Human placental lactogen (hPL), is a hormone secreted by the placenta during pregnancy, reaching a peak at term, the normal conclusion of pregnancy. HPL stimulates growth of the breasts to prepare the mother for production of milk, or **lactation** (lak-TA-shun). More importantly, it regulates

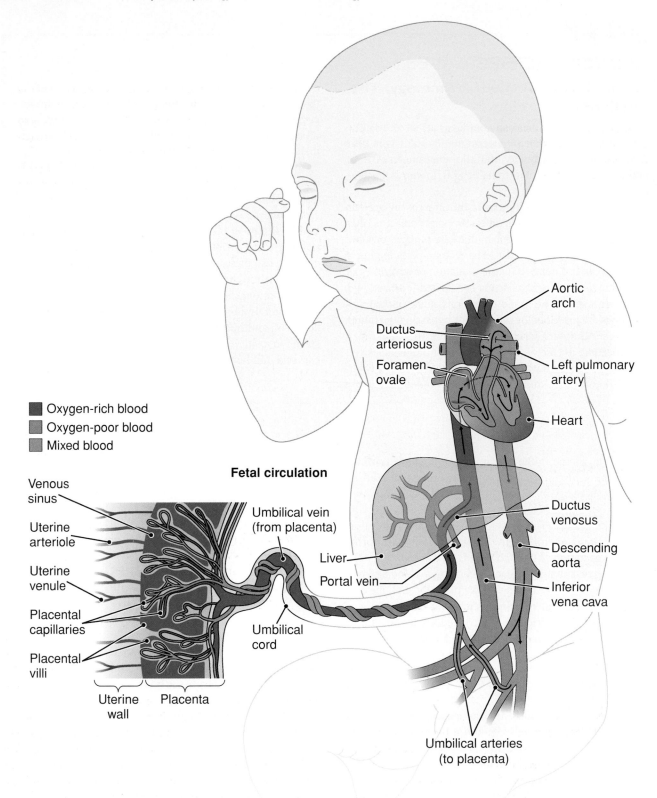

Oxygen-rich blood
Oxygen-poor blood
Mixed blood

Fetal circulation

Aortic arch

Ductus arteriosus

Foramen ovale

Left pulmonary artery

Heart

Venous sinus

Uterine arteriole

Uterine venule

Placental capillaries

Placental villi

Umbilical vein (from placenta)

Liver

Portal vein

Umbilical cord

Ductus venosus

Descending aorta

Inferior vena cava

Uterine wall   Placenta

Umbilical arteries (to placenta)

FIGURE 9-2.   Fetal circulation and section of placenta. Colors show relative oxygen content of blood.   *ZOOMING IN—What is signified by the purple color in this illustration?*

Box 9-2

A CLOSER LOOK
Fetal Circulation: Routing Blood to Miss the Lungs

The developing fetus has several adaptations in the cardiovascular system that change at birth. These adaptations serve to bypass the lungs, which in the fetus are not functional. Fetal blood is oxygenated instead by the placenta (see Fig. 9-2).

Oxygenated blood comes from the placenta to the fetus via the **umbilical vein**, which is contained in the umbilical cord. Most of this blood joins the inferior vena cava by way of a small vessel, the **ductus venosus**, and is carried to the heart. The rest is delivered to the liver. Once in the right atrium, some of the blood flows directly into the left atrium through a hole in the atrial septum called the **foramen ovale**. This blood bypasses the right ventricle and the pulmonary circuit. Blood that does enter the right ventricle is pumped into the pulmonary artery. However, most

of this blood shunts directly into the systemic circulation through a small vessel, the **ductus arteriosus**, which connects the pulmonary artery to the aorta. A small portion of blood remains in the pulmonary artery and is delivered to the lungs. Blood returns to the placenta through two **umbilical arteries**.

After birth, when the baby's lungs are functioning, these circulatory adaptations begin to close. The foramen ovale seals to become a depression called the fossa ovalis in the septum between the atria. The various vessels constrict into fibrous cords. Only the proximal parts of the umbilical arteries persist as arteries to the urinary bladder. Except for the foramen ovale, the circulatory adaptations close within 30 minutes after birth. The foramen ovale completely closes within one year. Certain congenital heart defects occur when the foramen ovale or ductus arteriosus fails to close.

---

the levels of nutrients in the mother's blood to keep them available for the fetus. This second function leads to an alternate name for this hormone: human chorionic somatomammotropin.

Relaxin is a placental hormone that softens the cervix and relaxes the sacral joints and the pubic symphysis. These changes help to widen the birth canal and aid in delivery.

Checkpoint Questions

2. What organ nourishes the developing fetus?
3. What is the function of the umbilical cord?

Development of the Embryo

The developing offspring is referred to as an embryo for the first 8 weeks of life (Figs. 9-3 and 9-4), and the study of growth during this period is called **embryology** (em-bre-OL-o-je). The beginnings of all body systems are established during this time. The heart and the brain are among the first organs to develop. A primitive nervous system begins to form in the third week. The heart and blood vessels originate during the second week, and the first heartbeat appears during week 4, at the same time that other muscles begin to develop.

By the end of the first month, the embryo is approximately 0.62 cm (0.25 inches) long, with four small swellings at the sides called **limb buds**, which will develop into the four extremities. At this time, the heart produces a prominent bulge at the anterior of the embryo.

By the end of the second month, the embryo takes on an appearance that is recognizably human. In male embryos, the

primitive testes have formed and have begun to secrete testosterone, which will direct formation of the male reproductive organs as gestation continues. Figure 9-3 shows illustrations of embryonic and early fetal development.

Checkpoint Question

4. All body systems originate during the early development of the embryo. At about what time in gestation does the heartbeat first appear?

The Fetus

The term *fetus* is used for the developing offspring from the beginning of the third month until birth. During this period, the organ systems continue to grow and mature. The ovaries form in the female early in this fetal period, and at this stage they contain all the primitive cells (oocytes) that can later develop in mature ova (egg cells).

For study, the entire gestation period may be divided into three equal segments or **trimesters**. The most rapid growth of the fetus occurs during the second trimester (months 4–6). By the end of the fourth month, the fetus is almost 15 cm (6 inches) long, and its external genitalia are sufficiently developed to reveal its sex. By the seventh month, the fetus is usually about 35 cm (14 inches) long and weighs approximately 1.1 kg (2.4 pounds). At the end of pregnancy, the normal length of the fetus is 45 to 56 cm (18–22.5 inches), and the weight varies from 2.7 to 4.5 kg (6–10 pounds).

The **amniotic** (am-ne-OT-ik) **sac,** which is filled with a clear liquid known as **amniotic fluid,** surrounds the fetus

Embryo

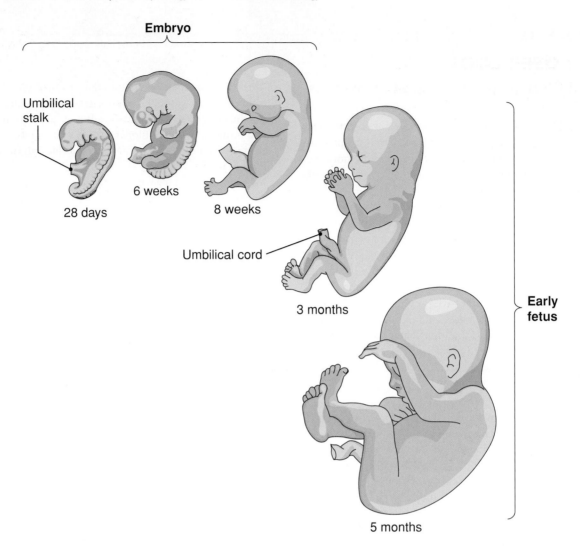

Umbilical
stalk

28 days

6 weeks

8 weeks

Umbilical cord

3 months

**Early
fetus**

5 months

FIGURE 9-3.   Development of an embryo and early fetus.

and serves as a protective cushion for it (Fig. 9-5). The amniotic sac ruptures at birth, an event marked by the common expression that the mother's "water broke."

During development, the fetal skin is protected by a layer of cheeselike material called the **vernix caseosa** (VER-niks ka-se-O-sah) (literally, "cheesy varnish").

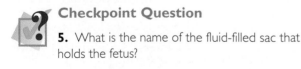

Checkpoint Question

5. What is the name of the fluid-filled sac that holds the fetus?

The Mother

The total period of pregnancy, from fertilization of the ovum to birth, is approximately 266 days, also given as 280 days or 40 weeks from the last menstrual period (LMP). During this time, the mother must supply all the food and oxygen for the fetus and eliminate its waste materials. To support the additional demands of the growing fetus, the mother's metabolism changes markedly, and several organ systems increase their output:

- the heart pumps more blood to supply the needs of the uterus and the fetus
- the lungs provide more oxygen by increasing the rate and depth of respiration
- the kidneys excrete nitrogenous wastes from both the fetus and the mother
- the digestive system supplies additional nutrients for the growth of maternal organs (uterus and breasts) and growth of the fetus, as well as for subsequent labor and milk secretion.

Nausea and vomiting are common discomforts in early pregnancy. These most often occur upon arising or during periods of fatigue, and are more common in women who smoke cigarettes. The specific cause of these symptoms is not known, but they may be a result of the great changes in hormone levels that occur at this time. The nausea and vomiting usually last for only a few weeks to several months.

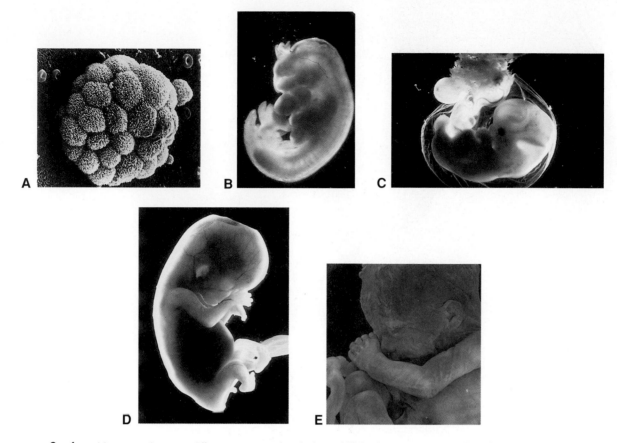

FIGURE 9-4. Human embryos at different stages and early fetus. **(A)** Implantation in uterus 7 to 8 days after conception. **(B)** Embryo at 32 days. **(C)** At 37 days. **(D)** At 41 days. **(E)** Fetus between 12 and 15 weeks. (Reprinted with permission from Pillitteri A. Maternal and Child Health Nursing. 4th ed. Philadelphia: Lippincott Williams & Wilkins, 2003.)

Urinary frequency and constipation are often present during the early stages of pregnancy and then usually disappear. They may reappear late in pregnancy as the head of the fetus drops from the abdominal region down into the pelvis, pressing on the rectum and the urinary bladder.

 Checkpoint Question

6. What is the approximate duration of pregnancy in days?

The Use of Ultrasound in Obstetrics

Ultrasonography (ul-trah-son-OG-rah-fe) is a safe, painless, and noninvasive method for studying soft tissue. It has proved extremely valuable for monitoring pregnancies and deliveries.

An ultrasound image, called a *sonogram,* is made by sending high-frequency sound waves into the body (Fig. 9-6). Each time a wave meets an interface between two tissues of different densities, an echo is produced. An instrument called a *transducer* converts the reflected sound waves into electrical energy, and a computer is used to generate an image on a viewing screen.

Ultrasound scans can be used in obstetrics to diagnose pregnancy, judge fetal age, and determine the location of the placenta. The technique can also show the presence of excess amniotic fluid and fetal abnormalities.

CHILDBIRTH

The exact mechanisms that trigger the beginning of uterine contractions for childbirth are still not completely known. Some fetal and maternal factors that probably work in combination to start labor are:

- stretching of the uterine muscle stimulates production of prostaglandin, which promotes uterine contractions
- pressure on the cervix from the baby stimulates release of **oxytocin** (ok-se-TO-sin) from the posterior pituitary. The uterine muscle becomes increasingly sensitive to this hormone late in pregnancy
- changes in the placenta that occur with time may contribute to the start of labor
- cortisol from the fetal adrenal cortex inhibits the mother's progesterone. Increase in the relative amount of estrogen as compared to progesterone stimulates uterine contractions.

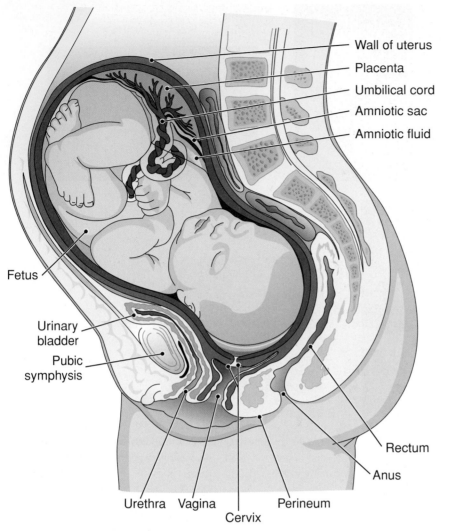

Fetus

Urinary bladder

Pubic symphysis

Urethra   Vagina

Cervix

Perineum

Rectum

Anus

Wall of uterus

Placenta

Umbilical cord

Amniotic sac

Amniotic fluid

FIGURE 9-5. Midsagittal section of a pregnant uterus with intact fetus. *ZOOM-ING IN—What structure connects the fetus to the placenta?*

After labor begins, stimuli from the cervix and vagina produce reflex secretion of oxytocin, which in turn increases the uterine contractions (an example of positive feedback).

The Four Stages of Labor

The process by which the fetus is expelled from the uterus is known as **labor** and **delivery**; it also may be called **parturition** (par-tu-RISH-un). It is divided into four stages:

1. The **first stage** begins with the onset of regular uterine contractions. With each contraction, the cervix becomes thinner and the opening larger. Rupture of the amniotic sac may occur at any time, with a gush of fluid from the vagina.
2. The **second stage** begins when the cervix is completely dilated and ends with the delivery of the baby. This stage involves the passage of the fetus, usually head first, through the cervical canal and the vagina to the outside.
3. The **third stage** begins after the child is born and ends with the expulsion of the **afterbirth**. The afterbirth includes the placenta, the membranes of the amniotic sac, and the umbilical cord, except for a small portion remaining attached to the baby's **umbilicus** (um-BIL-ih-kus), or navel.
4. The **fourth stage** begins after expulsion of the afterbirth and constitutes a period in which bleeding is controlled. Contraction of the uterine muscle acts to close off the blood vessels leading to the placental site. To prevent tissues of the pelvic floor from being torn during childbirth, as often happens, the obstetrician may cut the mother's perineum just before her infant is born and then repair this clean cut immediately after childbirth; such an operation is called an **episiotomy** (eh-piz-e-OT-o-me). The area between the vagina and the anus that is cut in an episiotomy is referred to as the *surgical* or *obstetrical perineum.*

 Checkpoint Question

7. What is parturition?

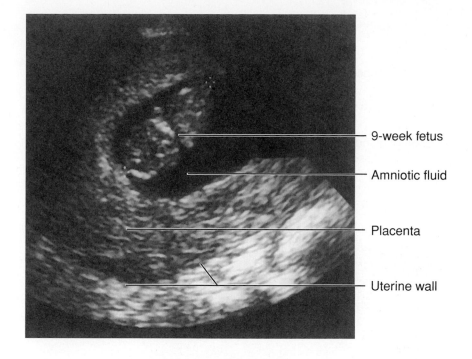

9-week fetus

Amniotic fluid

Placenta

Uterine wall

FIGURE 9-6. Sonogram showing a 9-week-old fetus. (Reprinted with permission from Erkonen WE. Radiology 101: Basics and Fundamentals of Imaging. Philadelphia: Lippincott Williams & Wilkins, 1998.)

Cesarean Section

A **cesarean** (se-ZAR-re-an) **section** (C section) is an incision made in the abdominal wall and in the uterine wall for delivery of a fetus. A cesarean section may be required for a variety of reasons, including placental abnormalities, abnormal fetal position, disproportion between the head of the fetus and the mother's pelvis that makes vaginal delivery difficult or dangerous, and other problems that may arise during pregnancy and delivery.

 Checkpoint Question

8. What is a cesarean section?

Multiple Births

Until recently, statistics indicated that twins occurred in about 1 of every 80 to 90 births, varying somewhat in different countries. Triplets occurred much less frequently, usually once in several thousand births, whereas quadruplets occurred very rarely. The birth of quintuplets represented a historic event unless the mother had taken fertility drugs. Now these fertility drugs, usually gonadotropins, are given more commonly, and the number of multiple births has increased significantly. Multiple fetuses tend to be born prematurely and therefore have a high death rate. However, better care of infants and newer treatments have resulted in more living multiple births than ever.

Twins originate in two different ways, and on this basis are divided into two types:

- **Fraternal twins** are formed as a result of the fertilization of two different ova by two spermatozoa. Two completely different individuals, as distinct from each other

as brothers and sisters of different ages, are produced. Each fetus has its own placenta and surrounding sac.
- **Identical twins** develop from a single zygote formed from a single ovum fertilized by a single spermatozoon. Sometime during the early stages of development, the embryonic cells separate into two units. Usually, there is a single placenta, although there must be a separate umbilical cord for each fetus. Identical twins are always the same sex and carry the same inherited traits.

Other multiple births may be fraternal, identical, or combinations of these. The tendency to multiple births seems to be hereditary.

Termination of Pregnancy

A pregnancy may end before its full term has been completed. The term **live birth** is used if the baby breathes or shows any evidence of life such as heartbeat, pulsation of the umbilical cord, or movement of voluntary muscles. An **immature** or **premature** infant is one born before the organ systems are mature. Infants born before the 37th week of gestation or weighing less than 2500 grams (5.5 pounds) are considered **preterm**.

Loss of the fetus is classified according to the duration of the pregnancy:

- the term **abortion** refers to loss of the embryo or fetus before the 20th week or weight of about 500 grams (1.1 pound). This loss can be either spontaneous or induced
  - **spontaneous abortion** occurs naturally with no interference. The most common causes are related to an abnormality of the embryo or fetus. Other causes include abnormality of the mother's reproductive organs, infections, or chronic disorders, such as kidney

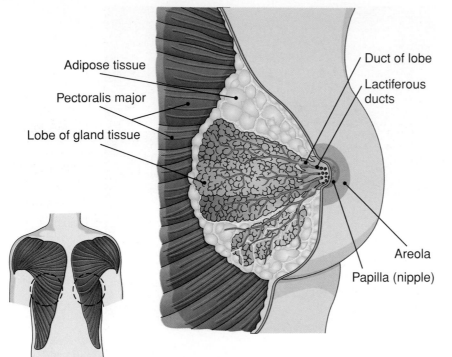

Adipose tissue

Pectoralis major

Lobe of gland tissue

Duct of lobe

Lactiferous
ducts

Areola

Papilla (nipple)

FIGURE 9-7.   Section of the breast (mammary gland).   *ZOOMING IN—What muscle underlies the breast?*

disease or hypertension. **Miscarriage** is the lay term for spontaneous abortion

- **induced abortion** occurs as a result of artificial or mechanical interruption of pregnancy. A **therapeutic abortion** is an abortion performed by a physician as a treatment for a variety of reasons. More liberal access to this type of abortion has dramatically reduced the incidence of death related to illegal abortion
- the term **fetal death** refers to loss of the fetus after the eighth week of pregnancy. **Stillbirth** refers to the delivery of an infant who is lifeless.

Immaturity is a leading cause of death in the newborn. After the 20th week of pregnancy, the fetus is considered **viable**, that is, able to live outside the uterus. A fetus expelled before the 24th week or before reaching a weight of 1000 grams (2.2 pounds) has little more than a 50% chance of survival. One born at a point closer to the full 40 weeks stands a much better chance of living. Increasing numbers of immature infants are being saved because of advances in neonatal intensive care.

Checkpoint Question

9. What does the term *viable* mean with reference to a fetus?

THE MAMMARY GLANDS AND LACTATION

The **mammary glands**, or breasts, of the female are accessories of the reproductive system. They provide nourishment for the baby after its birth. The mammary glands are similar in construction to the sweat glands. Each gland is divided into a number of lobes composed of glandular tissue and fat, and each lobe is further subdivided. Secretions from the lobes are conveyed through **lactiferous** (lak-TIF-er-us) **ducts,** all of which converge at the papilla (nipple) (Fig. 9-7).

The mammary glands begin developing during puberty, but they do not become functional until the end of a pregnancy. Placental lactogen (hPL) helps to prepare the breasts for lactation, and the hormone **prolactin (PRL)**, produced by the anterior pituitary gland, stimulates the secretory cells of the mammary glands. The first mammary gland secretion is a thin liquid called **colostrum** (ko-LOS-trum). It is nutritious but has a somewhat different composition from milk. Milk secretion begins within a few days following birth and can continue for several years as long as milk is frequently removed by the suckling baby or by pumping. Stimulation of the breast by the suckling infant causes oxytocin release from the posterior pituitary. This hormone causes the milk ducts to contract, resulting in the ejection, or *letdown*, of milk.

The digestive tract of the newborn baby is not ready for the usual adult mixed diet. Mother's milk is more desirable for the young infant than milk from other animals for several reasons, some of which are listed below:

- infections that may be transmitted by foods exposed to the outside air are avoided by nursing
- both breast milk and colostrum contain maternal antibodies that help protect the baby against pathogens
- the proportions of various nutrients and other substances in human milk are perfectly suited to the human infant. Substitutes are not exact imitations of human milk. Nutrients are present in more desirable amounts if the mother's diet is well balanced

Box 9-3

HOT TOPICS

The Human Genome Project: Reading the Book of Life

Packed tightly in nearly every one of your body cells (except the red blood cells) is a complete copy of your genome—the genetic instructions that direct all of your cellular activities. Written in the language of DNA, these instructions consist of genes parceled into 46 chromosomes that code for proteins. In 1990, a consortium of scientists from around the world set out to crack the genetic code and read the human genome, our "book of life." This monumental task, called the Human Genome Project, was completed in 2003 and succeeded in mapping the entire human genome—3 billion DNA base pairs arranged into about 30,000 genes. Now, scientists can pinpoint the exact location and chemical code of every gene in the body.

The human genome was decoded using a technique called sequencing. Samples of human DNA were fragmented into smaller pieces and then inserted into bacteria. As the bacteria multiplied, they produced more and more copies of the human DNA fragments, which the scientists extracted. The DNA copies were loaded into a sequencing machine capable of "reading" the string of DNA nucleotides that composed each fragment. Then, using computers, the scientists put all of the sequences from the fragments back together to get the entire human genome.

Now, scientists hope to use all these pages of the book of life to revolutionize the treatment of human disease. The information obtained from the Human Genome Project may lead to improved disease diagnosis, new drug treatments, and even gene therapy.

- the psychological and emotional benefits of nursing are of infinite value to both the mother and the infant.

Checkpoint Question

10. What is lactation?

HEREDITY

We are often struck by the resemblance of a baby to one or both of its parents, yet rarely do we stop to consider *how* various traits are transmitted from parents to offspring. This subject—heredity—has fascinated humans for thousands of years. The *Old Testament* contains numerous references to heredity (although, of course, the word was unknown in biblical times). It was not until the 19th century, however, that methodical investigation into heredity was begun. At that time, an Austrian monk, Gregor Mendel, discovered through his experiments with garden peas that there was a precise pattern in the appearance of differences among parents and their **progeny** (PROJ-eh-ne), their offspring or descendents. Mendel's most important contribution to the understanding of heredity was the demonstration that there are independent units of heredity in the cells. Later, these independent units were given the name **genes**.

Genes and Chromosomes

Genes are actually segments of DNA (deoxyribonucleic acid) contained in the threadlike **chromosomes** within the nucleus of each cell. Genes govern the cell by controlling the manufacture of proteins, especially enzymes, which are necessary for all the chemical reactions that occur within the cell. Other proteins regulated by genes are those used for structural materials, hormones, and growth factors.

When body cells divide by the process of mitosis, the DNA that makes up the chromosomes is duplicated and distributed to the daughter cells, so that each daughter cell gets exactly the same kind and number of chromosomes as were in the original cell. Each chromosome (aside from the Y chromosome, which determines sex) may carry thousands of genes, and each gene carries the code for a specific trait (characteristic). These traits constitute the physical, biochemical, and physiologic makeup of every cell in the body. (See Box 9-3 to learn about the Human Genome Project.)

In humans, every cell except the gametes (sex cells) contains 46 chromosomes. The chromosomes exist in pairs. One member of each pair was received at the time of fertilization from the offspring's father, and one was received from the mother. The paired chromosomes, except for the pair that determines sex, are alike in size and appearance. Thus, each body cell has one pair of sex chromosomes and 22 pairs (44 chromosomes) that are not involved in sex determination and are known as **autosomes** (AW-to-somes).

The paired autosomes carry genes for the same traits at exactly the same sites on each. The genes for each trait thus exist in pairs; each member of the gene pair that controls a given trait is known as an **allele** (al-LELE).

Checkpoint Question

11. What is a gene and what is a gene made of?

Dominant and Recessive Genes

Another of Mendel's discoveries was that genes can be either dominant or recessive. A **dominant** gene is one that expresses its effect in the cell regardless of whether its allele on the matching chromosome is the same as or different from the dominant gene. The gene must be received from only one parent to be expressed in the offspring. When the matching genes for a trait are different, the alleles are described as **heterozygous** (het-er-o-ZI-gus), or hybrid.

The effect of a **recessive** gene is not evident unless its paired allele on the matching chromosome is also recessive. Thus, a recessive trait appears only if the recessive genes for that trait are received from both parents. For example, the gene for brown eyes is dominant over the gene for blue eyes, which is recessive. Blue eyes appear in the offspring only if genes for blue eyes are received from both parents. When both the genes for a trait are the same, that is, both dominant or both recessive, the alleles are said to be **homozygous** (ho-mo-ZI-gus), or pure-bred. A recessive trait only appears if a person's genes are homozygous for that trait.

Any characteristic that can be observed or can be tested for is part of a person's **phenotype** (FE-no-tipe). Eye color, for example, can be seen when looking at a person. Blood type is not visible but can be determined by testing and is also a part of a person's phenotype. When someone has the recessive phenotype, his or her genetic make-up, or **genotype** (JEN-o-tipe), is obviously homozygous recessive. When a dominant phenotype appears, the person's genotype can be either homozygous dominant or heterozygous. Only genetic studies or family studies can reveal which it is.

A recessive gene is not expressed if it is present in the cell together with a dominant allele. However, the recessive gene can be passed on to offspring and may thus appear in future generations. An individual who shows no evidence of a trait but has a recessive gene for that trait is described as a **carrier** of the gene. Using genetic terminology, that person shows the dominant phenotype but has a heterozygous genotype for that trait.

Checkpoint Question

12. What is the difference between a dominant and a recessive gene?

Distribution of Chromosomes to Offspring

The reproductive cells (ova and spermatozoa) are produced by a special process of cell division called **meiosis** (mi-O-sis). This process divides the chromosome number in half, so that each reproductive cell has 23 chromosomes. Moreover, the division occurs in such a way that each cell receives one member of each chromosome pair that was present in the original cell. The separation occurs at random, meaning that either member of the original pair may be included in a given germ cell. Thus, the maternal and paternal sets of chromosomes get mixed up and redistributed at this time, leading to increased variety within the population. Children in a family resemble each other, but no two look exactly alike (unless

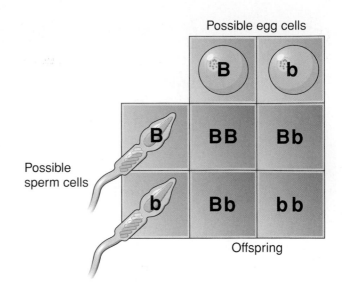

FIGURE 9-8. A Punnett square. Geneticists use this grid to show all the possible combinations of a given cross. *ZOOMING IN—What percentage of children will show the recessive phenotype blond hair?*

they are identical twins), because they receive different combinations of maternal and paternal chromosomes.

Geneticists use a grid called a **Punnett square** to show all the combinations of genes that can result from a given parental cross (Fig. 9-8). In these calculations, a capital letter is used for the dominant gene and the recessive gene is represented by the lower case of the same letter. For example, if B is the gene for the dominant trait brown eyes, then b would be the recessive gene for blue eyes. In the offspring, the genotype BB is homozygous dominant and the genotype Bb is heterozygous, both of which will show the dominant phenotype brown eyes. The homozygous recessive genotype bb will show the recessive phenotype blue eyes.

A Punnett square shows all the possible gene combinations of a given cross and the theoretical ratios of all the genotypes produced. Actual ratios may differ if the number of offspring is small. For example, the chances of having a male or female baby are 50-50 with each birth, but a family might have several girls before having a boy, and vice versa. The chances of seeing the theoretical ratios improve as the number of offspring increases.

Checkpoint Question

13. What is the process of cell division that forms the gametes?

Sex Determination

The two chromosomes that determine the offspring's sex, unlike the autosomes (the other 22 pairs of chromosomes), are not matched in size and appearance. The female X chromosome is larger than most other chromosomes and carries

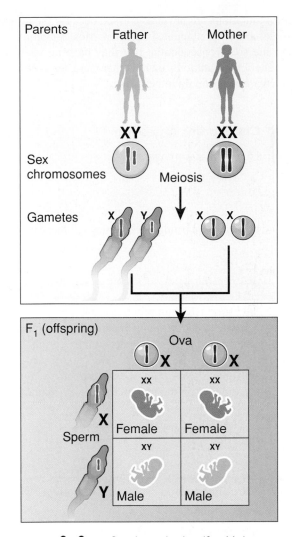

FIGURE 9-9. Sex determination. If an X chromosome from a male unites with an X chromosome from a female, the child is female (XX); if a Y chromosome from a male unites with an X chromosome from a female, the child is male (XY).

genes for other characteristics in addition to that for sex. The male Y chromosome is smaller than other chromosomes and mainly determines sex. A female has two X chromosomes in each body cell; a male has one X and one Y.

By the process of meiosis, each male sperm cell receives either an X or a Y chromosome, whereas every egg cell receives only an X chromosome (Fig. 9-9). If a sperm cell with an X chromosome fertilizes an ovum, the resulting infant will be female; if a sperm with a Y chromosome fertilizes an ovum, the resulting infant will be male (see Fig. 9-9).

Sex-Linked Traits

Any trait that is carried on a sex chromosome is said to be **sex-linked**. Because the Y chromosome carries few traits aside from sex determination, most sex-linked traits are carried on the X chromosome and are best described as

X-linked. Examples are hemophilia, certain forms of baldness, and red-green color blindness.

Sex-linked traits appear almost exclusively in males. The reason for this is that most of these traits are recessive, and if a recessive gene is located on the X chromosome in a male it cannot be masked by a matching dominant gene. (Remember that the Y chromosome with which the X chromosome pairs is very small and carries few genes.) Thus, a male who has only one recessive gene for a trait will exhibit that characteristic, whereas a female must have two recessive genes to show the trait. The female must inherit a recessive gene for that trait from each parent and be homozygous recessive in order for the trait to appear.

Checkpoint Questions

14. What sex chromosome combination determines a female? A male?

15. What term is used to describe a trait carried on a sex chromosome?

HEREDITARY TRAITS

Some observable hereditary traits are skin, eye, and hair color and facial features. Also influenced by genetics are less clearly defined traits, such as weight, body build, life span, and susceptibility to disease.

Some human traits, including the traits involved in many genetic diseases, are determined by a single pair of genes; most, however, are the result of two or more gene pairs acting together in what is termed **multifactorial inheritance**. This type of inheritance accounts for the wide range of variations within populations in such characteristics as coloration, height, and weight, all of which are determined by more than one pair of genes.

Gene Expression

The effect of a gene on a person's phenotype may be influenced by a variety of factors, including the individual's sex and the presence of other genes. For example, the genes for certain types of baldness and certain types of color blindness may be inherited by either males or females, but the traits appear mostly in males under the effects of male sex hormone.

Environment also plays a part in gene expression. One inherits a potential for a given size, for example, but one's actual size is additionally influenced by such factors as nutrition, development, and general state of health. The same is true of life span and susceptibility to diseases.

Genetic Mutation

As a rule, chromosomes replicate exactly during cell division. Occasionally, however, for reasons not yet totally understood, the genes or chromosomes change. This change may involve a single gene or whole chromosomes. Alternatively, it may consist of chromosomal breakage, in which there is loss or rearrangement of gene fragments. Often these changes occur during cell division (mitosis or meiosis) as chromosomes come together, re-assort, and get distributed to two new cells. Such changes are termed genetic **mutations**. Mutations may occur spontaneously or may be induced by some agent, such as ionizing radiation or chemicals, described as a **mutagen** (MU-tah-jen) or mutagenic agent.

If a mutation occurs in an ovum or a sperm cell, the altered trait will be inherited by the offspring. The vast majority of harmful mutations are never expressed because the affected fetus dies and is spontaneously aborted. Most remaining mutations are so inconsequential that they have no visible effect. Beneficial mutations, on the other hand, tend to survive and increase as a population evolves.

Checkpoint Question

16. What is a mutation?

Word Anatomy

Medical terms are built from standardized word parts (prefixes, roots, and suffixes). Learning the meanings of these parts can help you remember words and interpret unfamiliar terms.

Word part	Meaning	Example
Pregnancy		
zyg/o	joined	An ovum and spermatozoon join to form a *zygote*.
chori/o	membrane, chorion	Human *chorionic* gonadotropin is produced by the outermost cells (chorion) of the embryo and acts on the corpus luteum in the ovary.
somat/o	body	Human chorionic *somatomammotropin* controls nutrients for the body and acts on the mammary glands (mamm/o).
Childbirth		
ox/y	sharp, acute	*Oxytocin* is a hormone that stimulates labor.
toc/o	labor	See preceding example.
Genes and Chromosomes		
chrom/o	color	*Chromosomes* color darkly with stains.
aut/o-	self	*Autosomes* are all the chromosomes aside from the two that determine sex.
heter/o	other, different	*Heterozygous* paired genes (alleles) are different from each other.
homo-	same	*Homozygous* paired genes (alleles) are the same.
phen/o	to show	Traits that can be observed or tested for make a up a person's *phenotype*.
Hereditary Traits		
multi-	many	*Multifactorial* traits are determined by multiple pairs of genes.

Summary

I. Pregnancy (gestation)—lasts about 38 weeks
  A. Fertilization and the start of pregnancy
    1. Fertilization occurs in oviduct
    2. Zygote (fertilized egg)—formed by fusion of egg and sperm nuclei
      a. Divides rapidly
      b. Travels to uterus
      c. Implants in lining and becomes embryo
  B. The placenta
    1. Formed by tissue around embryo and in lining of uterus
    2. Functions
      a. Nourishment
      b. Gas exchange
      c. Removal of waste
      d. Production of hormones
        (1) Human chorionic gonadotropin (hCG)—maintains corpus luteum for 11–12 weeks
        (2) Human placental lactogen (hPL)
        (3) Relaxin—relaxes birth canal
    3. Umbilical cord—connects fetus to placenta
  C. Development of the embryo
    1. First 8 weeks
    2. All body systems begin to develop
  D. The fetus
    1. Third month to birth
    2. Amniotic sac

a. Surrounds fetus

b. Contains fluid to cushion and protect fetus

E. The mother

1. Increased demands on heart, lungs, kidneys

2. Increased nutritional needs

3. Ultrasound used to monitor pregnancy and delivery

II. Childbirth—initiated by changes in uterus, placenta, fetus

A. Four stages of labor

1. Contractions

2. Delivery of baby

3. Expulsion of afterbirth

4. Contraction of uterus

B. Cesarean section

1. Incision to remove fetus

C. Multiple births

1. Fraternal twins formed from two different ova

2. Identical twins develop from a single zygote

3. Larger multiples follow either pattern or a combination

4. Increased by fertility drugs

D. Termination of pregnancy

1. Immature (premature) infant—born before organ system mature

2. Preterm—born before 37th week or weighing less than 2500 grams

3. Abortion—loss of fetus before 20th week or weighing less than 500 grams

4. Fetal death—loss of fetus after 8 weeks of pregnancy

III. Mammary glands and lactation

1. Lactation—secretion of milk

a. Colostrum—first mammary secretion

2. Hormones

a. HPL—prepares prepares breasts for lactation

b. Prolactin—stimulates secretory cells

c. Oxytocin—promotes letdown (ejection) of milk

3. Advantages of breastfeeding

a. Reduces infections

b. Transfers antibodies

c. Provides best form of nutrition

d. Emotional satisfaction

IV. Heredity

A. Genes and chromosomes

1. Genes

a. Hereditary units

b. Segments of DNA

c. Control manufacture of proteins (*e.g.*, enzymes, hormones)

2. Chromosomes

a. Threadlike bodies in nucleus; 46 in humans

b. Composed of genes

c. 22 pairs autosomes (non-sex chromosomes)

d. 1 pair sex chromosomes

B. Dominant and recessive genes

1. Dominant gene—always expressed

a. May be heterozygous (two genes different)

b. May be homozygous dominant (two genes the same)

2. Recessive gene—expressed only if homozygous recessive (received from both parents)

a. Carrier—person with recessive gene that is not apparent but can be passed to offspring

b. Phenotype—characteristic that can be seen or tested for

c. Genotype—genetic make-up

C. Distribution of chromosomes to offspring

1. Meiosis

a. Cell division that forms sex cells with 23 chromosomes

b. Each cell receives one of each chromosome pair

c. Punnett square shows results of crosses

D. Sex determination

1. X chromosome larger and carries other traits

2. Y smaller and carries mainly gene for sex determination

3. Female cells have XX; male cells have XY

E. Sex-linked traits

1. Traits carried on sex chromosome (usually X)

2. Sex-linked traits appear mostly in males

a. Passed from mother to son on X chromosome

b. If recessive, not masked by dominant gene on Y

c. Examples—hemophilia, baldness, red-green color blindness

V. Hereditary traits

1. Genes determine physical, biochemical, and physiological characteristics of every cell

2. Some traits determined by single gene pairs

3. Most determined by multifactorial inheritance

a. Involves multiple gene pairs

b. Produces a range of variations in a population

c. Examples—height, weight, coloration, susceptibility to disease

A. Gene expression

1. Factors

a. Sex

b. Presence of other genes

c. Environment

B. Genetic mutation

1. Change in genes or chromosomes

2. May be passed to offspring if occurs in germ cells

3. Mutagenic agents

a. Factors causing mutation

b. Examples—ionizing radiation, chemicals

Questions for Study and Review

Building Understanding

Fill in the blanks

1. Fetal skin is protected by a cheeselike material called _____.
2. The first mammary secretion is called _____.
3. Sound waves can be used to safely monitor pregnancy with a technique called _____.
4. The basic unit of heredity is a(n) _____.
5. Chromosomes not involved in sex determination are known as _____.

Matching

Match each numbered item with the most closely related lettered item.

___ 6. A placental hormone that stimulates the ovaries to secrete progesterone and estrogen

    a. human placental lactogen

___ 7. A placental hormone that regulates maternal blood nutrient levels

    b. prolactin

___ 8. A placental hormone that softens the cervix, which widens the birth canal

    c. oxytocin

___ 9. A pituitary hormone that stimulates uterine contractions

    d. relaxin

___ 10. A pituitary hormone that stimulates maternal milk production

    e. human chorionic gonadotropin

Multiple choice

___ 11. For a few days after implantation, the embryo is nourished by the
  a. endometrium
  b. placenta
  c. yolk sac
  d. umbilical cord

___ 12. The total period of pregnancy, from fertilization to birth, is about
  a. 240 days
  b. 260 days
  c. 280 days
  d. 300 days

___ 13. With regard to identical twins, which of the following statements is incorrect?
  a. they develop from a single zygote
  b. they each have their own placenta
  c. they are always the same sex
  d. they carry the same inherited traits

___ 14. Genes govern the cell by controlling the manufacture of
  a. carbohydrates
  b. lipids
  c. proteins
  d. electrolytes

___ 15. Paired genes for a given trait are known as
  a. chromosomes
  b. ribosomes
  c. nucleotides
  d. alleles

Understanding Concepts

16. Distinguish among the following: *zygote*, *embryo*, and *fetus*.
17. Explain the role of the placenta in fetal development.
18. Is blood in the umbilical arteries relatively high or low in oxygen? In the umbilical vein?
19. What is the major event of each of the four stages of parturition?
20. List several reasons why breast milk is best for baby.
21. How many chromosomes are there in a human body cell? In a human gamete?
22. Dana has one dominant allele for brown eyes (B) and one recessive allele for blue eyes. What is Dana's genotype? What is her phenotype?
23. Describe the process of meiosis and explain how it results in genetic variation.

Conceptual Thinking

24. If mitosis were used to produce gametes, what consequences would this have on the offspring's genotype, phenotype, and chromosome number?
25. Jason and Nicole are expecting their first child and are wondering what their child's eye color might be. Jason has blue eyes (a recessive trait) and Nicole has brown eyes (a dominant trait). Both of Jason's parents have blue eyes. One of Nicole's parents has brown eyes, the other has blue eyes. What are Jason's and Nicole's genotype and phenotype? What are the possible genotypes and phenotypes of their children?

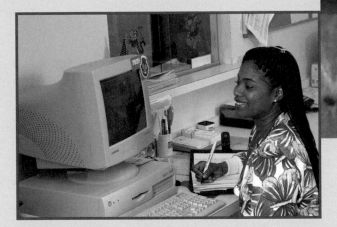

Human Behavior and Communication

10

Personality and Development

CHAPTER OBJECTIVES

In this chapter, you'll learn:

1. To define the concept of the personality.
2. To describe the forces that shape personality development.
3. To define what is meant by temperament.
4. To discuss the basic relationship between behavior and the personality.
5. To identify the basic concepts of the various theories of personality development.
6. To explain the relationship between cognitive and moral development.

KEY TERMS

accommodation
assimilation
behaviorism
concrete mental
  operations
conscious

defense mechanisms
ego
equilibration
formal operations
hierarchy
interpersonal

personality traits
postconventional
preconscious
preconventional
preoperational
psychosocial

reinforcement
secondary traits
sensorimotor
superego
temperament
unconscious

PERSONALITY DEVELOPMENT

Personality traits are defined as lasting patterns of perceiving, relating to, and thinking about the environment and oneself that are demonstrated in our social and personal interrelationships. Integrated into this personal portfolio are established characteristics and consistent behavioral responses that are unique to each person. This explains why everyone does not act the same in similar situations. **Central traits** are those general prominent features that are most often descriptive of the person, some of which are seen in all the behavior patterns. **Secondary traits** are those that may surface in some circumstances, such as in an anger-provoking situation.

From the moment of conception, our development is influenced by forces that ultimately shape the way in which we respond to the world around us. A person's natural tendencies are the result of a combined genetic transmission of personality traits from both parents. A unique blend of multigenerational family patterns is inherited through this genetic factor. There are also many societal and environmental forces that influence personality. Patterns of behavior are formed as one responds to the awareness and perception of the self as autonomous and capable of individual control. Abraham Maslow, a humanistic psychologist, theorized that one acts in response to a perceived internal or external force determined by certain needs that are unchanging and innate in origin. He defined these needs as a **hierarchy** in which some needs are more basic or more powerful than others, and as these needs are satisfied, we can move upward to meet other higher needs. It was his opinion that we cannot move to a higher level need unless the previous level of needs is satisfied. He believed that we have the unique ability to make conscious choices to seek certain things that provide value or meaning, which results in a personal identity. Life experiences may cause us to vacillate between levels and disrupt personal growth toward self-fulfillment.

JUST THE FACTS

Abraham Maslow—Hierarchy of Needs

- Basic physiologic needs
- Comfort and safety, stability and security
- Love and belonging, relationships
- Self-esteem, self-respect, competence
- Self-actualization, growth, and fulfillment

Humanistic theories view the developing person as a whole, a totality of the physical, emotional, spiritual, intellectual, and social aspects of life that influence us toward reaching our potential.

William Glasser, the founder of Reality Therapy and Control Theory, described four basic psychologic needs that determine our behavioral response in any given situation. He identified these as the need for love and belonging, power, freedom, and fun, which we must satisfy continually. The need to love and belong is internal, a hunger or void that may be filled by other people, pets, or even inanimate objects. Our drive for power often conflicts with our need for love as we seek to exert control over our world. Glasser asserts that we desire the freedom to exert this control over our lives and that when this drive is hampered, we respond or behave to regain the power that provides a psychologic homeostasis. He also theorizes that a measure of fun and playtime evens out the personality. In an effort to meet these needs, Dr. Glasser advocates that we have a choice regarding how to behave. From the moment of birth, we accumulate mental pictures from our experiences with the environment. This photo album provides the basis for our choices to behave in response to a given situation. Our behavior is a constant attempt to decrease the incongruence between what we want (pictures in our head) and what we have (our perception of the situation). Glasser asserted that we deny the reality of a situation instead of meeting our needs in a way that is responsible and within the boundaries of social norms and morality. He found that mental health is improved when we learn to meet our needs with responsible choices.

JUST THE FACTS

William Glasser—Reality Therapy and Control Theory

- Love and belonging
- Power and control
- Freedom and choice
- Fun and relaxation

We might ask why one person would respond to a situation with anger but diffuse it quickly, while another may show a milder emotional reaction and others no reaction at all. Variances in character, including intensity and extent of feeling such as these are ones of **temperament,** which influences the development of personality and our interpersonal relationships. Studies describe three types of temperament in babies. *Easy* babies, who comprise the largest group, are seen as playful and adaptable. In contrast, a smaller number of babies are seen as *difficult* or irritable and unable to adapt well. A third group of *slow-to-warm-up* babies shows lower activity levels and slower adaptation to any new situation. The child develops in an environment that grows increasingly more complex as the basic family unit expands to include the influence of society and the culture of their world. The change and growth in personality have been the focus of much research from which theories have been developed to provide a basis for understanding of this process.

JUST THE FACTS

Temperament

- Easy—playful and adaptable
- Difficult—irritable and unable to adapt well
- Slow-to-warm-up—slower adaptation

MEMORY JOGGER

What adult behaviors might reflect a difficult temperament? A slow-to-warm-up?

THEORIES OF PERSONALITY DEVELOPMENT

Have you ever wondered why you think and behave in the way you do? This very issue leads to an integral concept in the study of psychology. Sigmund Freud was the first of many who studied and developed theories about the human mind and behavioral response to environmental forces. These theories are the foundation of therapeutic approaches to the treatment of mental illness.

Sigmund Freud (Psychoanalytic Theory)

Freud proposed that the psyche is made up of three components: the **conscious** or present awareness; the **preconscious** or that which is below current awareness but easily retrieved; and the unconscious; which he cites as the largest body of material. The **unconscious** includes past experiences and the related emotions that have been completely removed from the conscious level. This level is largely responsible for contributing to the emotional discomfort and disturbances that threaten us. Freudian theory also divides personality formation into three parts (see Fig. 10-1). The id, which operates on the pleasure principle and demands instant gratification of drives, is present at birth and contains the instincts, impulses, and urges for survival. These drives include hunger, aggression, sex, protection, and warmth. The **ego** begins to develop during the first 6 to 8 months and is fairly well developed by

2 years of age. This is the conscious self, which develops in response to the wishes and demands of the id that require appropriate exchanges with the environment. It is here that sensations, feelings, adjustments, solutions, and defenses are formed. The **superego,** often referred to as the conscience, starts developing at about 3 to 4 years of age and is fairly well developed by the age of 10 to 11 years. It controls, inhibits, and regulates those impulses and instinctive urges whose unrestricted expression would be socially unacceptable. The values and moral standards of parents are incorporated into this control along with the norms and moral codes of the society in which one lives and grows. The superego operates at both the conscious and unconscious levels, decides right from wrong, and offers both critical self-evaluation and self-praise. The ego is the peacemaker and balance between the instinctual drives and societal demands.

EXAMPLE

Id—I want a piece of chocolate cake.
Superego—There are too many calories in that cake.
Ego—Be satisfied with a small piece.

The constant need for the ego to intercept the conflicts between the id and superego that are created in response to environmental stressors leads to increased anxiety. This anxiety creates a dilemma in which stability is needed to preserve our sense of self. Freud theorized that for the ego to remain in control, automatic psychologic processes called **defense mechanisms** are mobilized to protect us from anxiety and the awareness of internal or external stressors (see Box 10-1 on the next page.) Most of these mechanisms are mobilized at the unconscious level. High levels of anxiety can disturb perception and performance, which compromises the ability to problem solve and learn. These unconscious defense tools provide us with protection from unacceptable thoughts and

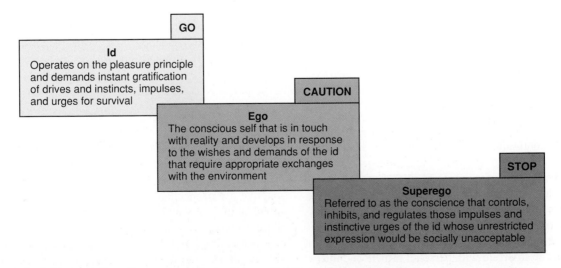

FIGURE 10-1. Freud's psychoanalytic theory: divisions of the personality.

Box 10-1

EGO DEFENSE MECHANISMS — FREUD

Mechanism	Description
Sublimation	Replacing a socially unacceptable behavior with one that is acceptable. Primitive impulses are not acceptable to the ego and are rechanneled into a constructive outlet. (Aggressive desire to attack another person is rechanneled into a sport activity such as football.)
Denial	Consciously rejecting reality or refusing to recognize facts of a situation. Ego refuses to see the truth because it causes severe mental pain. (Wife whose husband dies continues to set the table for two as if he will be present for dinner.)
Displacement	Transferring hostility or other strong feelings from the original cause of the feelings to another person or object. (Person who has a confrontation at his place of employment goes home and argues with his family.)
Fantasy	Consciously distorting unconscious wishes or needs by using imagination to solve problems. (Young child who sees father physically abuse mother may imagine he is attacking a wild animal and saves his mother from harm.)
Repression	Conscious distancing of events or thoughts that are too painful or unacceptable to one's ego into the unconscious level. These feelings can continue to influence behavior into adult years if unresolved. (Person who was sexually abused as a child is unable to achieve a meaningful intimate relationship as an adult.)
Regression	Returning to an earlier more comfortable and less stressful stage of behavior. (Child who is weaned returns to drinking from a bottle during hospitalization.)
Projection	Attributing or blaming emotionally unacceptable traits, feelings, or attitudes on something or someone else. Refusing to admit weakness or accept responsibility for own actions. (Person who drinks alcohol blames his wife for doing something to make him get drunk.)
Compensation	Emphasizing capabilities or strengths to make up for a lack or loss in personal characteristics. (Person who is not talented in athletics excels in scholastic achievement.)
Reaction-formation	Consciously attempting to make up for feelings or attitudes that are unacceptable to the ego by replacing them with the opposite feelings or beliefs. (Mother who secretly dislikes her child becomes overprotective and outwardly affectionate toward the child.)
Conversion	Transferring emotional conflicts into physical symptoms. (Person who dislikes her boss at work develops migraine headaches to avoid going to work.)
Undoing	Initiating a positive action to conceal a negative action or neutralizing a previously unacceptable action or wish. (Employer offers to take his secretary to lunch after verbally attacking her earlier in the day.)
Rationalization	Substituting false reasoning or justification for behavior that is unacceptable or threatening to the ego. Ignores the real reason for the behavior with falsehoods and avoids responsibility for the behavior. (Employee who is not given a promotion tells co-workers that he really did not want the position.)

impulses while continuing to meet personal and social needs in acceptable ways.

According to Freud, defenses are a major means of managing conflict and emotional response to environmental situations. These mechanisms differ from one another and may be adaptive as well as maladaptive. Maladaptive mechanisms may lead to distortion of reality and actual self-deception that can interfere with personal growth and interaction with society. For example, a person may continue to abuse alcohol using the mechanism of projection to blame his spouse and children for his behavior, while using denial to avoid self-blame and damage to his own ego. This maladaptive use of mechanisms interferes with an honest self-appraisal of reality and the detrimental effects of substance abuse. In contrast, a woman may temporarily deny her husband's extramarital affair by telling herself and others that he is just busy, yet project her feelings for her husband onto her children by punishing them for things they did not do.

When she sees her husband with the other woman, she realizes the reality of the situation and apologizes to her children for blaming them for the way she feels toward their father. The determinant for the effective use of defense mechanisms is based on the frequency, intensity, and length of time they are used.

Human beings sometimes behave in ways that provide a means of escape from the realities and responsibilities of life. These patterns of adjustment are common to everyone and are used to resolve conflicts and provide relief from the anxiety and stress of everyday existence. Most of the time, we are not aware that a defense mechanism is being used to adapt to a situation. However, when this escape becomes habitual, it becomes a dangerous inability to deal with reality and constitutes a psychiatric problem.

Theory of Psychosexual Development

Freud believed that as the personality develops, there is an increasing self-identification and changing self-perception of sexuality and sexual identification. In his psychosexual theory, he proposed four major stages of development. The oral stage occurs during the first 2 years as the child seeks pleasure from sucking and oral gratification of hunger. The anal stage takes place from 2 to 4 years of age, during which pleasure is achieved as the child develops an awareness and control of urination and defecation. In the phallic stage, around the age of 4 years, the child discovers pleasure in genital stimulation and also struggles to accept a sexual identity. According to Freud, this gives rise to the Oedipal conflict (boys) and the Electra conflict (girls) in which the child begins to feel romantic feelings for the parent of the opposite sex but fears the wrath of the parent of the same sex. The child resolves the conflict by identifying with the parent of the same sex and redirects the feelings for the opposite-sex parent into developing this gender role. Freud believed these feelings are put into **latency** during the period of middle childhood in which the sexual desires remain subdued. The genital stage occurs as the child enters puberty and adolescence. It is at this stage that Freud believed sexual feelings reemerge and become directed toward establishing a relationship with a person of the opposite sex. According to Freud, at any point during psychosexual development the child can become fixated and frustrated, resulting in exaggerated adult character traits that reflect the arrested growth. (See Box 10-2.) Although it has been the subject of much controversy regarding its sexual orientation, Freudian theory laid the groundwork for future developmental theories.

Box 10-2

ADULT BEHAVIORS OF STAGE THEORY DEVELOPMENT

Stage	Signs of Successful Resolution	Indicators of Developmental Problem
Freud (Psychosexual)		
1. Oral	Satisfaction—gratification	Dependent on and easily influenced by others, manipulative cocky attitude, gullible
2. Anal	Giving, openness, self-control	Stinginess and orderliness; stubborn and rigid meticulousness
3. Phallic	Sexual identity accepted	Vanity and brashness, flirtatious
4. Latency	Sexual urges suppressed—expansion of social contacts beyond family	Unsuccessful attempts at expanding social relationships
5. Genital	Sexual energy channeled toward peers of opposite sex	Unconscious sexual conflict and inability to form intimate sexual relationship
Erikson (Psychosocial)		
1. Trust versus mistrust	Hope	Suspicion and fear of people and relationships
		Extreme self-doubt and fear of independence
2. Autonomy versus shame and doubt	Will	Sense of inadequacy and defeat
3. Initiative versus guilt	Purpose	Inadequate problem-solving skills

(continued)

Box 10-2

ADULT BEHAVIORS OF STAGE THEORY DEVELOPMENT *(Continued)*

Stage	Signs of Successful Resolution	Indicators of Developmental Problem
4. Industry versus inferiority	Competence	Manipulation of others, no regard for the rights of others (such as in the workplace) Feelings of unworthiness, fear of failure
5. Identity versus role confusion	Fidelity	Uncertainty and loss of who one is in relationships with others
6. Intimacy versus isolation	Love and commitment	Emotional withdrawal into self
7. Generativity versus stagnation	Caring and giving	Inability to grow as an person
8. Integrity versus despair	Wisdom	Disillusionment with life and inability to view death as reality

Piaget (Cognitive)

Stage	Signs of Successful Resolution	Indicators of Developmental Problem
1. Sensorimotor	Growth of abilities related to senses and motor skill Goal-directed behaviors Egocentric thinking	Focus only on what one wants without regard to possible consequences of those actions
2. Preoperational	Exploration motivated by magical and imaginative thinking	Decisions based on intuition, fantasy, or superstition with inability to make choices rooted in reality
3. Concrete	Cognitive connections based on actual events or objects Logical thinking begins Thinking in terms of intentional moral response	Resistance to change with meager attempts at risk-taking strategies in which the outcome is an unknown
4. Formal operations	Abstract thinking Problem-solving ability Symbolic reasoning with conceptual theoretical thinking	Inability to visualize possibility or solution to a problem Unwillingness to formulate or accept reality-based decisions

Sullivan (Interpersonal)

Stage	Signs of Successful Resolution	Indicators of Developmental Problem
1. Infant	Satisfaction of needs	Anxiety develops as a result of unmet physiologic needs Lack of bonding between infant and caregiver
2. Childhood	Self-control in gratification of needs	Increasing anxiety experienced with delay in gratification of own needs
3. Juvenile	Successful relationships with peer group	Difficulty relating to others and developing interpersonal group relationships/workplace interaction
4. Preadolescence	Appropriate interactions with persons of opposite sex begins	Inability to relate in a meaningful way to persons of the opposite sex
5. Early adolescence	Sense of personal identity in heterosexual relationships	Fear and withdrawal of relationships with persons of the opposite sex
6. Late adolescence	Satisfying intimate relationship with another	Inability to form a long-term intimate relationship with another person

Erik Erikson (Psychosocial Developmental Theory)

Erikson proposed that we develop in a pattern of eight **psychosocial** stages throughout our lifespan. Each stage consists of a developmental crisis that must be faced, indicating a period of vulnerability. Resolution of this critical period could enhance a healthy continuation of the process. If unresolved, the progression to subsequent stages of development could be adversely affected. Erikson's view demonstrates, however, that failures at one stage can be corrected by successes at a later stage.

Stage I: Trust versus Mistrust (Birth to 1 Year)

A sense of trust results in a feeling of comfort and reassurance that the world is a safe and pleasant place in which the child can live with a minimum of fear and apprehension. The emphasis in this stage is on the oral-sensory gratification received during feeding through which the infant develops a trusting relationship with the parent or caregiver. Consistency and responsiveness by the parent in providing for the infant's needs of nourishment, comfort, and nurturing are essential to the development of trust. Babies who are not securely attached to their mothers are less responsive to the parent and show less effort in exploring the environment and world in which they exist.

Stage II: Autonomy versus Shame and Doubt (Ages 1 to 2)

According to Erikson, children begin a period of increased self-confidence and independent striving to do more on their own. The most important event during this stage is toilet training. Children also try to do new things such as feeding or dressing themselves. It is essential that the parents positively reinforce these efforts while avoiding the urge to be overprotective and critical. Erickson believed that if parents do not show a consistent and reassuring attitude during this stage, children would experience too much self-doubt and shame about their abilities, resulting in a lack of confidence that would persist throughout life.

Stage III: Initiative versus Guilt (2 to 6 Years)

During this period, children are challenged with increasing responsibility to take care of their physical needs, their behavior, toys, and pets. This requires children to be assertive and creative in assuming this responsibility. Children in this stage are eager to do things, and it is essential that parents praise and recognize the child's efforts no matter how small they may be. On the other hand, children must also learn to accept that in their quest for independence there are some things that are not allowed or safe for them to do. It is important they be reassured that being imaginative and pretending to take on adult roles is okay. If they are not given the chance to do things on their own and to be responsible, a sense of guilt may result. The child will learn to believe that what they want to do is not good enough or is always wrong.

Stage IV: Industry versus Inferiority (6 to 12 Years)

In this stage of development, children are learning to be productive and to accomplish things on their own, both physically and mentally. This is a period when they master their ability to succeed in peer relationships, school, and activities. It is essential for children to receive encouragement and support in their drive for success from parents and others. Children learn by repeated efforts driven by self-confidence in their own ability. If children have difficulty relating to others outside of the home or in achievement of skills, a sense of inferiority and self-doubt may result.

Stage V: Identity versus Role Confusion (12 to 18 Years)

During the stage of adolescence, there is a search for identity and answers to questions concerning our purpose in life. Erikson believed that a basic sense of trust and self-confidence in ourselves was necessary to provide the foundation for adolescents to make conscious choices about vocation, relationships, and life in general. Failure to resolve previous conflicts successfully would result in an inability to make these decisions and choices. As a result, adolescents may experience role confusion as to who they are and where they belong as they move into adulthood.

Stage VI: Intimacy versus Isolation (Ages 19 to 40 Years)

During young adulthood, the most important developmental goal is to form a committed relationship with another. A true intimate relationship requires sincerity and open sharing of feelings. Having a sexual relationship does not imply intimacy. A person can be sexually intimate without feelings for and commitment to the other person. Love relationships are strengthened by the ability of partners to relate on a deep personal level. The young adult who is unable to be open and committed to another may retreat into isolation and fear a giving and sharing relationship.

MEMORY JOGGER

How might failure to develop a sense of trust have implications in the establishment of adult relationships and interaction with society?

Stage VII: Generativity versus Stagnation (Ages 40 to 65 Years)

As we enter middle adulthood, the task is related to parenting and supportive involvement in providing for the next generation. This role includes being an active participant in issues that will make this world a safer and better place for the future. The inability to nurture and to give of whatever is ours to give in an attempt to ensure this progressive stability for our children may lead to stagnation and decreased meaning for one's life.

Stage VIII: Integrity versus Despair (Over 65 years)

The important event during these years is seen as a reflection on and acceptance of our life. According to Erikson, a positive outcome is demonstrated by a sense of fulfillment about a life lived and acceptance of death as an inevitable reality. This involves accepting responsibility for and being satisfied with choices that have been made over a lifetime. The older adult who has successfully reached this stage is able to put the past in perspective and achieve a sense of self-satisfaction with the present. Those who are unable to reach this sense of fulfillment and wholeness will despair about life accomplishments and fear death.

Erikson maintained that if each developmental crisis was not resolved in sequence, the personality would continue to manifest this conflict into the adult years. Although critics of the stage theory say that psychologic development may be influenced and altered by experiences throughout life, many have found Erikson's theory useful for continued study of personality development.

JUST THE FACTS

Erik Erikson—Eight Stages of Psychosocial Development

1. Trust versus mistrust
2. Autonomy versus shame and doubt
3. Initiative versus guilt
4. Industry versus inferiority
5. Identity versus role confusion
6. Intimacy versus isolation
7. Generativity versus stagnation
8. Integrity versus despair

Jean Piaget (Cognitive Development Related to Personality)

Piaget proposed that personality is the result of increasing intellectual ability to organize and integrate experiences into behavior patterns. His observations led him to conclude that this organization tended to occur at certain age groups. Movement forward relies on four interdependent factors. Physical and psychologic growth or maturation occurs in the child during a specific stage as the child thinks and *experiences* interaction with the environment. As the child begins to distinguish the self as a separate being, social experiences become a part of this learning. According to Piaget, **equilibration** occurs as the child brings all these factors together to build mental schema or connections that lead to a cognitive balance. Children are motivated to seek this balance by a perceived imbalance between what they already know (existing schema) and something new. Piaget refers to the ability to incorporate new ideas and experiences as **assimilation,** while **accommodation** is the ability to alter existing schema to incorporate the new information.

Piaget theorized that cognitive development occurs in four stages. In the first two years of life, the **sensorimotor** stage involves the growth of abilities related to the five senses and motor functions. Early responses are primarily reflexive in nature, with a gradual increase in skill as children adapt to their environment. These responses tend to reflect only a perception of that which is visible to the child. The perception that what is gone from view still exists (object permanence) begins to develop at about 9 months of age and is well developed by 1 year.

The **preoperational** stage of development occurs from 2 to 7 years. The mental schema developed during the earlier stage emerge into communication of thoughts that is largely egocentric without regard for another point of view. Language and actions reflect a focus on thinking that the world exists solely to meet the demands of the child's ego. As children grow, they explore and try out many new activities motivated by increasing magical and imaginative thinking.

From 7 to 12 years of age, Piaget saw children as able to perform **concrete mental operations** on their accumulated thoughts and memories. The phrase "seeing is believing" is descriptive of the child's need to base these cognitive connections on actual events or objects. Facts and routines with one way of doing things are a characteristic of this age group. The child begins to think logically, classify objects, and recognize that combinations are reversible. (For example: Daddy can also be a husband, brother, and uncle all at the same time.) Although they are capable of thinking more logically, children of this age still depend on concrete cues to develop these thoughts.

According to Piaget, the person moves into the stage of **formal operations** during the years of 11 to 12 and up. This period of growth involves abstract thought processes, problem solving, and systematic, purposeful mental relationships. The adolescent is capable of symbolic thinking and comprehension of theoretical concepts. They are able to visualize beyond what is known and formulate hypothetical reasoning.

Piaget maintains that once the child has entered a new stage, the process is irreversible, with each stage building on the previous level of development.

Box 10-3

OTHER THEORETICAL APPROACHES TO PERSONALITY AND BEHAVIOR

Behavioristic Theory—B. F. Skinner

- **Behaviorism** is based on the concept that thinking, feeling, and interpersonal relationships are irrelevant and that all behavior is observable or learned behavior in response to a stimulus from the environment.
- Behavior is the result of conditioning shaped by a system of reward, punishment, and **reinforcement**.
- Human personality is formed in response to these stimulus-response situations. The personality may include both adaptive and maladaptive behavior as the result of reinforcement.
- People show consistent patterns of behavior that will continue if the action is rewarded by a response. If no reinforcement is given, the behavior will decline.
- Positive reinforcement of a negative behavior can lead to continuation of the very behavior we wish to negate.
- Conditioning strengthens and weakens behaviors automatically without regard to the conscious thought processes.

Social Learning Theory—Albert Bandura

- Personality is largely shaped through learning by actively seeking out and processing information about the environment in response to a need for a positive outcome.
- People can act to change their surroundings as a result of both internal and external forces that influence each other.
- Social learning is based on observation and imitation of others. Both children and adults tend to imitate people they like or respect more than those whose persona is less appealing.
- Models whose behavior leads to an approved outcome are also more likely to be copied.
- Self-confidence develops as the belief that performance of behaviors should lead to the expected outcome becomes reality in the actions of that person.

Cognitive-Behavioral Theory—Aaron Beck

- Focus is on the person's abilities to think, analyze, and decide on certain behavior rather than acting on feelings.
- Actions are the result of distorted perceptions, and thoughts that can be changed. This is unlike Freud who saw mental disturbances as being the result of childhood experiences.
- Self-defeating behaviors are maintained because of irrational thoughts and erroneous beliefs.
- Self-concept and evaluation of social image is affected by how people think others see them. Self-talk is used to praise or criticize and interpret situations. This is reflected in both normal behaviors and mental disorders as well.
- Negative self-talk can be changed into more positive thoughts, leading to a more positive self-image and more productive outcomes.

JUST THE FACTS

Jean Piaget—Theory of Cognitive Development
Sensorimotor: Birth to 2 years
Preoperational: 2 to 7 years
Concrete: 7 to 11 years
Formal operations: 11 years and up

Lawerence Kohlberg (Theory of Moral Development)

In his research on cognitive development, Piaget concluded that changes in the child's level of thinking also affect the moral decisions the child makes. Motivated by Piaget's studies, Lawerence Kohlberg developed his own theory based on six stages of moral reasoning included in three levels. Basic to his theory is his belief that the choices one makes do not determine the stage of moral reasoning, but the reasons one gives to justify the behavior determine the moral stage. Like Piaget, he believed that the intellect and the child's emotional development occur in a parallel pattern of stages during which the child changes his or her concept of self in relation to interaction with others. The level of cognitive development determines how the child perceives a situation and what is learned from that experience. Each of the three levels builds on the previous with increasing complexity in the individual view of a moral issue.

> **MEMORY JOGGER**
>
> What do the stage theories have in common? How do they differ? What influence does each aspect of development have on the personality?

Preconventional Level: Values indicate environmental pressure
    Stage 1: Acts or behaves to avoid punishment
    Stage 2: Is motivated by personal reward (What's in it for me?)
Conventional Level: Influenced by societal pressure
    Stage 3: Values and acts to meet the expectations of others (peer group)
    Stage 4: Is motivated by the laws of society/legal system
Postconventional Level: Influenced by standards and shared principles
    Stage 5: Acts for the good of society or the most people (e.g., U.S. Constitution)
    Stage 6: Bases actions on moral principles and ethical values (the right thing to do)

SUMMARY

The formation of our personality is essentially the formation of who we are over the continuum of a lifetime. Our drives, our thought processes, and our behavior are all integral parts of this holistic human system. The established theoretical models for the study of human cognition and behavior have provided current studies with an eclectic view of development. Research continues to uncover the many mysteries inherent in the human mind and personality.

Personality is a combination of characteristic patterns of how we perceive, relate to, and think about ourselves and the world in which we exist. These patterns are the result of genetics and the influence of social and environmental forces throughout the lifespan. The development of personality is most often described by stage theories that divide the lifespan into age-related periods. These theories provide an approach to personality and psychologic development that correlates with the physical growth and development.

Other theories have developed that reflect the various ways in which the human component can be studied and viewed. Since human behavior is most often seen as how we interact with one another and the social environment, it is most often studied within this context. Our patterns of behavior are established as a result of these interrelationships. The self-concept is developed as behaviors are reinforced or threatened by reprisal. As environmental situations confront us, we view them from the perspective of past encounters with similar occurrences. The way in which we respond is reflective of established patterns. It is also theorized that we have the ability to think, analyze, and decide on certain behaviors rather than just reacting to the environmental stimuli.

Knowledge of the various theories provides the basis for understanding the various therapeutic approaches to the treatment of mental illness. The dynamics that combine and develop over generations make us who we are. We cannot undo the past, but to understand it is an invitation to repair the present and the future.

Bibliography

American Psychiatric Association (2000). *Diagnostic and statistical manual of mental disorders text revision* (4th ed.). Washington, DC: American Psychiatric Association.

Johnson, B. S. (1993). *Psychiatric-mental health nursing* (3rd ed.). Philadelphia, PA: Lippincott.

Sternberg, R. J. (1995). *In search of the human mind*. Ft. Worth, TX: Harcourt Brace.

Weiten, W. (1995). *Psychology themes and variations* (3rd ed.). Boston, MA: Brooks/Cole.

Student Worksheet

Fill in the Blank

Fill in the blank with the correct answer.

1. Patterns of perceiving, relating to, and thinking about ourselves and the world around us define the concept of _____.
2. _____ describes the variances in character that influence the development of personality and interpersonal relationships.
3. The process by which we bring factors together to build mental schema or connections that lead to a cognitive balance is called _____.
4. According to Piaget, _____ is the ability to incorporate new ideas and experiences into our existing mental schema.
5. Once new experiences are encountered, the ability to alter the existing schema to incorporate this new information is referred to as _____.
6. The concept that all behavior is observable or learned in response to a stimulus from the environment is the basis for the theory of _____.
7. The theory of development that states that the reasons we give to justify our choices and the behavior that results from those choices determine the level of moral development was the work of _____.
8. B. F. Skinner theorized that the human personality is formed in response to a conditioned stimulus-response of reward and punishment called _____.

Matching

Match the defense mechanism with the appropriate behavior.

a. Unhappy with her boss for his criticism, Clara turns around and takes her anger out on her husband.
b. David is unable to remember a boating accident in which his friend was killed.
c. After going to the movie the night before an exam, Molly states that she failed the exam because she did not study the right chapter.
d. An adolescent wants his mother to stay with him during a hospital stay.
e. Confined to a wheelchair, Jack becomes a computer specialist.
f. A young man who secretly desires to harm his wife appears on a television show against spousal abuse.
g. When Martha is confronted about her alcohol problem, she states she can quit anytime she chooses.
h. After taking funds out of their savings account to buy golf clubs, Hank tells his wife that the bank must have made a mistake.

   1. _____ Rationalization
   2. _____ Denial
   3. _____ Repression
   4. _____ Regression
   5. _____ Projection
   6. _____ Displacement
   7. _____ Reaction-formation
   8. _____ Sublimation

Multiple Choice

Select the best answer from the multiple-choice items.

1. A 70-year-old person states, "My life is a pile of shambles with nothing to show for it." The person is demonstrating what Erikson would term:
   a. Doubt
   b. Inferiority
   c. Despair
   d. Stagnation
2. A 4-year-old boy states, "When I grow up I am going to marry Mommy." Which stage of psychosexual development is portrayed by this statement?
   a. Phallic
   b. Anal
   c. Latency
   d. Genital
3. According to Piaget, children who seek to control their world from a concentrated point of view would be in which stage of cognitive development?
   a. Sensorimotor
   b. Preoperational
   c. Concrete
   d. Formal operations
4. To avoid hurting his friend, John refrains from telling the truth to a friend whose partner is having an affair with a co-worker. According to Kohlberg, this demonstrates which level of moral development?
   a. Preconventional—stage 2
   b. Conventional—stage 3
   c. Postconventional—stage 5
5. Al has been arrested for physical assault. He has a history of previous aggressive offenses. Behavioral theory would explain this behavior as:
   a. Feelings of repressed hostility
   b. A diminished sense of self-esteem
   c. An innate impulsive drive for survival
   d. Reinforcement of early learning experiences
6. Surveys show that cigarette smoking and alcohol consumption are common among the adolescent population. These results reflect peer behavior and provide support for which of the following theories?
   a. Social learning theory
   b. Conditioning theory
   c. Psychosexual theory
   d. Human needs theory

Seek and Find

Find the incorrect information in the statements below.

1. According to Freudian theory, the division of the personality that is most closely in touch with reality is the superego.
2. The theory of psychosexual development suggests that during the latency stage, the child is discovering pleasure in genital stimulation while struggling to accept a sexual identity.
3. According to Erikson, the child begins a period of increased self-confidence and striving to become more independent in the preschool years during the stage of initiative versus guilt.
4. The person who is unable to be open and committed to a giving and sharing relationship with another is said by Erikson to be stalled in the stage of identity versus role confusion.

Grief and Loss

CHAPTER OBJECTIVES

In this chapter, you'll learn:

1. To define grief as a process.
2. To describe the relationship between loss and grief.
3. To discuss adaptive versus maladaptive responses to grief and loss.
4. To identify factors that may contribute to dysfunctional grief.
5. To assess signs and symptoms that indicate unresolved grief.

KEY TERMS

anticipatory grief	conventional grief	depression	unresolved grief
bereavement	denial	grief	

DEFINING GRIEF AND LOSS

Grief is defined as the emotional process of coping with a loss. Instinctively, we associate this process with the death of a loved one, such as a spouse, parent, or child, or of any person who is important in our life. In a broader sense, the reality of loss can be applied to the absence of anything that is significant or meaningful to our existence. This can include a separation or divorce, loss of a body part, loss of a job or source of income, and losses that result from a natural or imposed disaster. All of these events or circumstances may leave the person with a sense of emptiness, hopelessness, and detachment from the meaning that previously was found in life. The extent to which emotional energy was previously invested in these objects, persons, and relationships will determine the intensity with which an individual responds to the absence of that object. Although a person may experience sadness or sorrow in response to making a mistake or doing something that is hurtful to another, the grief felt as the person adjusts to the absence of the endeared person or object is a deeper and longer lasting emotion that involves time and emotional energy.

Loss can be an actual or perceived change in the status of one's relationship to a valued object or person. This concept is easily associated with the death of a valued person or pet. There is also a major loss when losing a home to fire or natural disaster with a lifetime of memories suddenly gone from view and reality. The loss may be seen as the lack of certainty that a goal or desired outcome will be achieved, such as not receiving a job promotion or an academic failure. The attachment bond that is seen as strong and secure is suddenly shattered, making a person vulnerable to an unstable emotional response. Grief is the emotion encountered when an individual is confronted with a loss. It is a feeling of sadness and despondency centered on the experience itself. These feelings may lead to behaviors such as forgetfulness and crying at unpredictable times. It is helpful for the person to be reassured that this is a common reaction to grief. Tears are accepted as a part of the healing that takes place in the months after the loss.

Anticipatory grief may be seen in individuals and families who are expecting a major loss in the near future. This concept is helpful in understanding the reaction of the terminally ill client and the family who will be left to mourn the death of their loved one. In this case, death is inevitable and there is a time of preparation and closure that can ease the emotional pain at the actual time of death. This is the premise for hospice care, which provides patient care and supportive interventions to assist the client and family members in coping with the imminent loss.

JUST THE FACTS

Anticipatory grieving: Entering the grieving process in anticipation of a loss
Conventional grieving: Feelings expected after a loss

Conventional grief is primarily associated with the grief that is experienced following a loss. This process of **bereavement** or adapting to loss may take days, weeks, or years, depending on the sense of loss for the person involved. Each person responds to loss in a personal and unique way and time. This response is based on the person's level of development, past experiences, and current coping strategies.

Children and adolescents respond according to the level at which they understand the concept of death or loss (see Box 11-1). The response will reflect the age-related cognitive and psychologic development of the child. A toddler may respond to separation from a parent or attachment figure with anxiety but has no concept of loss. Should that attachment figure not return, the child will usually adapt to another attachment figure who is nurturing. The preschool child reacts with magical thinking, such as in a 5-year-old child who says, "Grandpa is sleeping. Will he wake up in time to take me to the park?" The concept of death as a finality is not yet understood. Associated with the growing moral concept of right and wrong, the school-age child may feel a sense of

---

Box 11-1

AGE-RELATED CONCEPTS OF LOSS

Toddlers

- Egocentric and concerned with themselves
- Do not understand concept of loss

Preschool

- Use magical thinking, and may feel shame or guilt when thinking is associated with loss (i.e., belief that the child's behavior is the reason a parent is gone, such as in divorce)
- Primitive coping mechanisms result in more intense response
- Do not understand death as permanent

School-Age

- Still feel guilt and responsibility in associating negative actions with loss
- Respond to concrete, simple, and logical explanation of death (often explained by death of a pet)

Age 9 to 10

- Understand permanence of death and that some losses are temporary

Adolescent

- Able to understand the concept of death, but have difficulty accepting loss
- Perceive loss as a threat to their identity

Memory Jogger

How might failure to achieve one's ambition be seen as a positive experience?

Memory Jogger

How might environmental factors during childhood affect a person's ability to cope with loss?

guilt or responsibility for a loss, such as when a parent is absent following a divorce. Although the adolescent understands the concept of death as finality, it is difficult for this age group to fit death or loss into their search for an identity.

Adults may view loss as temporary or permanent, and most are able to accept their losses and grow from these situations. Acceptance often opens the door of opportunity for new and expanded life experiences. It is important to remember that regardless of age, bereavement is a natural, healthy, and healing process that emerges in response to a significant loss.

GRIEF AS A PROCESS

The grieving process describes a series of occurrences in the resolution of loss. This process provides support as an individual works through the feelings of anger, hopelessness, and futility that accompany loss. It provides time to put things into perspective, to place into memory that which is gone, and to emerge with a newly developed embrace of life. Life is an evolving challenge of events that inevitably requires us to cope with disappointment and loss. Learning to deal with these situations in small increments better prepares us to deal effectively with a major loss. We can learn to accept loss as part of living, or we can choose to react with hostility, often suppressing the anger into hidden feelings that eventually may erupt in negative or maladaptive patterns of behavior such as substance abuse or suicide. Learning to cope or adapt to loss involves giving ourselves the right to grieve in whatever timeframe is needed to go through the process. It is important to recognize and accept the feelings, such as anger, fear, and guilt, that are normal and appropriately a part of grieving.

Just the Facts

Steps of Grieving

- Shock and denial
- Anger and pain
- Negotiation and bargaining
- Withdrawal and depression
- Acceptance and resolution

Growth occurs as the bereaved person comes to the point of letting go of the past. This does not reduce the importance of the loss but allows the person to continue living with new perspective. In time, the sadness and loneliness felt as a result of the void left by the cherished object are replaced with hopefulness as one is freed from the previous relationship. This acceptance indicates that the grief process is coming to a close.

Just the Facts

Grief is a process of working through the emotional response to loss, reorganizing one's life, and accomplishing some degree of resolution or closure.

Stages of Grief

Perhaps the best known theory of bereavement is that of Dr. Elisabeth Kübler-Ross, a German psychiatrist, who described the stages that a person who is facing death, either their own or that of a loved one, encounters before coming to actual acceptance of death as a final stage of life. Dr. Kübler-Ross believed that the dying process is a lifelong process and that we repeat the stages each time we are confronted by loss.

Dr. Kübler-Ross identified five stages that we go through in reaction to loss or death. The first step is shock, disbelief, and **denial** that the event is happening. We want to avoid the reality of the loss and may act as if nothing has occurred, or as though the lost object or person is still present. Denial actually allows us an adjustment period in which to gather coping strategies for the grieving work ahead. As we realize that the loss is real, the denial gives way to feelings of bitterness, anger, and turmoil. Anger is expressed in many ways, often demonstrated openly in behaviors such as crying or expressions of self-blame and guilt. Some may turn the anger inward, resulting in physical illness and/or psychologic dysfunction.

Anger may be followed by bargaining as we attempt to postpone acceptance of the loss. As is often seen with terminal illness, this is a time when deals with God are attempted as a way to prolong the inevitable. Frequent labile moods are common and are often intermingled with continued anger and unwillingness to accept the loss. This period is gradually followed by a deep sense of loss as the reality of what has happened or is anticipated settles. At this point we may withdraw from social interaction, choosing to spend hours and days alone in the depth of loneliness for that which is gone. **Depression** is a normal response in this process as we adjust to life without the loved object and the full impact of the emptiness. For some people this period is overwhelming and recovery from the depth of sorrow felt is unlikely without professional support and guidance. The final stage is that of acceptance when the person begins to experience peace and serenity. This is the time of letting go and allowing life to provide new experiences and relationships.

MEMORY JOGGER

What objective signs might indicate a person has reached acceptance?

JUST THE FACTS

Other Grief Reactions
Anxiety: Related to future without loved object
Panic: Related to inability to control the outcome
Blame: Self-blame for doing or not doing something to cause the loss

There are several theories that have evolved concerning the grief process, and while not absolute, the stages of grief supply a basis for understanding this process. A person may experience all stages in rapid succession or rally back and forth between stages, remaining in some longer than others. When the process of grieving becomes prolonged it may be seen as abnormal or maladaptive with symptoms of a major depressive episode such as extreme sadness, insomnia, anorexia, and weight loss. The person may consider these symptoms normal but may seek professional help for the insomnia or appetite loss. The diagnosis of major depressive disorder is not generally assigned unless the symptoms are still present 2 months after the loss.

Dysfunctional Grief

The psychologic process of grieving involves an emotional separation from the valued person or object. The loss is felt as a break in the continuity of the person's life and sense of security. Even as life itself involves a series of separations in the search for autonomy and independence, the ability to cope with each loss poses a challenge in adaptive strategy. Coping skills are most often learned through observation of the social environment around us. If an individual has developed the psychologic tools to deal with loss and failure in an adaptive way, these resources will help the person to deal with a major loss in a similar way. However, if an individual has a lifelong pattern of inadequate coping skills, the chances are greater that a resolution to the grieving process will be delayed.

Dysfunctional grief is a failure to complete the grieving process and cope successfully with the loss. Chronic sorrow describes the feelings a person has while attempting to deal with the loss. Those factors that may contribute to **unresolved grief,** which then leads to the dysfunction, include:

- Socially unacceptable death such as suicide or homicide
- Missing person related to war or mysterious disappearance or abduction
- Multiple losses or losses in close succession (loss of several family members in short period with financial loss or disaster loss)
- Ambivalent feelings toward the lost person or object
- Unresolved grieving from a previous loss
- Guilt with regard to circumstances at or near the time of death
- Feelings of the survivor that he or she should have died with or instead of the deceased
- Consuming feelings of worthlessness with suicidal tendencies
- Physiologic response to the loss with marked decrease in functioning
- Delusional thinking or hallucinations of seeing the image or hearing the voice of the deceased

Because the intensity of feelings at this level is often desperate, it is essential that the person with prolonged bereavement receives treatment.

SUMMARY

Grief is defined as the emotional process of coping with loss. Loss can occur with the death of a loved one or any person or object that is a needed and cherished entity in our lives. Loss of a job and income, a home, or other important parts of our lives are likely to elicit the same emotions of grief. Grief is the response that is experienced in anticipation of or as a result of a loss. Bereavement includes that process one goes through in adapting to life without the cherished object. Reaction to loss changes with the growth and maturation of cognitive ability. By the age of 9 or 10, the child is able to view death or termination with adult understanding of permanent or temporary loss.

Grief in itself is a process of mourning for the loss, coming to terms with the reality of the loss, and putting it into perspective as we move beyond the period of bereavement. Several theories have evolved that propose that this process involves stages. Dr. Elisabeth Kübler-Ross defined five stages of dying or grief that occur with loss: denial, anger, bargaining, depression, and acceptance. Once the loss is accepted, we are ready to adapt to a new period of growth without the esteemed object. If a person is not able to emerge from the grieving process and remains in a state of unresolved loss, it may fall into the category of maladaptive or dysfunctional grieving. Counseling and treatment may be required for the person with this level of grief.

Bibliography

American Psychiatric Association (2000). *Diagnostic and statistical manual of mental disorders text revision* (4th ed.). Washington, DC: American Psychiatric Association.

Barry, P. D. (1996). *Psychosocial nursing* (3rd ed.). Philadelphia, PA: Lippincott.

Milliken, M. E. (1998). *Understanding human behavior* (6th ed.). Albany, NY: Delmar.

Student Worksheet

Fill in the Blank

Fill in the blank with the correct answer.

1. _____ is defined as the emotional process of coping with a loss.
2. Those who may be expecting a major loss in the near future will usually experience _____ grief.
3. The period of time involved in the process of adapting to loss is often referred to as _____.
4. _____ describes an actual or perceived change in a relationship between a person and a valued object or other person.
5. The 5-year-old child reacts to separation from a loved person or object with _____ thinking.
6. A lack of resolution to the grief process is referred to as _____.

Matching

Match the following stages of grief with the appropriate description.

a. Deep sense of loss with withdrawal from social interaction.
b. Adjustment period in which the reality of the loss is avoided.
c. Labile moods and attempts to make deals to postpone the loss.
d. Time of peaceful letting go and allowing life to move forward.
e. Feelings of bitterness, self-blame, guilt, and hostility.

1. _____ Denial
2. _____ Anger
3. _____ Bargaining
4. _____ Depression
5. _____ Acceptance

Multiple Choice

1. Maria has been in a comatose state for the past 8 months as a result of an automobile accident. Although he has been told that there is no brain function, her husband, Reuben, insists that she is showing purposeful response. Which of the following stages of grief is Reuben experiencing?
   a. Bargaining
   b. Anger
   c. Denial
   d. Depression

2. Which of the following describes how 9-year-old Jeremy would most likely respond to the death of his grandfather?
   a. Feels death happened because he went skating with a friend instead of visiting his sick grandfather.
   b. Sees the loss as interfering with his ability to determine a sense of who he is.
   c. Believes that angels took his grandfather in a chariot and went riding into the sky.
   d. Would not understand the concept of permanent loss.

Scenario: Lost and Alone

Art, whose wife died 6 months ago, describes himself as "lost, forgetful, and unable to concentrate." He also states, "I seem to cry at the most inconvenient moments, so I just stay to myself."

What feelings might be responsible for Art's symptoms?

_____

_____

What stage of the grief process is Art most likely experiencing?

_____

_____

12

Fundamental Communication Skills

CHAPTER OBJECTIVES

In this chapter, you'll learn:

1. To spell and define the key terms.
2. To list two major forms of communication.
3. To explain how various components of communication can affect the meaning of verbal messages.
4. To define active listening.
5. To list and describe the six interviewing techniques.
6. To give an example of how cultural differences may affect communication.
7. To discuss how to handle communication problems caused by language barriers.
8. To list two methods that you can use to promote communication among hearing-, sight-, and speech-impaired patients.
9. To list five actions that you can take to improve communication with a child.
10. To discuss how to handle an angry or distressed patient.
11. To discuss your role in communicating with a grieving patient or family member.
12. To discuss the key elements of interdisciplinary communication.

KEY TERMS

anacusis	discrimination	messages	presbyacusis
bias	dysphasia	mourning	reflecting
clarification	dysphonia	nonlanguage	stereotyping
cultures	feedback	paralanguage	summarizing
demeanor	grief	paraphrasing	therapeutic

COMMUNICATION IS SENDING and receiving **messages** (information), verbally or otherwise. The ability to communicate effectively is a crucial skill for allied health professionals. In your role, you must accurately and appropriately share information with physicians, other professional staff members, and patients. When communicating with patients you must be able to receive messages correctly, interpret them, and respond to the sender appropriately. The allied health professional is usually the first person the patient meets in the health care facility. Thus, your positive attitude, pleasant presentation, and use of good communication skills will set the tone for future interactions.

BASIC COMMUNICATION FLOW

Communication requires the following elements:

- a message to be sent
- a person to send the message
- a person to receive the message

During the act of communicating, two or more people will alternate roles as sender and receiver as they seek **feedback** (responses) and **clarification** (understanding) regarding the message. The process of message exchange is a swing moving back and forth between two people.

As an allied health professional, you will primarily be communicating in a therapeutic manner. This means that your communication will focus on conversations regarding pertinent topics relating to facility procedures, policies, and patient care. Your other responsibilities for ensuring good communication include the following:

- clarifying confusing messages
- validating (confirming) the patient's perceptions
- adapting messages to the patient's level of understanding
- asking for feedback to ensure that the messages you sent were received by the patient or other persons as intended

 Checkpoint Question

1. What three elements must be present for communication to occur?

FORMS OF COMMUNICATION

Verbal Communication

Verbal communication involves an exchange of messages using words or language; it is the most commonly used form and is usually the initial form of communication.

You need good verbal communication skills when performing such tasks as making appointments, providing patient education, making referrals, and sharing information with other health care professionals.

Oral communication is sending or receiving messages using spoken language. As a professional, you should use a pleasant and polite manner of speaking. Use proper English and grammar at all times; lapsing into slang and colloquialisms projects an unprofessional image.

Gear your conversation to the patient's educational level. A well-educated patient may resent your using other than the correct terms, yet a less educated patient may be confused and intimidated by the same phrases. Avoid using elaborate terminology if you think it might confuse or frighten a patient. Will this patient understand "myocardial infarction," or should you say heart attack? Do not talk down to the patient, but do phrase your communication appropriately.

Be aware, too, that the meaning of spoken messages may be affected by other components of oral communication, including paralanguage and nonlanguage sounds. The cliché that it's not what you say but how you say it is true. Research shows that the primary message is transmitted more by the way it is said than by the words that are used. This refers to paralanguage. **Paralanguage** includes voice tone, quality, volume, pitch, and range. Nonlanguage sounds include laughing, sobbing, sighing, grunting, and so on. Other **nonlanguage** clues to understanding can be found in a speaker's grammatical structure, pronunciation, and general articulation, which can indicate regional or cultural background and level of education. Knowing this information can help you adapt responses and explanations to the patient's level of understanding.

Written communication uses written language to exchange messages. The ability to write clearly, concisely, and accurately is important in the health care profession. Typically, patients receive oral instructions first, as you or the health care provider explain key points of concern. These verbal instructions are then reinforced with written instructions (Box 12-1) on the next page.

If the instructions, oral or written, are not clear, the patient may misinterpret them. This misunderstanding can hinder treatment and recovery. Here is an example of unclear instruction: "Return to the office if you don't feel better." This provides the patient with no details. Clearer instructions would state, "If your fever and sore throat are not better in 24 hours, call the office to schedule a revisit." Even the most clearly outlined instructions can be misunderstood, particularly by those with deficient hearing or reading abilities. As an allied health professional, you are responsible for asking questions to verify that the patient has correctly understood the information. To verify that the patient understood these instructions, a good question to ask would be, "When should you call the office if you don't feel better?"

Box 12-1

EXAMPLE OF WRITTEN DISCHARGE INSTRUCTIONS

Main Street Pediatric Group
343 Main Street, Suite 609
Philadelphia, PA 19106

Discharge Instructions for Otitis Media

Your child has an ear infection. It is easily treated with antibiotics. Get the prescription filled immediately. The first dose should be given as soon as you arrive home. Read the attached information on the antibiotic.

Here are some other important things to remember:

• ear infections are not contagious
• symptoms usually resolve within 24 hours of beginning antibiotics. It is very important to make sure your child takes all of the prescription
• if the pain persists for more than 48 hours, call the office
• if you see any blood in the ear canal, call the office.

Make an appointment for a follow-up visit in 2 weeks.

_____   _____
Patient's signature   Physician's signature

Checkpoint Question

2. List five examples of paralanguage.

Nonverbal Communication

Nonverbal communication—exchanging messages without using words—is sometimes called body language. Body language includes several types of behaviors, such as kinesics, proxemics, and the use of touch. Kinesics refers to body movements, including facial expressions, gestures, and eye movements. A patient's face can sometimes reveal inner feelings, such as sadness, happiness, fear, or anger, that may not be mentioned explicitly during a conversation (Fig. 12-1). Gestures also carry various meanings. For instance, shrugging the shoulders can mean simple lack of interest or hopeless resignation. Eyes can often hint at what a person may be thinking or feeling. For example, a patient whose eyes wander away from you while you are talking may be impatient, lack interest, or not understand what you are saying.

Nonverbal communication may more accurately reflect a person's true feelings and attitude than verbal communication. In other words, people may say one thing but show a completely different response with their body language. For example, if the patient says, "The pain in my foot is not too bad," but the patient's face shows pain with each step, the nonverbal clues demonstrate an inconsistent message. Many patients mask their feelings, so you must learn to read their

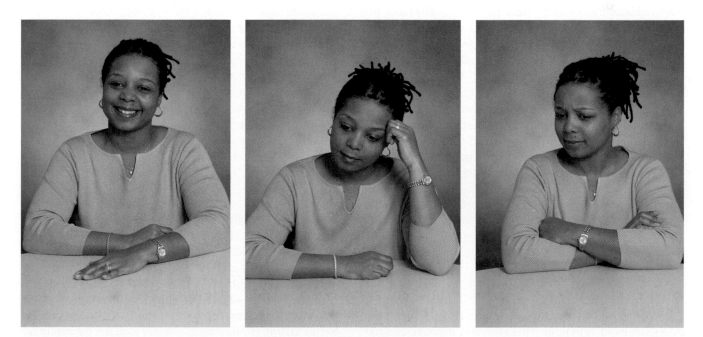

FIGURE 12-1. Different facial expressions convey different messages.

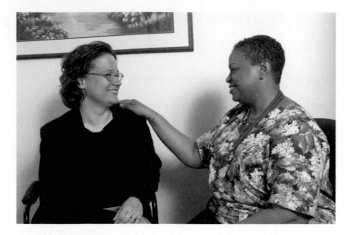

Figure 12-2. Therapeutic touch conveys caring and concern.

actions and nonverbal clues in addition to what they tell you. Be aware that patients are also acutely attuned to your facial and nonverbal reactions. Responding with an expression of disgust or shaking your head in a negative way can jeopardize communication and rapport between you and the patient.

How and where individuals physically place themselves in relation to others can affect communication as well. Proxemics refers to spatial relationships or physical proximity tolerated by humans. Generally, the area within a 3-foot radius around a person is considered personal space and is not to be invaded by strangers, although this area varies among individuals and people of various **cultures** (societies). To deliver care to a patient, an allied health professional must enter a patient's personal space. After a patient task is completed, it is appropriate to take a few steps back and allow for more space between you and the patient. **Because some individuals become uncomfortable when their space is invaded, it is essential to approach the patient in a professional manner and explain what you plan to do.** Explanations help ease patient anxiety about what will happen.

Related to proxemics is the use of touch, which can be **therapeutic** (beneficial) for some patients. It can indicate emotional support and convey concern and feeling. For some patients, however, being touched by a stranger is an uncomfortable or even a negative experience. Many patients perceive touch in a health care setting as a prelude to something unpleasant, such as an injection. To change this negative perception, try offering a comforting touch when nothing invasive or painful is imminent (Fig. 12-2). Before comforting a patient by touching, assess the patient's **demeanor** (expressions and behavior) for clues indicating that touch would be acceptable.

ACTIVE LISTENING

Active listening is important to ensure that messages are correctly received and interpreted. Failure to do so can result in poor patient care. To listen actively, you must give your full attention to the patient with whom you are speaking. Interruptions should be kept to a minimum. You need to focus not only on what is being said but also on what is being conveyed through paralanguage, body language, and other aspects of communication. Occasionally, a patient's verbal messages may seem to conflict with the nonverbal messages. For example, a patient who is wringing his hands while telling you that everything is fine is sending conflicting signals that require further exploration. If a patient's verbal response does not correspond to your observations, convey your concern to the physician.

Active listening is a skill that develops with practice. To test your listening ability, try this exercise: Ask another student to speak continuously for 1 to 2 minutes while you listen. (The student should discuss a topic with which you are unfamiliar.) When he or she finishes, wait silently for the same amount of time. Then try to repeat the message. If you have trouble doing this exercise, you need to practice listening.

INTERVIEW TECHNIQUES

As an allied health professional, you are typically responsible for gathering initial information and updating existing information about the patients. This task is accomplished by interviewing the patient. The interview will consist of you asking certain questions and then interpreting the patient's responses. The main goal is to obtain accurate and pertinent information.

To conduct an interview, you must use effective techniques: listen actively, ask the appropriate questions, and record the answers. During the interview, you must demonstrate professionalism. Begin by introducing yourself. Always conduct the interview in a private area. Know what questions you need to ask and in what order to ask them before you begin the interview. Be organized. It is also helpful to have an extra pen. And most important, do not answer phone calls or attend to other distractions until you have finished the interview. Last, when you leave the room, let patients know who will be in to see them and the approximate time, for example, "Dr. Sanchez will be in to see you in about 10 minutes."

The six interviewing techniques are reflecting, paraphrasing, clarification, asking open-ended questions, summarizing, and allowing silences.

Reflecting

Reflecting is repeating what you have heard the patient say, using open-ended statements. With this technique, you do not complete a sentence, but leave it up to the patient to do so. For example, you might say, "Mrs. Rivera, you were saying that when your back hurts you. . . ." **Reflection encourages the patient to make further comments.** It also can help bring the patient back to the subject if the conversation begins to drift. (Reflecting is a useful tool, but be careful not to overuse it, because some patients find it annoying to have their words constantly parroted back.)

Paraphrasing or Restatement

Paraphrasing or restatement means repeating what you have heard, using your own words or phrases. **Paraphrasing can help verify that you have accurately understood what was said.** It also allows patients the opportunity to clarify their thoughts or statements. Typically, a paraphrased statement begins with "You are saying that . . . ," or "It sounds as if . . . ," followed by the rephrased content.

Asking for Examples or Clarification

If you are confused about some of the information you have received, ask the patient to give an example of the situation being described. For instance, "Can you describe one of these dizzy spells?" The patient's example should help you better understand what the patient is saying. It also may give you an insight into how the patient perceives the situation.

Asking Open-Ended Questions

The best way to obtain specific information is to ask open-ended questions that require the patient to formulate an answer and elaborate on the response. Open-ended questions usually begin with what, when, or how. For example, "What medications did you take this morning?" "When did you stop taking your medication?" "How did you get that large bruise on your arm?" **Be careful about asking "why" questions, because they can often sound judgmental or accusing.** For example, asking "Why did you do that?" or "Why didn't you follow directions?" may imply to patients that you have already made a negative value judgment about their behavior, and they could become defensive and uncooperative. Instead you might ask, "What part of the instructions did you not understand?" or "How can we help you follow these instructions?"

Avoid closed-ended questions that allow the patient to answer with one word, such as yes or no. For example, suppose you ask the patient, "Are you taking your medications?" The patient can easily say yes but may not be taking all of them. However, suppose you ask, "What medications do you take every day?" The patient's answer will give you a clearer understanding of whether the patient is taking the correct medications.

Summarizing

Briefly reviewing the information you have obtained, or **summarizing**, gives the patient another chance to clarify statements or correct misinformation. This technique can also help you organize complex information or events in sequential order. For example, if the patient has been feeling dizzy and stumbling a lot, you might summarize by saying, "You told me that you have been feeling dizzy for the past 3 days and that you frequently stumble as you are walking."

Allowing Silences

Periods of silence sometimes occur during the interview. These can be beneficial. Some people are uncomfortable with prolonged silences and feel a need to break the silence with words in an effort to jump-start a stalled conversation. **Silences are natural parts of conversations and can give patients time to formulate their thoughts, reconstruct events, evaluate their feelings, or assess what has already been said.** During moments of silence, gather your thoughts and formulate any additional questions that you may have.

Checkpoint Question

3. What are the six interviewing techniques?

FACTORS AFFECTING COMMUNICATION

Sometimes, despite your best efforts, others may not receive your message accurately. A common occurrence that causes messages to be misinterpreted is the use of a cliché. For example, suppose you are teaching a patient to use crutches and she is having difficulty managing them. A cliché comment may be, "Don't worry. Rome wasn't built in a day. This takes time." The cliché is innocent and not meant to be demeaning, but the patient may misinterpret it to mean that she is slow, ancient. A more positive message would be, "I can see that you are making progress. Let's try walking down the hallway."

Here are some reasons for miscommunication:

1. The message may have been unclear or inappropriate to the situation. For example, "I have scheduled you for a PET scan in radiology tomorrow at 8 A.M." Keep in mind that most of your patients do not understand medical abbreviations and terms. Since positron emission tomography (PET) is newer technology, they may confuse it with computed tomography (CT). Also, where is radiology? A better message would be, "The doctor wants you to have a test done tomorrow. It is called a PET scan; here is a brochure that explains it. Go to the second floor of the outpatient center on Main Street. Do you know how to get there?"

2. The person receiving the message may have been distracted, anxious, or confused. A common cause of distraction is pain. For example, teaching a patient how to use crutches cannot be done if the patient's ankle or knee still hurts. The concentration will be on the pain, not on what you are saying. Patients who have just received positive news can also be anxious to contact loved ones. This is commonly seen with patients who have just been told that they are pregnant. The patient's focus is on calling family members and not on your conversation.

3. Environmental elements, such as noise or interruptions, may also distort messages. Environmental noises from staff lounges or break rooms can easily be overheard. Keep the doors to these areas closed. Cleaning staff should not be vacuuming or emptying trash while patients are present.

In addition to these three items, other factors may affect communication. They are discussed next.

Cultural Differences

The way a person perceives situations and other people is greatly influenced by cultural, social, and religious beliefs or firmly held convictions. Personal values (principles or ideals) are commonly developed from these same beliefs. As an allied health professional, you will interact with people from varied ethnic backgrounds and cultural origins who bring with them beliefs and values that may differ from your own. Understanding those differences can aid communication and thereby improve patient care. It is very important that you not form preconceived ideas about a given culture. Remember that each patient is unique and that their health care needs differ.

Some cultures may be offended by the types of intensely personal questions necessary for a patient history and may perceive them as an inexcusable invasion of privacy. If this occurs, your supervisor may be required to intervene to allay the patient's concerns.

Looking someone else directly in the eyes, or eye contact, is also perceived differently by people of various backgrounds. Eye contact occurs more often among friends and family members than among acquaintances or strangers. In the United States, someone who maintains good eye contact is usually perceived as being honest, believable, and concerned. In contrast, in some Asian and Mideastern cultures, direct eye contact is perceived as sexually suggestive or disrespectful. In other cultures, lack of eye contact or casting the eyes downward is a sign of respect.

In addition to cultural differences in values, many differences occur among individuals. Some people are just more reserved or shy than others and may feel less comfortable in health care settings. To help avoid miscommunication and offending patients, you must be sensitive to these differences in all of your patient interactions.

Stereotyping and Biased Opinions

Allied health professionals deal with people of differing ages, races, and sexual orientation. Sometimes, your values may be in stark contrast to those held by a patient, but you should not let your personal values or **bias** (opinions) affect your communication or treatment of a patient. **All patients must be treated fairly, respectfully, and with dignity, regardless of their cultural, social, or personal values.** To treat them in any other fashion is **discrimination**.

Stereotyping is holding an opinion of all members of a particular culture, race, religion, age group, or other group based on oversimplified or negative characterizations. It is a form of prejudice. Stereotyping and prejudice are deterrents to establishing therapeutic relationships because they do not allow for patients' individuality and can prevent quality care from being given to everyone on an equal basis.

As a health care professional, you are expected to treat all patients impartially, to guard against discriminatory practices, remain nonjudgmental, avoid stereotypes, and have a professional demeanor. By doing so, you communicate to patients that you accept human differences and that quality health care will be provided to all those who seek it.

Language Barriers

Effective communication depends on the use of language, but some patients cannot speak or understand English well enough for good communication. **Because it is crucial for you to give and receive accurate information, you will need to use an interpreter to help bridge any language barriers.** A staff person might serve as the interpreter, or an English-speaking member of the patient's family may be able to help. In either case, be sure the interpreter fully understands what you are saying. In the absence of a reliable interpreter, a phrase book may be of help. If your area has a large population of non–English-speaking patients, your office should be equipped with an appropriate phrase book.

When choosing an interpreter, try to find someone of the same sex as the patient, because certain cultures prohibit members of the opposite sex (even family members) from discussing personal issues about the body. Some cultures follow religious guidelines dictating how members of the opposite sex should interact with each other.

Use the following suggestions for communicating with non–English-speaking patients:

1. Do not shout. Raising your voice will not increase their understanding.
2. Demonstrate or pantomime as needed. Gestures are usually relatively universal.
3. If you are using an interpreter, speak directly to the patient, with the interpreter in your line of vision, so that the patient can read your facial expressions.
4. Speak slowly with simple sentences and phrases that require simple answers. The patient may comprehend some simple English.
5. Avoid slang; it may not translate well.
6. Avoid distractions and provide a relaxed, quiet interview space.
7. Learn some basic phrases of the most common languages used in your area. Patients appreciate your effort.

ñ *Spanish Terminology*

Hable despacio, por favor.	Please speak slowly.
Sí, hablo español un poco.	Yes, I speak Spanish a little.
No, no comprendo.	No, I don't understand.
¿Comprende?	Do you understand?
¿Cuándo?	When?
¿Qué clase?	What kind?
¿Porqué?	Why?
¿Cuántos?	How many?
¿Qué, Qué tal?	What?
¿En qué puedo ayudarlo?	What can I help you with?
¿Dígame porque esta aquí?	Tell me why you are here?
¿Cómo?	How?

WHAT IF

You need to call a hearing-impaired patient. What should you do?

Hearing-impaired patients can make and receive calls using a special telephone with a service called converse communication center, which uses a system called telecommunication device for the deaf (TDD) or a text telephone (TTY). If your office has either of these types of phones, you call the patient and type in your message. The patient reads your message and types a response. If your office does not have one of these phones, your local telephone company can communicate with TDD/TTY users and nonusers. Check your telephone directory for more information. Most hospitals have TDD/TTY phones available.

SPECIAL COMMUNICATION CHALLENGES

Many situations present special communication challenges. For instance, hearing- or sight-impaired patients, young children, patients with limited understanding, those who are too ill or sedated to comprehend, and those who are frightened or anxious require particular attention. In each instance, you will need to assess the situation and the patient's ability to comprehend. In some cases, a responsible family member will be with the patient and can be included in the communi-

cation process. Never exclude the patient from the exchange, but do ensure that all needed information is communicated, whether you obtain the information through questions about the patient's condition or you give instructions for further care. Patients must feel that they are part of the process even if their condition requires involvement by family members or other caregivers.

Hearing-Impaired Patients

There are many forms of hearing impairments. Impairments can vary from a partial loss to **anacusis**, complete hearing loss. The two types of impairments are conductive and sensorineural. Conductive hearing loss is caused by interference with sound in the external canal or the middle or inner ear. Sensorineural hearing loss is caused by lesions or problems with either nerves or the cochlea. The cochlea is a coiled tubular structure that turns vibrations into sounds. Most patients with anacusis are adept with communicating through sign language, interpreters, or other tools. However, patients with **presbyacusis**, a common hearing impairment in older patients, often have a more difficult time communicating and tend to be in denial about their hearing abilities. Patients with presbyacusis benefit from hearing aids and other amplification devices.

To communicate with patients who cannot hear what you are saying, you need tact, diplomacy, and patience. These suggestions may help.

1. Touch the patient gently to gain his or her attention.
2. Talk directly face-to-face with the patient, not at an angle and certainly not with your back turned.
3. Turn to the most prominent light so that your face is illuminated.

4. Lower the pitch of your voice, since higher pitches are frequently lost with nerve impairment, but speak distinctly and with force. In most instances, shouting does not help and will only distort what might be heard.

5. Use note pads or demonstration as needed.

6. Pictograms are very helpful and should be readily available. A pictogram is a flash card that shows basic medical terms.

7. Use short sentences with short words. Enunciate clearly but do not exaggerate your facial movements.

8. Eliminate all distractions. Extraneous noises may confuse the patient.

Checkpoint Question

4. What is the term for complete hearing loss?

Sight-Impaired Patients

Sight impairments range from complete blindness to blurred vision. The changes in vision tend to be slow and progressive. Box 12-2 has a list of conditions that can cause visual impairment. Patients who can't see lose valuable information from nonverbal communication. To improve communication with a sight impaired patient, try these suggestions.

1. Identify yourself by name each time the patient comes into the office.

2. Do not raise your voice; the patient is not hearing impaired.

3. Let the patient know exactly what you will be doing at all times and alert him or her before touching.

Box 12-2

CONDITIONS THAT CAN CAUSE VISUAL IMPAIRMENT

Below are some common conditions that can cause visual impairment:

Cataract
Hyperopia (farsightedness)
Glaucoma
Macular degeneration
Myopia (nearsightedness)
Nyctalopia (night blindness)
Presbyopia
Retinal detachment
Retinopathy
Strabismus

---

4. Orient the patient spatially by having him or her touch the table, the chair, the counter, and so forth.

5. Assist the patient by offering your arm and escorting him or her to the interview room.

6. Tell the patient when you are leaving the room and knock before entering.

7. Explain the sounds of machines to be used in the examination (e.g., buzzing, whirring) and what each machine will do.

Speech Impairments

Speech impairments can come from a variety of conditions. The medical term for difficulty with speech is **dysphasia**. Dysphasia is usually the result of a neurological problem. A common neurological condition that can result in dysphasia is a stroke. **Dysphonia** is a voice impairment that is caused by a physical condition, such as oral surgery, cancer of the tongue or voice box, or cleft palate. Stuttering is another condition that can impair the patient's ability to communicate.

Here are some suggestions to help you communicate with a patient who has a speech impediment:

- Allow such patients time to gather their thoughts.
- Allow plenty of time for them to communicate.
- Do not rush conversations.
- Offer a note pad to write questions.
- Discuss with the physician the potential benefits for getting a speech therapist referral for the patient.

Checkpoint Question

5. What is the medical term for difficulty with speech? What does dysphonia mean?

Mental Health Illnesses

Many mental illnesses and psychiatric disorders can impair a patient's ability to communicate. These illnesses produce a broad range of communication challenges. Some illnesses can lead the patient to have uncontrollable outbursts, while others can cause a mute condition in which the patient will not communicate at all. Patients may hear voices that direct their communication to a given topic, while others may see objects that do not exist and will want confirmation from you that you see the objects. Communicating with patients with moderate to severe psychiatric disorders requires in-depth training. It is important to stress that not all patients with mental illnesses will be challenges. Most mental illnesses can be controlled and treated with medications and other therapies. Here are a few suggestions for communicating with patients who have mental illnesses:

- Tell the patient what to expect and when things will happen.
- Keep conversations focused and professional.
- Do not force or demand answers from patients who are withdrawn or mute.
- If you feel unsafe communicating with a given patient, speak to your supervisor regarding your concerns.
- Do not confirm hearing voices or seeing nonexistent objects.
- Orient the patient to reality as appropriate.

Patients with a history of substance abuse, alcoholism, and other addictions can also present a communication challenge. Patients may have euphoria and communicate with a flight of ideas. Or they may demonstrate aggression and agitation while they are withdrawing from the addiction. Your responsibility in communicating with patients who have any of these conditions is to identify the reasons for the day's visit and follow your regular assessment duties. It is not the role of the allied health professional to recommend treatments or counseling for these patients. Your communication should be professional, nonjudgmental, and encouraging when appropriate.

Angry or Distressed Patients

Patients' emotions can run the spectrum from polite and cordial to angry and upset. There are numerous reasons for the latter. Prolonged waiting times, financial issues, and illness can spark untoward emotions. At some time in our lives we all have had a cold, felt terrible, and have snapped angrily at an innocent bystander. The key to communicating with upset patients is to prevent an escalation of the problem. Keep your patients informed about waiting times, billing and insurance changes, and other facility policies that might trigger untoward emotions.

It is understandable that patients will become upset on hearing sad or unfortunate news about their health. Most patients take sad news in a calm manner. It is important to offer assistance as needed. Provide written instructions and information for the patient to read later. This material should consist of information on the diagnosis, causes of the illness, treatment options, and phone numbers that the patient may call for additional information.

Here are some suggestions that will help you communicate with an angry or distressed patient:

- Be supportive.
- Be open and honest in all communication.
- Do not provide false reassurances.
- Do not belittle the problem or concern.
- Ensure your own safety if the angry patient becomes aggressive or threatening.

Children

Levels of comprehension vary greatly during childhood, and therefore communication needs must be tailored to the specific child's needs. The following suggestions will help facilitate communication:

1. Children are responsive to eye-level contact. Either raise them to your height or lower yourself to theirs.
2. Keep your voice low-pitched and gentle.
3. Make your movements slow and keep them visible. Tell children when you need to touch them.
4. Rephrase your questions until you are sure that the child understands.
5. Be prepared for the child to return to a lower developmental level for comfort during an illness. For example, a child may revert to thumb sucking during a stressful event.
6. Use play to phrase your questions and to gain the child's cooperation. (For example, if the child appears shy and does not want to talk, start by asking the child how a stuffed animal feels today. "How does Teddy feel today?" Follow up on the child's answer with "And how do you feel?" Offering to take the teddy's temperature first may lessen any fear of thermometers.
7. Allow the child to express fear, to cry, and so on.
8. Many adolescents resent authority. During the interview, some teenagers may not want a parent in the room. Assess the situation before including the parent.
9. Never show shock or judgment when dealing with adolescents; this will immediately close communication.

Communicating With a Grieving Patient or Family Member

Occasionally, you will need to support patients who are in **grief** or great sadness caused by a loss. Grieving starts when a person has a significant loss, such as the loss of a loved one through death or the loss of a relationship, a body part, or personal health. Grief includes such emotional responses as anger, sadness, and depression, and each emotion may trigger certain behaviors. For example, anger may result in outbursts, sadness may cause crying, and depression may lead to unusual quietness or isolation.

Grieving occurs in stages: denial, anger, bargaining, depression, and acceptance. Here are some examples of what a patient in denial may say: "The doctor must have read the test wrong." "I don't have cancer; I feel fine." Anger may be voiced by, "I hate the doctor." "This is a terrible place." Bargaining is a stage in which the patient or family member tries to trade off the sad news, for example, "God, I will be the best person I can be if you take away this disease." Depression is often expressed through quiet, withdrawn behaviors. The patient may state, "I don't care if I live anymore." Acceptance is the last stage. The patient may state, "I understand that I have terminal disease and am going to die." It is very important to stress that each person grieves in his or her own way and at his or her own pace. These stages may spread over months or years. It is possible to go through stages more than once. Sometimes, the collective signs of grief are referred to as **mourning**.

In health care settings, expect to see grief displayed in many ways. Know, too, that several factors can influence how a patient demonstrates grief and that different cultures and individuals demonstrate their grief in a variety of ways ranging from stoic, impassive responses to loud, prolonged wailing and fainting. Other responses may reflect religious beliefs about the meaning of death. Grieving is a unique and personal process. There is no set time period for grieving, and there is no "right" way to grieve.

Grieving patients may want to talk about their feelings and review events. Terminally ill patients may want to discuss their fears of dying and concerns for surviving loved ones. To support grieving patients, allow time for them to express themselves and actively listen to what they say. When appropriate, consider using touch to convey your understanding. If patients' concerns stem from a lack of understanding about their condition, provide pertinent education for them and for their caregivers (if appropriate). You should also become familiar with available community resources, such as

---

Box 12-3

COMMUNICATING WITH A GRIEVING FAMILY MEMBER OR PATIENT

Patients and families faced with great loss can be helped through a variety of community resources. Hospice is a national program that offers support to patients and family members dealing with a loss. Hospice deals with all types of medical conditions and with people of all ages. The earlier the patient is introduced to a hospice program, the more beneficial. Hospice does have a palliative component. Hospice staff and volunteer grief counselors are trained to answer the questions, acknowledge the fears and anger, ease the transition, and offer respite for caregivers. A patient must never be forced to join hospice or other community resources. Grieving is an individual experience. Your local hospital may also have grief counselors or social workers who can help your patients. Other community resources may be available. The knowledgeable medical assistant will, with the physician's permission, direct the patient and the family to the proper organization.

---

grief or other counseling services and hospice care, so you can suggest these services when necessary.

It is normal for you to feel sad when a patient dies. It is important that your communication focus on empathy, not sympathy. Many psychologists describe sympathy as feeling *for* someone and empathy as feeling *with* someone. In the health care setting, empathy means trying to understand what patients are feeling so you can help them. **Empathy can help you recognize a patient's fear and discomfort so you can do everything possible to provide support and reassurance.** Sympathy, or pitying your patient, may compromise your professional distance and cause you to become personally involved. Box 12-3 offers suggestions for helping grieving patients.

Checkpoint Question

6. What are the five stages of grieving?

ESTABLISHING POSITIVE PATIENT RELATIONSHIPS

Your approach to patients conveys a message about who you are and how you feel about yourself and your profession. Allied health professionals can be role models, earning the trust and admiration of patients. **To establish and maintain positive relationships with patients, speak respectfully and exhibit an appropriate demeanor during all interactions.**

Proper Form of Address

The way you address patients provides clues about your attitude and how you will likely provide care. When greeting patients, use a proper form of address, for example, "Good morning, Mr. Jones!" or "How are you feeling, Mrs. Smith?" This type of address shows respect and sets a professional tone. In contrast, calling patients by pet names, such as sweetie, granny, gramps, or honey, can offend the person. These terms denigrate the individual's dignity and put the interaction on a personal, not professional, level.

Other inappropriate forms of address include referring to the patient as a medical condition, such as "the gallbladder in room 2" or "the broken arm in the waiting room." Patients often come to the health care facility feeling anxious, so they may be particularly sensitive to everything they see and hear (or overhear). **Referring to the patient as a condition sends the message that the staff values the patient as nothing more than an illness, which can lead to heightened anxiety.**

Professional Distance

How people interact with each other is influenced by the level of emotional involvement between them. For instance, communication between a husband and wife is more intimate than the personal level of communication between friends or the social level of communication between acquaintances. In the health care setting, you must establish an appropriate level of communication to deliver direct patient care, make objective assessments, and provide quality patient teaching. You should not become too personally involved with patients because doing so may jeopardize your ability to make objective assessments. It is easy to become overattached, especially to elderly patients who are lonely. For example, do not offer to drive patients to appointments, pick up prescriptions, or do their grocery shopping. Keeping a professional distance allows you to deal objectively with patients while creating a therapeutic environment. To keep this distance, avoid revealing intimate information about yourself (e.g., marital woes, financial troubles, family conflict) that might shift the dynamics of the relationship to a more personal level. Often, in an attempt to help a patient, we might say, "My grandmother was diagnosed with cancer too, but she is fine; it's not a big deal. You will be okay too." Every situation is different. The patient may misinterpret this to mean that you don't think that his or her diagnosis of cancer is a big deal. But at that moment it is a very big deal to the patient!

TEACHING PATIENTS

One of the fundamental communication skills you will need is the ability to teach patients about their conditions. Teaching patients might involve something as relatively simple as explaining how often they should take a medication or instructing a newly diagnosed diabetic patient about self-injection. The guidelines listed below incorporate such key communication skills as interviewing and active listening. Follow these to provide effective patient education.

1. Be knowledgeable about current health care issues, discoveries, and trends.
2. Be aware of special services available in your area.
3. Have pertinent handouts or information sheets available.
4. Allow enough teaching time so that you are not interrupted or rushed.
5. Find a quiet room away from the main office flow if at all possible.
6. Give information in a clear, concise, sequential manner; provide written instructions as a follow-up.
7. Allow the patient time to assimilate this new information.
8. Encourage the patient to ask questions.
9. Ask questions in a way that will allow you to know whether the patient understands the material.
10. Invite the patient to call the office with additional questions that may arise.

ETHICAL TIPS

All patient communication is confidential. Patient information is sometimes discussed unintentionally, however. To avoid breaching confidentiality, follow these guidelines:

- Do not discuss patients' problems in public places, such as elevators or parking lots. A patient's friends or family members might overhear your conversation and misinterpret what is said.
- The glass window between the waiting room and the reception desk should be kept closed.
- Watch the volume of your voice.
- When calling coworkers over the office intercom, do not use a patient's name or reveal other information. Avoid saying something like, "Bob Smith is on the phone and wants to know if his strep throat culture came back." Instead, say "There's a patient on line 1."
- Before going home, destroy any slips of paper in your uniform pockets that contain patient information (e.g., reminder notes from verbal reports).

PROFESSIONAL COMMUNICATION

Communicating With Peers

Communication among your peers must remain professional and appropriate throughout the workday. Discussions of non–work-related topics should be kept to a minimum and occur only during designated break times. It is not appropriate to discuss last night's TV shows, arguments with boyfriends, shopping lists, and so on in front of patients. Excessive laughing, high-pitched voice tones, and whispering can produce an unprofessional atmosphere.

During your career, you may come across a situation that requires communication with your supervisor about another peer's actions. Your communication must always be honest and accurate when reporting facts to a supervisor. Embellishing or hiding information can result in termination of your employment.

An excellent way to promote communication among your peers is to become active in your local professional organization. Your involvement at the local level can spread to national exposure. Involvement in local community organizations and support groups is also beneficial to promoting you and your profession.

Communicating With Other Facilities

The facility staff often makes referrals to other facilities or doctors. Box 12-4 has examples of various referrals you might make. No matter whom you are contacting, follow these key points:

- Patient confidentiality is always foremost. Make sure you have appropriate patient consent.
- Observe all legal requirements for dispensing patient data.
- Use caution with fax machines, e-mail, and other electronic devices. Make sure the intended receiver is the one who gets the communication.
- Provide only the facts. Do not relay suspicions or assumptions.
- Always be nonjudgmental.
- Confirm that the message was received and that the referral will be handled.

Box 12-4

TYPES OF REFERRALS

Numerous types of referrals can be made. Here are some of the most common examples:

Cardiac rehabilitation
Diabetes education
Dietitian
Home care services
Laboratory studies
Occupational therapy
Physician specialties (cardiologist, pulmonologist, podiatrist)
Physical therapy
Psychotherapy
Radiology
Social worker
Speech therapy

Procedure 12-1

Recognizing and Responding to Verbal Communications

Equipment/Supplies: Paper, writing utensil.

Steps

1. Identify possible communication barriers, and obtain resources to help overcome these barriers.

2. Begin the interview by properly greeting and addressing the patient.

3. Begin the conversation with an open-ended question.

4. Ask for clarification or examples as needed.

5. Allow time for thought formation (for yourself and the patient).

6. Paraphrase what the patient is saying to help clarify their message.

7. Watch for and identify any paralanguage and nonverbal cues that may indicate incongruence with the verbal message.

8. Ask closed-ended questions to get specific information.

9. Summarize the interview for the patient and ask if there is anything else you need to discuss.

10. Terminate the interview once you have satisfactorily discussed all of the patient's concerns.

Procedure 12-2

Recognizing and Responding to Nonverbal Communications

Equipment/Supplies: Paper, writing utensil.

Steps

1. Be aware of the nonverbal cues that you are conveying to the patient. Use your body language and facial expressions to show care and concern for the patient.

2. Identify the nonverbal communication cues that the patient is conveying.

3. Ask appropriate questions to help verify your assumption.

4. If the nonverbal cues do not correspond with the verbal message, convey your concern to the physician.

SUMMARY

Communication is a complex and dynamic process involving the sending and receiving of messages. It includes verbal and nonverbal forms of expression and is influenced by personal and societal values, individual beliefs, and cultural orientation. In a health care facility, important aspects of patient communication are interviewing and active listening. You will need to overcome many communication challenges to communicate with all patients. These challenges include patients with hearing, sight, and speech impairments. Children, or angry or distressed patients, and patients with mental illnesses can also present a challenge to communication. To communicate effectively, you must understand the various factors that can affect the exchange of messages and use the communication techniques that are most appropriate for each individual situation.

Critical Thinking Challenges

1. List five common clichés. Then select one and draw a picture illustrating how it may be misinterpreted.
2. List five local resources that can assist a grieving patient or family member. Include the name of the agency, type of help that it offers, any special information, and its phone number.

Answers to Checkpoint Questions

1. For communication to occur, these three elements must be present: a message to be sent, a person to send the message, and a person to receive the message.

2. Voice tone, quality, volume, pitch, and range are five examples of paralanguage.
3. When interviewing patients, you can use six different techniques. These include reflecting, paraphrasing or restatement, asking for examples or clarification, asking open-ended questions, summarizing, and allowing silences.
4. The medical term for complete hearing loss is anacusis.
5. The medical term for difficulty with speech is dysphasia. Dysphonia is a voice impairment.
6. The five stages of grieving are denial, anger, bargaining, depression, and acceptance.

 ## Websites

Here are some websites that can give you some additional information:

National Institute of Deafness and Other Communication Disorders
    www.nidcd.nih.gov
American Speech-Language-Hearing Association
    www.asha.org
Hearing, Speech and Deafness Center
    www.hsdc.org
National Hospice and Palliative Care Organization
    www.nhpco.org

13

Patient Education

CHAPTER OBJECTIVES

In this chapter, you'll learn:

1. To spell and define the key terms.
2. To explain the allied health professional's role in patient education.
3. To define the five steps in the patient education process.
4. To identify five conditions that are needed for patient education to occur.
5. To explain Maslow's hierarchy of human needs.
6. To list five factors that may hinder patient education and at least two methods to compensate for each of these factors.
7. To discuss five preventive medicine guidelines that you should teach your patients.
8. To explain the kinds of information that should be included in patient teaching about medication therapy.
9. To identify the components of a healthy diet, and explain how to use a food guide pyramid.
10. To explain the importance of teaching range-of-motion exercises to patients.
11. To explain your role in teaching patients about alternative medicine therapies.
12. To list and explain relaxation techniques that you can teach patients to help with stress management.
13. To list three national organizations that can help patients with smoking cessation.
14. To identify a national organization that can assist patients with treating alcoholism.
15. To describe how to prepare a teaching plan.
16. To list potential sources of patient education materials.

KEY TERMS

alternative	detoxification	learning objectives	planning
assessment	documentation	noncompliance	psychomotor
carbohydrates	evaluation	nutrition	range-of-motion
coping mechanisms	implementation	placebo	stress

EDUCATING PATIENTS ABOUT HEALTH care issues will be one of your most challenging and rewarding roles as an allied health professional. Of course, you will not be responsible for teaching patients everything they need to know about health care. Patient education will likely be performed under the direction of your supervisor. The amount and types of education that you will be expected to do will vary greatly depending on your facility. This chapter will give you the foundation needed for providing patient education.

THE PATIENT EDUCATION PROCESS

Patient education involves more than telling patients which medications they need to take or which lifestyle behaviors they need to change and expecting them to follow these instructions blindly. To educate patients effectively, you need to help them accept their illness, involve them in the process of gaining knowledge, and provide positive reinforcement. Ultimately, that knowledge should lead to a change in behavior or attitudes.

The process of patient education involves five major steps:

- Assessment
- Planning
- Implementation
- Evaluation
- Documentation

These five steps collectively produce the teaching plan. The plan may be formally written as the process is occurring or may be documented after the event. You must follow all these steps to achieve effective patient education.

Assessment

Before you begin to teach, you must assess your feelings and attitudes about the patient and the topic to be taught. Sometime in your career as an allied health professional, you may encounter situations or patients that make you feel uncomfortable. Your role as an educator, however, requires that you set aside your own personal feelings and life experiences to instruct the patient objectively and to the best of your ability. Always consider how your responses and actions will affect the patient and be sure to treat each patient impartially.

Assessment requires gathering information about the patient's present health care needs and abilities. In addition to knowing the present health care needs, you must also look at these other areas:

- Past medical and surgical conditions
- Current understanding and acceptance of health problems
- Need for additional information
- Feelings about their health care status
- Factors that may hinder learning (covered in detail later in the chapter)

You may obtain this information from a number of sources. The most comprehensive source will be the health record. The patient's health record consists of all information regarding current diagnoses, treatments, medications, past medical history, and a variety of other documentation. Most health records have a problem list on the inside cover. This will provide you with a snapshot of the patient and save you time from reading the entire document. Other sources of information will be the doctor, family members, significant others, and other members of the health care team. When you have collected all of the assessment data, you are ready to start the next step of the education process: planning.

 Checkpoint Question

1. What is the purpose of the assessment step during patient education?

Planning

Planning involves using the information you have gathered during the assessment phase to determine how you will approach the patient's learning needs. If possible, involve the patient in this part of the process. Learning goals and objectives that are established with input from the patient are most meaningful. A patient's learning goal is what the patient and educator want to be the outcome of the program. The patient's **learning objectives** include procedures or tasks that will be discussed or performed at various points in the program to help achieve the goal. Make certain the objectives you establish are specific for each individual patient and are measurable in some manner. If the objectives are measurable, you will be able to evaluate when or whether the patient successfully completed them.

For example, consider a patient who needs to limit his fluid intake. Which of the following objectives is more specific and would allow you to evaluate the patient's progress: (1) the patient understands why he should limit his fluid intake, or (2) the patient is able to prepare a schedule for daily fluid intake and explain why it is important that he limits his fluids? The second objective is more specific and not only evaluates the patient's understanding but also requires the patient to demonstrate understanding. Having patients prepare their own schedule gets them involved in their health care. It allows them to customize the schedule to fit their lifestyle, which is likely to increase compliance.

Implementation

After you establish the need for patient teaching and agree on the goals and objectives, you begin implementation. **Implementation** is the process used to perform the actual teaching. The teaching usually is carried out in several steps. Box 13-1 presents some commonly used teaching strategies. For example, you may start by telling the patient how to use crutches, followed by a demonstration, and finally, the

Box 13-1

IMPLEMENTATION STRATEGIES

Implementing the learning process should be individualized to the patient's best method of comprehension and retention. These may include:

1. *Lecture and demonstration.* This method presents the information in the most basic form but requires no patient participation for reinforcement and retention.
2. *Role playing and demonstration.* The patient watches you perform a medical procedure, then performs it to ensure understanding. Information is more likely to be recalled if the patient actively participates in the process.
3. *Discussion.* This two-way exchange of information and ideas works well for lifestyle changes (e.g., making dietary changes to lower cholesterol) rather than for medical procedures.
4. *Audiovisual material.* Audiocassettes or videos can often be taken home and reviewed by the patient and family members as needed. This allows for reinforcement of teachings and provides both visual and auditory stimulation.
5. *Printed material and programmed instructions.* All information should be discussed with the patient to clarify points and to elicit questions before assuming that the instructions are understood.

patient may do a return demonstration. Patients also benefit from the use of teaching aids (drawings, charts, graphs, pamphlets) that they can take home and use as reference material. You can also use videos and audiocassettes to supplement the implementation process.

Miscommunication or misinterpretation can lead to serious complications or injury. For example, assume you are teaching a patient to use crutches. It is very important that you stress to the patient that the crutch must not press directly into the axilliary area. (There should be a two-finger distance between the crutch and the armpit.) If the patient does not comprehend the dangers of nerve damage to the axillary area from pressing the crutch into the armpit, a serious complication to the patient could occur. Miscommunication about medications can have fatal consequences.

The implementation stage may occur once or over a longer period. The disease process and the patient's ability to comprehend information will dictate the length of teaching. For example, teaching a patient about diabetes takes place over multiple sessions. The first session may focus on what diabetes is, while subsequent teachings may include topics such as diet, foot care, glucose monitoring, and insulin injection.

After implementation of a given skill or knowledge, you must determine whether your teaching was effective. This step is called evaluation.

Evaluation

Is the patient progressing? Did the teaching plan work? Does the plan need any changes? These are a few of the questions you may ask yourself when you begin to evaluate. **Evaluation** is the process that indicates how well patients are adapting or applying new information to their lives.

In the medical setting, where contact with patients is limited, part of the evaluation may have to be done by patients at home. For example, if facility visits for direct observation are not scheduled, patients will be responsible for telephoning and reporting their status. In other words, can patients do the task they were taught, or are they having troubles? If they voice concern or appear unclear about their instructions, you should either redirect them on the phone or schedule them for an office appointment.

During the evaluation, you may discover noncompliance. **Noncompliance** is the patient's inability or refusal to follow a prescribed order. After determining that the given order is not being followed, your first step is to determine why the order is not being followed. It may be a misunderstanding. For example, a patient who is to take a certain medication twice a day may be taking it only twice a week because that is what he or she thought you said. If the noncompliance is because the patient refuses to follow these orders, however, you must notify the physician. Remember that the patient has the right to refuse medical treatment unless the patient is determined to be mentally incompetent. A doctor will determine the next appropriate action in these cases. Evaluation is an ongoing process, so you should expect to update and modify your plan periodically.

 Checkpoint Question

2. What is the purpose of evaluation during patient education?

Documentation

Documentation includes recording of all teachings that have occurred. It should consist of the following information:

- Date and time of teaching.
- What information was taught, e.g., "Diabetes foot care was discussed. It consisted of the proper method for toenail cutting and regular examination by a podiatrist."
- How the information was taught, e.g., "ADA [American Diabetes Association] foot care video shown to the patient."
- Evaluation of teaching. For example, "Patient verbalized the need to make an appointment with a podiatrist."

Box 13-2

CHARTING EXAMPLE

11/27/04

    Patient arrived in the office for teaching on the glucose meter; brought meter from home. Following steps were demonstrated by me: calibration of meter strips, battery change, finger sticks, strip insertion into machine, use of the patient logbook. Normal BGM ranges were reviewed along with the treatment of low blood sugar. Pt. returned demonstration without problem. Reviewed glucose meter instructions manual with pt. Pt. instructed to bring logbook to each MD appointment.—Bea Zame, CMA

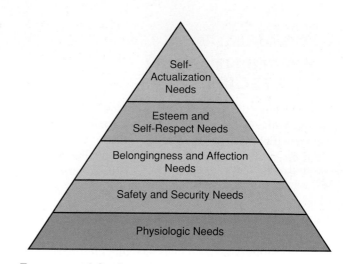

FIGURE 13-1.   Maslow's hierarchy pyramid.

- Any additional teaching planned, e.g., "Patient will return on Monday to the office with his wife for glucose monitoring instructions."

Box 13-2 has a charting example for patient education.

Your signature implies that you performed the teaching. If this is untrue or if another staff member assisted you in teaching, make sure that information is clearly noted. Also include the names of any interpreters who were used.

You must also document all telephone conversations, e.g., "I spoke with this patient via the telephone today and he said he is testing his blood sugar every morning without problem."

Documentation is essential because from a legal viewpoint, procedures are only considered to have been done if they are recorded.

CONDITIONS NEEDED FOR PATIENT EDUCATION

Learning is the process of acquiring knowledge, wisdom, or skills through study or instruction. This process does not occur without certain conditions. Learning cannot occur without motivation or a perceived need to learn. For example, suppose you want to teach a patient about the need to adopt a low-sodium diet because of hypertension. Patients who feel that hypertension is not a problem, however, will not be motivated to learn the diet because they have not accepted the need for the teaching. For such patients to be taught, the following steps must occur:

1. The patient must accept that the hypertension has to be managed.
2. The patient must accept that there is a correlation between high sodium intake and hypertension.
3. The patient must accept and be willing to make this dietary change.

Only then can teaching begin.

    In addition to patient motivation, basic human needs must be met first.

Maslow's Hierarchy of Needs

Abraham Maslow, an American psychiatrist, recognized that people are motivated by needs and that certain basic needs must be met before people can progress to higher needs, such as taking personal responsibility for their health (self-actualization). Maslow arranged human needs in the form of a pyramid, with basic needs at the bottom and the higher needs at the top (Fig. 13-1). The patient progresses upward, fulfilling different levels of needs toward the highest level, which results in a state of health and well-being. In your responsibility as an educator, you need to be aware that patients must have the basic needs satisfied before they are willing or able to learn to take care of their own health. Not everyone will start at the bottom of the pyramid. Some patients will never reach the top, while others may be at the top and slide backward as a result of unfortunate circumstances.

Physiologic needs are air, water, food, rest, and comfort. If these basic needs are unmet, the patient cannot begin the process. Everyone has a different tolerance and expectation for these needs. For example, one person may expect that their food is served over three meals with full courses, while another person may accept that they will have one meal a day from a soup kitchen. If the patient perceives that these needs are met, we need to accept that and not judge the situation.

Safety and security needs include a safe environment and freedom from fear and anxiety. Patients are susceptible to fear and anxiety that accompany many medical conditions. For example, patients diagnosed with cancer may be so frightened that they are unable to think of anything but dying. Patients who have undergone some sort of trauma or disaster (hurricane, fire, motor vehicle accident) may place the need to feel safe above all other needs.

Affection needs, or the need for love and belonging, are essential for feeling connected and important to others. A sense of love or belonging can often be a powerful motivation for patients to try to regain good health.

Esteem needs involve our need to feel self-worth. Esteem can be self-generated, or it can come from those who admire us. If others value us or if we value ourselves, we are more likely to strive to maintain good health. Patients who lack self-esteem are less likely to want or accept education that targets improving their health. Thus, they will not see this as important information and will not be motivated to learn.

Self-actualization is the pinnacle of the pyramid, at which a person has satisfied all the other basic needs and feels personal responsibility and control over his or her own life. Self-actualized patients will strive to control their state of wellness by following all health directives and may even help others to achieve wellness. Not all patients will reach this level. Patients who have met this level will be ready to learn a multitude of health care skills and will strive to follow preventive health care maintenance guidelines.

After determining where on the pyramid the patient is, you can determine the appropriateness of education. For example, if the patient has not met the basic physiologic needs, you should help the patient meet these needs before beginning to teach. Patients who are in the middle levels may be able to focus and learn certain skills but may not be ready for complex teachings. If possible, you should involve family members or significant others in the teaching process.

Checkpoint Question

3. What are the basic physiologic needs outlined in Maslow's pyramid?

Environment

The environment where you teach must be conducive to learning. The room should be quiet and well lit and have limited distractions. It is not appropriate to teach patients a skill in a hallway, waiting room, or other high-traffic area. These areas produce distractions and prohibit confidentiality. For patients to acquire knowledge, they must feel relaxed and comfortable.

Equipment

A common type of education is teaching patients to perform a **psychomotor** skill. A psychomotor skill requires the participant to physically perform a task. Some examples include crutch walking, glucose monitoring, eyedrop instillation, and dressing changes. The equipment for the skill must be present and functional. If possible, the equipment should be from the patient's home or be the exact replica of it.

The steps to teach a psychomotor skill are as follows:

1. Demonstrate the entire skill.
2. Demonstrate the skill step by step, explaining each step as you complete it.
3. Have the patient demonstrate the skill with your help.
4. Have the patient demonstrate the skill without your help.

Provide positive reinforcement throughout the steps. Always provide written step-by-step instructions along with the equipment. Always include instructions on maintenance of the equipment.

Knowledge

The person teaching the skill must have a solid knowledge of the material. Imagine how difficult it would be to learn to ski from an instructor who did not know how to put skis on. The same is true in allied health. If you are not comfortable or do not feel knowledgeable about the topic, ask for help before starting to teach a patient. Be reassured that you do not have to be an expert on the topic, but you do need to feel comfortable with the information. If you start teaching a given topic and the patient asks you a question that you are not able to answer, state that you are not sure about that specific piece but you will get the answer. Then either research the answer or ask for help from another health care professional. Never guess or imply that you know something that you do not know.

Resources

For patient education to be effective, it must consist of multiple techniques or approaches. The more techniques that are used, the more the patient will learn and retain. The three ways that we can learn are through hearing, seeing, and touch. If you can apply at least two of these senses in your teaching, your patient will be more stimulated to learn and will learn more information. For example, if you were teaching a patient about the dangers of smoking, which of the following would be more effective: (1) giving the patient a pamphlet that explains the dangers of smoking along with statistical data, or (2) showing a patient a diagram of how what a nonsmoker's lung looks like versus a smoker's and providing the patient with pamphlets about local smoking cessation programs? The teaching in the second approach would be more beneficial. The patient sees and hears the dangers of smoking and receives a brochure that contains practical hands-on information. Box 13-3 on the next page lists types of resources that you can use to help you teach patients.

In addition to the five conditions already discussed, these factors will be necessary for the patient to learn:

- Family or significant others should be present if the information is complex or if it will require their assistance. Family members are essential if the patient is confused or unreliable.

Box 13-3

TEACHING RESOURCES

Here are some teaching tools that you can use to help teach patients:

Audiocassettes	Models (heart, lungs)
Compact discs	Plastic food settings
Food labels	Pamphlets
Internet and websites	Videos
Manikins	

- Patients should be wearing any sensory devices that they need (glasses, hearing aids).
- Qualified interpreters should be present if needed.

FACTORS THAT CAN HINDER EDUCATION

Many factors or circumstances can hinder learning. It is important to recognize these factors and intervene as appropriate. In certain cases, teaching may have to be delayed, or your teaching plan may have to be revised.

Existing Illnesses

The type of illness that patients have will play a large role in their ability and willingness to learn. Generally, patients with acute short-term illnesses will be motivated to learn a skill that will accelerate healing. Examples of short-term illnesses are orthopedic injuries (uncomplicated fractures, sprains), colds, and viruses.

These are six examples of illnesses or conditions that will affect learning:

- *Any illness in which the patient has moderate to severe pain.* Examples of these illnesses include neuropathies, bone cancer, kidney stones, and recent surgical procedures. The patient's pain level must reach a tolerable stage before teaching can start and the patient can concentrate on learning.
- *Any illness or condition with a poor prognosis or limited rehabilitation potential.* Examples include progressive neurologic disorders, certain cancers, and large traumatic events. It is important that you assess such patients' readiness to learn and their level of acceptance of their illness before you proceed with your teaching.
- *Any illness or condition that results in weakness and general malaise as a primary symptom.* Examples include gastrointestinal disorders that cause vomiting and diarrhea, anemia, Lyme disease, and recent blood transfusion. For these patients, teaching should be lim-

ited to the essential information and expanded on as the patient regains strength.

- *Any illness or condition that impairs the patient's mental health or cognitive abilities.* Examples of these conditions include brain tumors, Alzheimer's disease, substance abuse, and psychiatric disorders. In these patients, education should be provided to patients at their ability level. Family members or significant others should be brought in to complement the learning process.
- *Any patient who has more than one chronic illness.* For example, patients with diabetes often have cardiac, renal, and integumentary complications. In patients with multiple system failures, it is important to prioritize the learning needs. Focus your education on the main problem and work from there.
- *Any illness or condition that results in respiratory distress or difficult breathing.* Examples of these conditions include chronic obstructive pulmonary disease, pneumonias, lung cancer, and asthma. The priority goal is first to establish optimal oxygenation for the patient. Once this is met, you can begin teaching. These patients tend to become exhausted easily during acute exacerbations of their illnesses. Keep the teaching time short and to the point and expand teachings as their activity tolerance allows.

 Checkpoint Question

4. List six types of conditions or illnesses that may hinder your ability to educate patients effectively.

Communication Barriers

Effective communication skills are essential for patient education. Any barriers to communication must be resolved before you can start teaching the patient. If an interpreter is needed for language translation or for hearing-impaired patients, schedule a time convenient to all parties.

Age

The age of the patient plays a very important part in the amount and type of education that you can do. Small children need to be educated at an age-appropriate level. For example, it would be inappropriate to teach a 2-year-old child how to assemble an asthma nebulizer. The parent or caregiver must be taught. It would be appropriate, however, to explain to the 2-year-old that the nebulizer is not a toy and that it contains medication. Safety education is a prime teaching focus for small children and their parents. Box 13-4 presents some tips for communicating with and teaching children.

As children mature at different speeds, you should assess what information this child can handle and what information should not be shared with the child. Communication with the

Box 13-4

TIPS FOR TEACHING CHILDREN

Children require special communication skills and different teaching strategies. Here are a few tips to help you:

- Encourage the child to be part of the teaching process.
- Speak directly to the child.
- Avoid confusing medical terms.
- Avoid using baby language.
- Teach only age-appropriate information.
- Discuss with the parents the child's knowledge base about the illness and any feelings the parent may have regarding what they want the child to know. (This should not be done in front of the child.)
- Demonstrate skills on stuffed animals or dolls.

parents is essential. They know the child's developmental stage. For example, a 7-year-old child who has just been diagnosed with diabetes needs to know the signs and symptoms of low blood sugar and how to treat it. The child may not be ready, however, to learn about the long-term complications (e.g., blindness, renal failure). It is important to teach the child that the disease must be well controlled to prevent future problems, but not to the extent that the child develops fear.

The challenge in teaching adults is that they often have multiple responsibilities to their children, spouses, or aging parents. Obligations at work, school, church, and other activities may also limit their free time. These obligations and responsibilities can interfere with willingness to learn and attentiveness. Your teaching may have to occur in short sessions over long periods. This age group may benefit from electronic resources that they can access on their own time schedule.

Elderly patients can be a challenge to teach for a variety of reasons. These reasons include confusion, lack of interest, and overall poor health. Some older patients, however, can be the most attentive and curious learners. It is fairly common for this age group to address items that they have heard on the news. For example, a patient may hear an advertisement for a new medication and request clarification from you regarding its effectiveness.

 Checkpoint Question

5. What is the primary teaching focus for small children and their parents?

Educational Background

Most initial health assessment forms ask patients what level of education they have obtained. This information may help you to determine the patient's ability to read. Caution is essential, because graduation alone does not guarantee that the patient can read. You will need to use your tact and diplomacy to evaluate the situation.

Patients who have completed some college courses, however, are likely to be interested in preventive health care. Patients with an educational background in health care will still need the same attention and teaching from you. Do not assume that since the patient is a nurse or a doctor, you can skip teaching a skill. Their specialty may be in an unrelated area.

Physical Impairments

Numerous physical impairments may hinder learning. For example, patients with severe arthritis in their hands may have difficulty performing certain psychomotor skills, like giving themselves insulin. An occupational therapist is the best resource for assistance.

Other Factors

Other factors may hinder your ability to teach patients. The patient's culture may affect willingness to learn or the family's involvement in learning. Patients with financial troubles may not be ready to focus on learning new skills or knowledge. It is important that you assess the patient's readiness to learn and remove any obstacles that may be present.

TEACHING SPECIFIC HEALTH CARE TOPICS

Your role in patient education will vary greatly. The topics that you will teach will depend on the patient and type of facility.

Preventive Medicine

Preventing health problems is the key to living a long, healthy life. But the advantages to good preventive medicine extend much further. There are huge economical benefits to preventing illnesses. According to the American Hospital Association, approximately 34 million people are hospitalized each year. Caring for sick patients at home costs Medicare $200 billion annually. These statistics affect everyone. They lead to higher taxes, higher health insurance premiums, and limited programs for low-income families.

These are some commonly recommended preventive health care tips that you should teach all of your patients:

- Regular physical examinations for all age groups
- Annual flu and regular pneumonia vaccinations
- Adult immunizations for tetanus and hepatitis B
- Childhood immunizations
- Regular dental examinations
- Monthly breast self-examinations for women and regular physician examinations

- Mammograms on a regular basis for certain groups of women
- Annual Papanicolaou tests
- Prostate-specific antigen blood tests for all men, along with need for regular digital rectal examinations

The frequency and age at which these procedures will be recommended to patients vary with the patient's medical history and genetics and the physician's preference. Some insurance will pay for these procedures, while others will not pay unless the procedure is deemed diagnostic. Many hospitals and clinics offer free preventive screenings to patients. Your facility may have a list of which free screenings are available. Public health departments may also have this information available for your patients.

Another large part of preventive medicine is teaching safety tips. Preventable injury is the leading cause of death in persons aged 1 to 21. Approximately 25% of children will require at least one emergency room visit for treatment of a preventable accident during their childhood. Preventable injuries can arise from bicycle and car accidents, poisoning, fires, choking, falls, drownings, firearms, and lawn mowers. Toys can lead to injuries when they are broken or used by a child of an inappropriate age. The American Academy of Pediatrics offers injury prevention tips for parents and health care providers. You will find valuable teaching tips to give to parents from their website. The AAP also provides numerous educational materials that can be mailed to physician offices and given to your patients.

One in three adults over age 65 will fall. These falls account for most of the 340,000 patients who are admitted to hospitals each year for hip fractures. Hip fractures require long hospitalizations and often rehabilitation in a nursing home. Most falls occur at home and are preventable. Fall prevention tips should be taught to all older patients or any patient who has a problem with maintaining balance or uses an ambulation device (cane, walker). Here are some tips that you can use to teach fall prevention:

- Encourage the patient to remove all scatter rugs in their home. Remind patients to keep hallways clutter free.
- Instruct the patient to ensure adequate lighting in all rooms and hallways.
- Encourage the patient to avoid steps. Encourage one-floor living.
- Ensure that the patient has well-soled shoes or sneakers. Advise the patient to avoid wearing heels.
- Instruct the patient to place nonskid surfaces in bathtubs or purchase a shower chair.
- Instruct the patient to install handrails or grab bars in hallways and stairwells.
- Encourage smoke detector installation and remind the patient to change the batteries twice a year.
- Advise patients taking medications that lower their blood pressure to stand up slowly and get their balance, then begin to walk.

- Advise patients to have regular eye examinations and have their glasses adjusted as needed.
- Encourage patients to have a plan for power outages and severe storms.

 Checkpoint Question

6. Which patients should you teach fall prevention tips?

Medications

With the increasing number of medications available, the possibilities for teaching patients in this area are virtually endless. Pharmaceutical companies offer in-depth medication information for health care providers and patients concerning the chemical makeup of the drug, physiologic reactions in the body, prescribed dosage and route, and possible side effects. This information comes from the pharmaceutical companies either by mail or from the sales support team. In addition, some of this information will come in package inserts. If this information is not available, the patient may not understand the importance of the medication therapy, and this could lead to noncompliance, drug interactions, or other serious side effects. You may be responsible for gathering the information needed and preparing teaching materials for your patients to help prevent such complications.

When preparing a medication therapy teaching tool, you must consider such factors as the patient's financial abilities, social or cultural demands, physical disabilities, and age. Be sure to include the following information in any teaching:

- Medication name (generic or brand)
- Dosage
- Route
- What the medication is for
- Why the medication must be taken as prescribed
- Possible changes in bodily functions (e.g., colored urine)
- Possible side effects
- Other medications (including over-the-counter ones) that might interfere with the action of this medication
- Foods or liquids to be avoided
- Activities to be avoided
- Telephone number to call for any questions or concerns

Figure 13-2 on the next page shows a medication therapy teaching tool that incorporates all of these elements.

Medication teaching should also include any over-the-counter medications the patient is taking. This information should consist of the same items listed above. Many patients have the misconception that over-the-counter medications (e.g., aspirin, ibuprofen, cough syrup) are 100% safe and no dangers are associated with them. Some of these medications may interact with their prescribed medications.

Medication Therapy Teaching Tool

Trade name/Brand name: _____

Circle the one that applies:
Take by mouth   Apply to affected area   Drop into ear
Insert rectally   Place under tongue   Insert vaginally
Drop in eye   Other _____

The dosage of this medication is:
This medication was ordered for you because:
It may cause:
You should not take this medication if:
If you notice any of the following, you should call Dr. Smith's office at 555-1111.

The above information has been explained to me, and I understand the importance of following the prescribed treatment.

_____   _____
(patient's signature)   (date)

_____
(signature of person teaching patient)

FIGURE 13-2. Medication therapy teaching tool.

After assessing patients' understanding of all of their medications, you may find that scheduling is a prime concern. For example, the patient may be taking several types of medications at different times of the day or week. Before developing a medication schedule, evaluate the patient's daily routine to see how adhering to the schedule may affect the patient's lifestyle. For instance, you might ask the patient:

- How late do you sleep each morning?
- What time do you go to bed?
- When do you usually eat?

Once you have collected this information, you can create a scheduling tool to serve as a reminder to the patient about what medications to take when. Pillboxes can also help to remind patients to take their medication. Pillboxes are plastic containers prelabeled with the days of the week and times. You may instruct the patient in how to fill them. Pillboxes are sold in most pharmacies.

Another patient education area that falls under the category of medication therapy includes how to administer medications—orally, vaginally, rectally, and so on.

For more patient teaching information regarding safe and effective use of medications, you can contact the National Council on Patient Information and Education (NCPIE), a nonprofit organization, at 666 Eleventh Street, NW, Suite 810, Washington, DC 20001. NCPIE can provide you with literature and referrals to other sources.

Nutrition

Patients seen in the medical office have numerous reasons for being concerned about their nutrition. **Nutrition** is focused not only on what people consume but also on how the body uses the food it ingests to maintain and repair itself. Everyone needs to understand nutrition, not just people who are ill. People often turn to the medical profession to sort through the large amount of media hype pertaining to diets that bombards them each day. Whether the information pertains to the values of fast food or fad diets to lose weight, the media should not be the only source of guidelines for your patients. Materials are available to help you instruct patients about healthy eating.

Here are a few basic facts that you can teach all patients:

- There are no quick fixes to weight loss.
- Moderation is key. Total elimination of favorites (chips, ice cream, candy) is not necessary.
- A good dinner or meal will consist of a rainbow of colors.
- Limit salt and sodium intake.
- Eat three balanced meals a day.
- Avoid eating at least 2 hours before going to bed.
- Drink plenty of water. Avoid excessive soda and caffeine ingestion.

The Food Guide Pyramid

The U.S. Department of Agriculture (USDA) has developed a basic food group system and the Food Guide Pyramid (Fig. 13-3 on the next page). The pyramid consists of five main food group categories and one "other" category:

1. Bread, cereal, grains, and pasta
2. Vegetables
3. Fruits
4. Milk, yogurt, and cheese (dairy)
5. Meat, poultry, fish, dry beans, eggs, and nuts (protein)
6. Fats, oils, sweets (other)

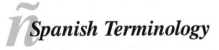

Ñ Spanish Terminology

Tres veces al día.	Three times a day.
Antes/después de las comidas.	Before/after meals.
Al acostarse.	At bedtime.
Tómela con la comida.	Take this with food.
Dele la medicina cada cuatro horas.	Give him the medicine every 4 hours.

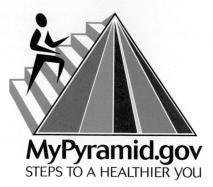

FIGURE 13-3. General food pyramid.

Next are listed some teaching tips for each of these categories.

Bread, Cereal, Grains, and Pasta

- Eat darker breads; avoid white. Avoid croissants, biscuits, sweet rolls, and pastries.
- The best cereals are oat, bran, and whole grain cereal. Avoid frosted or sweet types.
- Graham crackers, melba toast, and saltines are good cracker choices. Avoid cheese and butter crackers.
- Pasta and rice in limited portions are fine, but avoid the sauces.

Vegetables and Fruits

- Fresh or frozen is the best. Avoid dried fruits.
- Eat vegetables without butter or cream sauces.
- Limit boiling time for vegetables to prevent draining out the nutrients.

Milk, Yogurt, and Cheese

- Milk: skim or 1%. Avoid creams and buttermilks.
- Yogurt: low fat or nonfat.
- Eat low-fat cheeses, 1% or 2% cottage cheese.

Meat, Poultry, and Fish

- Use USDA-select grade beef. Avoid beef with large amounts of marbling (indicates fat).
- Limit bacon to small serving sizes and limit its frequency.
- Fish should be fresh. Cook unbreaded and avoid sauces.

Fat, Oil, and Sweets

- Use oil sparingly.
- Avoid mayonnaise and salad dressings (unless low fat).
- Low-fat snacks: air-popped popcorn, pretzels, and rice cakes are good choices.

In addition to the traditional food pyramid, the USDA has formed a variety of other pyramids to meet the needs of various groups. There is a special pyramid for children aged 2

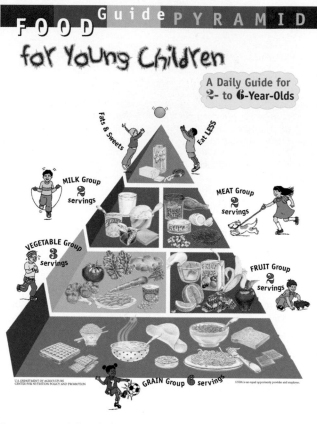

FIGURE 13-4. Food guide pyramid for children.

to 6 (Fig. 13-4). This pyramid is visually appealing to children and provides parents with realistic serving size portions. The pyramid for people over age 70 focuses on the nutritional needs of older patients. A variety of ethnic pyramids have also been created to meet the needs of various cultures. For example, the Mediterranean diet pyramid (Fig. 13-5 on the next page) varies in its recommended daily servings of the basic food groups. When you are teaching nutritional guidelines, provide the patient with a copy of the appropriate pyramid. Copies of pyramids can be obtained from the USDA website.

Checkpoint Question

7. What are the five main food groups listed in the USDA pyramids?

Dietary Guidelines

The USDA and U.S. Department of Health and Human Services also have guidelines to help improve our diets:

1. Eat a variety of foods from each of the five food groups.
2. Maintain a healthy weight by balancing the food you eat with physical activity.
3. Choose a diet low in fat, saturated fat, and cholesterol.

ñ Spanish Terminology

¿Qué comidas le gustan?	What foods do you like?
De dos a cuatro porciones de leche.	Two to four servings of milk.
De dos a tres porciones de carne, pescado o aves de corral.	Two to three servings of meat, fish, poultry.
De tres a cinco porciones de vegetales.	Three to five servings of vegetables.
Pan de trigo y cereales.	Wheat bread and cereals.

4. Choose a diet with plenty of vegetables, fruits, and grain products.
5. Use sugar and salt (sodium) in moderation.
6. Drink alcoholic beverages in moderation.

Encourage patients to read the labels on food containers; these labels provide important information on the nutritional value of the food, specific ingredients used, or any additives. All information on labels is based on the portion size. If you eat double the portion, you will need to double the nutritional facts. The serving size is at the top of the label. Below the serving size is the number of servings per container.

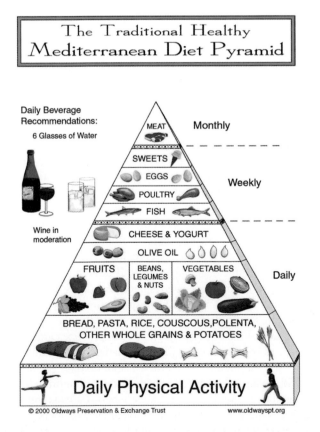

FIGURE 13-5. Food guide pyramid for a Mediterranean diet.

Total fat will be the first nutritional fact listed. This will give you the total grams of fat in a serving. The average diet consists of 2000 calories per day. On a 2000-calorie diet, the maximum grams of fat per day should be less than 65, with less than 20 g of saturated fat. Teach patients to add their total grams of fat per day. The label will list a percentage number as well. The percentage refers to what percent of the daily allowed fat is contained in one serving. Most patients find it easier to add up their total grams ingested. Explain that an item may be fat free or low fat but not healthy. Food manufacturers often add extra **carbohydrates** to low-fat foods to give them extra flavor and taste.

Total carbohydrates is the next fact listed on labels that patients should understand. This number tells the patient how many carbohydrates are in each serving. Carbohydrates are the prime energy source for our bodies. Carbohydrates are turned into sugar in the body. The unused portion of sugar is stored as fat. Based on a 2000-calorie diet, the total carbohydrates per day should not exceed 300 g. Again, patients should add their total carbohydrate intake for 24 hours. It is essential that patients with diabetes learn to count carbohydrates.

Sodium, cholesterol, and protein facts are also listed on food labels. Large fast food chains, like McDonald's and Dunkin' Donuts, will have this information available at each of their stores. Patients should be encouraged to read this information.

In certain foods it is easy to determine the serving size. The label may say two cookies or one slice of bread. In other cases, however, it may be more difficult. Generally, serving sizes are listed in ounces. Here is a simple way to teach measuring: A thumb equals 1 ounce, the palm equals 3 ounces, a handful is 2 ounces, and a fist is approximately 1 cup.

After discussing healthy foods, give patients information about healthy food preparation. Here are a few guidelines on how to prepare healthy foods that you can teach your patients:

- Encourage patients to broil, boil, bake, roast, or grill.
- Trim the fat off of beef.
- Use a cooking rack so that fat drips away from the meat.
- Remove the skin from chicken. Use caution with raw chicken. Wash hands and cutting surfaces immediately.

Box 13-5

CALCIUM TEACHING TIPS

Calcium is an essential mineral in everyone's diet. Here are a few teaching tips that you can your patients:

- Calcium keeps the bones and teeth strong. It is also necessary for muscle contraction and blood clotting.
- Calcium supplements are highly recommended for all women to prevent osteoporosis.
- Calcium is found in milk, yogurt, cheese, ice cream, dried beans, broccoli, and kale. Also, it can be added to cereals and some energy bars.
- Vegetables should be boiled in the least amount of water and for the shortest time to ensure nutrients are not lost.
- Daily recommended dosage is based on age: Children 1–3 should get 500 mg/day; children 4–8 should get 800 mg/day; children 9–18 should get 1200–1500 mg/day; adults should get 1000 mg/day; and people over age 50 are recommended to get 1200 mg/day.
- Supplements can come in pills, chewable tablets, or antacids.
- Calcium carbonate should be taken with meals. Vitamin D is needed to absorb calcium into the body.

- Homemade soups or gravies should be cooked, then chilled. Skim the fat off and then reheat.
- Use unsaturated oils (canola, corn, safflower). Use nonstick spray when possible. Avoid saturated oils (butter, lard).

Patients may ask you about vegetarian diets. There are three types of vegetarian diets. Lacto-ovovegetarian means that a diet of vegetables is supplemented with milk, eggs, and cheese. Lactovegetarian means the diet is supplemented only with milk and cheese; pure vegetarian is only vegetables and excludes all foods of animal origin. It is possible to eat healthy and obtain necessary nutrients with all three vegetarian diets. The USDA has created a vegetarian pyramid that will provide necessary education to your patients regarding serving sizes and meal planning.

Patients may ask you about vitamin and mineral supplements. If the patient maintains an appropriately balanced diet, adequate vitamins and minerals will be included in the foods consumed. A daily multipurpose vitamin can offer many benefits to patients. A common mineral supplement that patients are urged to take is calcium. Box 13-5 presents some important teaching tips on calcium supplements.

As with any patient teaching, you must consider many factors before sending the patient home with a preprinted diet form. The patient's age, culture, religion, geographic background, and social and financial circumstances may influence how well the patient complies with the diet modification. If necessary, the physician may refer the patient to a registered dietitian for in-depth nutritional education. Patients with diabetes, heart disease, and eating disorders are generally referred to dietitians. Remember to check your patient's progress during each return visit.

Exercise

Exercise is an activity using muscles, voluntary or otherwise, that helps maintain fitness. It is beneficial to the body for several reasons. If done in moderation, exercise can help relieve stress, maintain healthy body weight, and increase circulation and muscle tone. All patients should actively participate in some form of exercise on a regular basis. Box 13-6 on the next page discusses some common myths associated with exercising.

Patients who are under age 35 and in good health usually do not need a medical clearance before starting a routine exercise program. A physician consultation is recommended, however, for patients aged 35 or older who have not been active in several years. Patients with known medical disorders (e.g., hypertension, cardiovascular problems, or a family history of strokes) should check with the physician before exercising. Pregnant patients should consult their obstetrician prior to starting an exercise program.

The American Heart Association (AHA) offers information on exercise. The AHA has numerous frequently updated pamphlets available on various exercise activities and

WHAT IF

A patient asks you about "crash" or "fad" diets. What should you say?

Patients often want to try fad diets, but they need to be taught about the potential dangers of these diets. Fad diets are advertised as "quick weight loss" fixes. These diets require precise meal plans and adherence to unhealthy portions and food selections. They are not balanced to meet all food group requirements. Most plans are targeted to a specific food, such as the grapefruit diet. Some of these diet plans can produce cardiac, renal, and digestive complications. Patients who want to lose weight should be instructed about eating regular small, balanced meals, counting calories, monitoring fat intake, and reading food package labels. Patients must also be taught that diet modification alone will not result in a significant long-term weight loss; regular exercise must also be included in any weight reduction plan.

Box 13-6

MYTHS ABOUT EXERCISE

Here are some common myths about exercising that you can correct for your patients:

- "No pain, no gain." Patients should be instructed never to exercise to the point of exhaustion and pain. This can produce serious musculoskeletal injuries and cardiac complications.
- "I'm too old to exercise." Exercising at any age can help improve muscle tone, maintain joint flexibility, and prevent injuries.
- "Weight lifting is a man's sport." Weight lifting has been proved to help with weight reduction and limit the progression of osteoporosis.
- "The only good exercise is aerobic." Although aerobic exercise has many cardiovascular benefits, it can also lead to joint injuries. A combination of weight training, strength and resistance training, and a moderate aerobic workout is often most beneficial.

---

programs such as swimming, running, jogging, walking, and biking. Pamphlets cover the following information:

- Benefits of the specific exercise
- How to get started
- How to choose a time to exercise
- How to choose a partner
- What clothing is best suited for the exercise
- How to warm up
- What a target heart rate zone is and how to achieve it
- Training program
- Calories used
- Checklist (a review of highlights from all of the above topics)

After physician clearance (if needed), you should review the information on the pamphlets with the patients. Answer any questions and document the teaching. Patients should be able to take the information in the AHA pamphlets and continue exercising on their own.

If patients are unable to perform exercises without assistance, it may be necessary to instruct them or their family members on **range-of-motion** (ROM) exercises. To perform ROM exercises, the patient moves the affected limb and joint through all of the movements that the joint is capable of making, until resistance is met. In most cases, ROM exercises are ordered by the physician to prevent further loss of motion or disfigurement after a musculoskeletal injury, surgery, or neurological damage.

When a stroke or other type of paralyzing injury is involved, ROM exercises are performed several times a day on each involved joint. If the patient is unable to perform the exercise on the affected area, passive ROM is per-

formed. This requires someone else to perform the exercises on the patient. Remember, ROM exercises are needed to promote circulation and maintain muscle tone. If they are not performed as ordered, the patient may not be able to regain use of the affected area. Patients with significant loss of motor skills will often be referred to physical therapy or occupational therapy for intense ROM teachings.

 Checkpoint Question

8. Why is teaching range-of-motion (ROM) exercises important?

Alternative Medicine

Many ancient remedies that were once considered voodoo and dismissed by Western medicine have proven to be beneficial. Approximately $300 billion a year is spent on **alternative** medicine, and surveys have shown that about 50% of all Americans have used some form of unconventional medicine. In 1998, a federal agency was created to evaluate and monitor alternative medicine therapies. The name of the agency is National Center for Complementary and Alternative Medicine (NCCAM). The NCCAM also conducts clinical trials and training programs for practitioners of alternative medicine.

There are numerous types of alternative medicine therapies. Below is a discussion of four of the most common therapies.

Acupuncture

Acupuncture is one of the oldest forms of Chinese medicine. Acupuncture works on the principle that there are 2,000 acupuncture points in the human body. These 2,000 points are connected throughout the body by 12 pathways called meridians. The meridians conduct energy, or qi, in the body when they are triggered. The trigger comes in the form of a needle. When the meridian is stimulated, it prompts the brain to release certain chemicals and hormones.

Acupuncture is primarily used to treat addictions, fibromyalgia, osteoarthritis, asthma, and chronic back pain. It is sometimes used in treating children with attention-deficit/hyperactivity disorder.

In 1996, the Federal Drug Administration (FDA) required that all acupuncture needles be labeled single use. Only 40 states require that acupuncturists be licensed to practice. Training requirements vary among states.

Acupressure

Acupressure is a similar practice except that it does not use needles. The practitioner applies pressure to the meridians through direct touch. This method has shown great success in treating nausea and vomiting associated with chemotherapy. Some hospitals and clinics offer acupressure on an outpatient basis to cancer patients. Studies have shown that acupressure may help alleviate chronic pains and may even boost the immune system. Requirements for licensure and training vary among states.

Hypnosis

Hypnosis is portrayed on television as a magical method for reaching the inner workings of the brain. There is proof, however, that when conducted properly, it may provide some health care benefits. It is primarily used for weight reduction, for treatment of obsessive-compulsive disorders, and for smoking cessation. The training requirements vary greatly from state to state, and in most areas licensure is not required.

Yoga

Yoga has proved to be very beneficial for relieving stress and improving flexibility. Yoga consists of a comprehensive discipline of physical exercise, posture, breathing exercises, and meditation. There are a variety of types of yoga. Iyengar consists of motionless poses that emphasize posture and form. Once this method is learned, patients are able to practice this at home. This method may help patients who are recovering from injuries. Bikram consists of 26 poses that are conducted at 100°F. This method promotes muscle relaxation and stretching. Perspiration is thought to help cleanse the body of various toxins. Sivananda is a 5-step system that focuses on breathing exercises, relaxation, diet, and meditation.

Herbal Supplements

The use of herbal supplements is a multibillion-dollar business in the United States. The general public views herbal supplements as "natural," hence safe. This is a misconception. Herbal supplements, vitamins, and similar substances are not regulated by the FDA. The patient or consumer must understand that since there has been no formal government testing or approval of these substances, their dosages, side effects, interactions, and possible benefits are unclear. A classic example of an herbal supplement that has been shown to have dangerous side effects is ephedrine. This supplement was once thought to be the weight-loss miracle. It can, however, cause heart attacks and strokes. The FDA has issued many warnings about ephedrine and its dangers.

Furthermore, since these products are not regulated, there is no guarantee that what the label claims is in the bottle is actually there. The quality and the purity of the herbal supplements have been shown to vary greatly from manufacturer to manufacturer. Patients should be advised to purchase only supplements that are stamped with a U.S. Pharmacopeia bar code. This bar code means that the manufacture site has met certain standards for distribution but does not mean that the supplement has been tested for health care benefits. Box 13-7 provides some general teaching tips for any patient using an herbal supplement.

Box 13-7

GENERAL TEACHING TIPS FOR HERBAL SUPPLEMENTS

Here are a few general teaching points on herbal supplements:

- Explain to patients the importance of always telling the physician or other health care provider about any herbal supplements that they are taking.
- Explain to patients that the fact that a product is "natural" does not mean it is safe. A good example is mushrooms. All mushrooms are natural, but some are very poisonous.
- Teach patients the importance of looking for the USP (United States Pharmacopeia) label. Teach patients to look for expiration dates on all supplements.
- Advise patients not to ask health store clerks for information on supplements but to speak to physicians or pharmacists.
- Advise patients to distrust advertisements that use words like magical or breakthrough or that claim to detoxify the whole body.
- Instruct patients to stop taking all herbal supplements at least 2 weeks prior to surgery and to tell their surgeon what supplement they have been using and how long. (Some supplements can increase bleeding time.)
- Warn diabetic patients that many supplements will interfere with blood sugar levels.
- Advise parents to avoid giving herbal supplements to their children unless approved by a physician.
- Advise pregnant or breast-feeding patients to consult with a pharmacist or physician before taking any supplements.

Some of these substances have evolved through folklore, various cultures, or clinical research. In some cases, there is an element of **placebo** action involved. Placebo is the power of believing that something will make you better when there is no chemical reaction that warrants such improvement. Other supplements actually have scientific studies to document their effects. Table 13-1 on the next page lists some commonly used herbal supplements and their reported benefits.

Your role as an allied health professional may require you to assess whether patients are using any alternative therapies. Your assessment should include the length of time they have used these treatments and any side effects or benefits that the patient has noted. Patients should be advised to verify the training and credentials of the practitioner they are using and to ascertain that the practitioner is appropriately licensed. Patients should be encouraged to look at the NCCAM website for safety updates and for more detailed information

Table 13-1 HERBAL SUPPLEMENTS^a

Supplement	Reported Benefits
Alfalfa	Relief from arthritis pain; strength
Anise	Relief of dry cough; treatment of flatulence
Black cohosh root	Relief of premenstrual symptoms; rheumatoid arthritis
Camomile	Treatment of migraines, gastric cramps
Cholestin	Lowers cholesterol and triglycerides
Echinacea	Treatment of colds; stimulates immune system; attacks viruses
Garlic	Treatment of colds; diuretic; prevention of cardiac diseases
Ginkgo	Increased blood flow to brain; treatment of Alzheimer's disease
Ginseng	Mood elevator, antihypertensive
Glucosamine	Treats arthritis symptoms; improves joint mobility
Kava	Treatment of anxiety, restlessness; tranquilizer
Licorice	Soothes coughs, treats chronic fatigue syndrome
St. John's wort	Treats depression, premenstrual symptoms; antiviral

^a This table lists some commonly used herbal supplements and their reported benefits. Research is an ongoing process to document these findings. Some of these herbal supplements may have side effects or may interact with prescribed medications.

about alternative medicine. You should never recommend that a patient start taking herbal supplements or other alterative medicine therapies without a doctor's approval.

Checkpoint Question

9. What is a placebo?

Stress Management

Everyone is affected by an illness or injury at some time. Along with this often comes stress. **Stress** can come from forces such as fear, anger, anxiety, crisis, and joy. The stress may produce physiologic changes as well as psychologic effects. When faced with illness or injury, a patient usually must confront:

- Physical pain
- Inability to perform self-care
- Stress of treatments, procedures, and possible hospitalization
- Changes in role identity and self-image
- Loss of control and independence
- Changes in relationships with friends and family

Patients with chronic conditions may need more time to adjust than patients with acute illnesses. If patients are able to deal with stress factors, they are more likely to adapt and adjust to lifestyle changes.

Many other causes besides illness or injury can place patients under stress. The best way to cope with stress is by living a healthy lifestyle. When the body is healthy, it can handle stress more easily. Unfortunately, most of the reasons that hinder learning are the same factors that hinder patients' ability to comply with patient education.

Positive and Negative Stress

Two types of stress affect all of us daily: positive stress and negative stress. Positive stress motivates individuals to work efficiently and perform to the best of their abilities. Examples of positive stress include working on a challenging new job or assignment, getting married, and giving a speech or performance. In fact, many people work best under positive stress. Under positive stress the brain releases chemicals that increase the heart rate and breathing capacity. The body also releases stored glucose that gives an energy boost. Once the job (or wedding) is over, though, time must be taken to relax and prepare for the next project. If relaxation techniques are not incorporated into the daily routine, positive stress can become negative stress.

Negative stress is the inability to relax after a stressful encounter. Left unchecked, it can lead to such physiologic responses as

- Headache
- Nausea, diarrhea
- Sweating palms

- Insomnia
- Malaise
- Rapid heart rate

Long-term physical effects of unrelieved stress include increases in blood pressure, glucose levels, metabolism, intraocular pressure, and finally exhaustion. There is also an increased risk of heart attack, stroke, diabetes, certain cancers, and immune system failure. If the stress is not relieved, patients will progress to higher anxiety levels and will require all of their energy and attention to focus solely on the problem at hand. Most mental and physical activity will be directed at relief of the stress to avoid the ultimate anxiety level known as panic—a sudden, overwhelming state of anxiety or terror.

Most people have developed methods of alleviating intense stressors called **coping mechanisms**, which are usually beyond our conscious ability to direct. Coping mechanisms are a psychologic defense against unpleasant situations. Some common coping mechanisms are repression, denial, and rationalization.

It may be difficult to escape completely from stress-causing factors, but management of them is possible. For a patient suffering from the physiologic effects of negative stress, you can offer the following coping strategies:

- Encourage patients to attempt to reduce stressors, but emphasize that it is not possible to remove all stressors. Warn them to avoid attempting to make everything perfect; perfectionism adds its own stress.
- Encourage patients to organize and limit activities as needed.
- Try to lessen patients' fear of failure so they just do the best they can.
- When they are feeling anxious, encourage them to talk to someone about their problems and let off steam.

Any one of these tips may help patients to regain control over stressors. In addition, a number of relaxation techniques described in the following sections may help.

Relaxation Techniques

Patients can use any of several types of relaxation techniques. To determine what works best for them, they must first consider how much time they have and what type of relaxation they need. Next are three examples of relaxation techniques.

Breathing techniques.   Breathing exercises can be done anywhere. Most people are shallow breathers and need to be instructed on deep-breathing techniques. To perform these breathing exercises, the patient should sit up straight with hands placed on the stomach and take a deep breath in through the nose, feeling the hands being pushed away by the stomach. (This may feel awkward because most people do just the opposite.) The patient holds the breath for a few

seconds, then exhales through pursed lips as the hands are felt being pulled in. This exercise allows for good control of the rate of exhalation. Sometimes, getting the oxygen flowing through the body at a faster rate is all that is needed to relieve boredom, tension, and stress.

Visualization.   Visualization is a relaxation technique that involves allowing the mind to wander and the imagination to run free and focus on positive and relaxing situations. It is similar to daydreaming. It can "remove" the patient from a stressful situation and put him or her in a place where, if nothing else, the mind can relax. Instruct the patient to find a quiet place, close the eyes, and then visualize a soothing scene. Sometimes, background music helps. Remind the patient that it is important to choose appropriate times for this daydreaming technique. For example, it would be dangerous to use this technique when driving a car or operating heavy equipment.

Physical exercise.   There is no better tranquilizer than physical exercise. Most people who exercise regularly say that it helps them reduce tension, relax, and rest better at night.

Smoking Cessation

The health risks associated with smoking have been well documented for many years. Nicotine is highly addictive whether ingested by inhaling or chewing. This drug reaches the brain in 6 seconds, damages the blood vessels, decreases heart strength, and is associated with many cancers. The withdrawal symptoms include anxiety, progressive restlessness, irritability, and sleep disturbances. There are numerous methods to try to stop smoking. The methods vary greatly. Some programs have the patient gradually stop, while other programs seek a total, abrupt stoppage. There is research data to support both methods.

Here are some suggestions to help patients stop smoking:

- Find local smoking cessation support groups. Provide phone numbers and contact names of these groups to your patients.
- If you do not have a local connection, the American Heart Association, American Lung Association, or American Cancer Society may help. Websites are provided at the end of this chapter.
- Encourage patients to discuss options of prescription patches, gums, or other interventions. Some products have side effects, and the physician may opt not to order them based on the patient's age or other medical illnesses.

Substance Abuse

Substance abuse is excessive use of and dependency on drugs. Some abused substances are legal (e.g., alcohol, nicotine), whereas others are illegal (e.g., marijuana, cocaine). Patients affected by commonly abused substances usually work with trained specialists or counselors. Substance abuse can be highly detrimental to your patients' health, so it is important that you give them information about substance abuse if they should ask. This information may come from various national organizations. You should have information available for patients on any local chapters or organizations that may help these patients. Following is a brief outline of abused drugs and some of the consequences of using them.

Alcohol is the most commonly abused drug in our society. Alcohol is chemically classified as a mind-altering substance because it contains ethanol, which has the chemical power to depress the action of the central nervous system. This depression affects motor coordination, speech, and vision. In large amounts, alcohol can affect respiration and heart rate. The long-term effects of excessive alcohol use are liver failure, certain cancers, strokes, and nutritional deficiencies.

Alcoholics Anonymous (AA) was founded in 1935 and has approximately 2 million members. It is the leading organization in treating alcoholism. The success of the AA program is based on the patient's completion of a 12-step program. Recovering alcoholics provide many of the support services. AA has numerous chapters and support services throughout the country for both the patient and the family. There are also special services for teenage alcoholics.

Marijuana and hashish impair short-term memory and comprehension. They alter the user's sense of time and reduce the ability to perform tasks requiring concentration and coordination. They also increase the heart rate and appetite. Long-term users may develop psychologic dependence. Because these drugs are inhaled as unfiltered smoke, users take in more cancer-causing agents and do more damage to the respiratory system than with regular filtered tobacco smoke.

Cocaine and crack cocaine stimulate the central nervous system and are extremely addictive. Crack cocaine is particularly dangerous because this pure form of cocaine is usually smoked and absorbed rapidly in the bloodstream. It can cause sudden death. Use of cocaine can cause psychologic and physical dependency. Side effects include dilated pupils, increased pulse rate, elevated blood pressure, insomnia, loss of appetite, paranoia, and seizures. It can also cause death by disrupting the brain's control of the heart and respiration.

Stimulants and amphetamines can have the same effect as cocaine, causing increased heart rate and blood pressure. Symptoms of stimulant use include dizziness, sleeplessness, and anxiety; these substances can cause psychosis, hallucinations, paranoia, and even physical collapse. The long-term effects of these substances include hypertension, heart disease, stroke, and renal and liver failure.

Depressants and barbiturates can cause physical and psychologic dependence. Abuse of these drugs can lead to respiratory depression, coma, and death, especially when they are taken with alcohol. Withdrawal can lead to restlessness, insomnia, convulsions, and death.

Hallucinogens such as lysergic acid diethylamide (LSD), phencyclidine ("angel dust" or PCP), mescaline, and peyote all interrupt brain messages that control the intellect and keep instincts in check. Large doses can produce seizures, coma, and heart and lung failure. Chronic users complain of persistent memory problems and speech difficulties for up to a year after discontinuing use. Because hallucinogens stop the brain's pain sensors, drug experiences may result in severe self-inflicted injuries.

Narcotics such as heroin, codeine, morphine, and opium are addictive drugs. These drugs can produce euphoria, drowsiness, and blood pressure and pulse fluctuations. An overdose can lead to seizures, coma, cardiac arrest, and death.

Any of these substances can impair a fetus's health. Two such common illnesses are fetal alcohol syndrome and infant cocaine dependency. You will learn more about these conditions in the clinical portion of your program. It is important to teach all pregnant women the damage substance abuse may do to their unborn child and to refer pregnant patients to support services.

Patients with a substance abuse problem may require **detoxification** before counseling. Detoxification is the process of clearing drugs out of the patient's body and treating the withdrawal symptoms. This process varies with the type of substance, length of abusing the substance, and the patient's overall health. In certain cases, hospitalization will be needed.

The most important role of the allied health professional in educating patients about any type of substance abuse is to be supportive. Provide positive reinforcement as appropriate. Offer services to patients for cessation programs. Never condemn a patient for not seeking help. Always be nonjudgmental.

Checkpoint Question

10. What is the most commonly abused drug in our society? What does the term detoxification mean?

PATIENT TEACHING PLANS

Developing a Plan

You may often find yourself teaching without a written plan. To ensure that teaching is done logically, always use the education process to help you formulate a plan in your mind. Also remember to document in the patient's record whatever teaching you perform and the patient's response.

Many facilities use preprinted teaching plans for common problem areas, such as "Controlling Diabetes," "Living With Multiple Sclerosis," and "Coping With Hearing Loss." Although these save time, they are not individualized to the patient. If you use preprinted teaching plans, be sure to adapt them to your particular patient's learning needs and abilities.

If preprinted plans are not an option, consult teaching plan resource books, which contain the necessary information in outline form. You can take the plans from these sources and transfer them as needed to your facility-approved teaching plan format, adding your own comments to fit the patient's needs.

All teaching plans, no matter what the design, should contain the following elements:

- *Learning goal.* A description of what the patient should learn from implementation of the teaching plan.
- *Material to be covered.* All major topics to be discussed.
- *Learning objectives.* Steps or procedures the patient must understand or demonstrate to accomplish the learning goal.
- *Evaluation.* Appraisal of the patient's progress.
- *Comments.* Remarks concerning circumstances that may be preventing successful completion of the objectives.

Teaching plans must also include an area for documenting when the information was presented to the patient and when the patient successfully completed each objective. Figure 13-6 is an example of a teaching plan.

Selecting and Adapting Teaching Material

An enormous amount of teaching material is available. Although your facility may select much of the material you will use, you may be responsible for selecting some teaching aids. Assess your patients' general level of understanding to choose materials appropriately. When using preprinted material, consider the format, headings, illustrations, vocabulary, and writing style for overall clarity and readability. Also, ensure that the information provided on commercial materials is truthful and in agreement with the policies and procedures of your facility. A good rule of thumb is to use commercial material only from nationally recognized organizations or government agencies.

Teaching Plan: 32-year-old female with Iron Deficiency Anemia
Patient Learning Goal: Increase patient's knowledge of Iron Deficiency Anemia, its complications and treatments
Material to be Covered: Description of disorder, complications, diet, medications, procedures

Learning Objectives Comments	Teaching Methods/Tools	Procedure Explained/Demonstrated Date/Initial	PT Demonstrated/ Objectives Met Date/Initial
1. Patient describes what happens when body's demand for oxygen is not met. a. oxygen and hgb concentration decrease b. signs/symptoms of anemia c. anemia occurs only after body stores of iron are depleted	Instruction		
2. Patient describes complications caused by decrease of oxygen concentration a. chronic fatigue b. dyspnea c. inability to concentrate, think d. decrease in tissue repair e. increase of infection f. increase in heart rate	Instruction		
3. Patient discusses importance of diet in prevention of iron deficiency anemia a. including iron-rich foods in diet (beef, poultry, green vegetables) b. including foods that contain ascorbic acid to assist in absorbing iron in body (fruits) c. importance of limiting large meals if fatigued; stress importance of several small meals	Instruction/Video: "Your Diet: Why It Is Important"		
4. Patient describes prescribed medication, its purpose, dosage, route, and side effects	Instruction/Pamphlet: *Taking Your Iron Supplements*		
5. Patient aware of importance of follow-up appointments for evaluation of prescribed plan of treatment	Instruction/Appointment slip with next scheduled appointment		

FIGURE 13-6. Teaching plan.

Many patient education textbooks are available in the library, local bookstores, or through the Internet. Many of these sources list addresses for other patient education materials available from companies or associations. These materials commonly include printed items as well as videos, audiocassettes, and compact discs.

Developing Your Own Material

Sometimes, you may need to create your own teaching materials. Review available resources and teaching aids and adapt the information to benefit your patients. When developing teaching material, remember to do the following:

- Indicate the objective of the information.
- Personalize the information so the patient wants to learn.
- Make sure information is clear and well organized.

- Use lists and outlines, which are easier to read and remember than paragraphs.
- Avoid medical jargon as much as possible.
- Focus on the key points.
- Select appropriate printing type.
- Use diagrams that are simple, clear, and well labeled.
- Include the names and telephone numbers of people or organizations that patients can call with further questions or concerns.

After patients have been using the material for a while, periodically evaluate its effectiveness and modify your teaching plan as needed.

Not all of the patient teaching materials you create will have to be in print form. Patients must be motivated to read, but many will be more receptive to audiovisual instruction. Take advantage of any opportunity to develop teaching materials in other media.

Procedure 13-1

Identifying Community Resources

Equipment/Supplies: Paper, writing utensil, access to local community resource book, telephone book, or internet.

Steps

1. Locate a support group for patients needing help with alcohol or drug abuse and determine the contact information, services provided, hours of operation, associated fees, location and frequency of meetings, and any other pertinent information.

2. Locate a support group for cancer patients and determine the contact information, services provided, hours of operation, associated fees, location and frequency of meetings, and any other pertinent information.

3. Locate a food delivery program for home-bound patients and determine the contact information, services provided, hours of operation, associated fees, location and frequency of meals, and any other pertinent information.

4. Locate area homeless shelters and determine the contact information, location, services provided, hours of operation, associated fees, and any other pertinent information.

5. Locate financial resources for patients who do not have insurance or have financial problems affecting their ability to get appropriate medical care and determine the contact information, location, services provided, hours of operation, and any other pertinent information.

SUMMARY

Your role in teaching depends on the setting in which you work. Some facilities hire professional staff to teach patients. If that is the case in your facility, your teaching role may be limited. Even so, never pass up an opportunity to teach. Encourage patients to ask questions. Always provide a telephone number that patients can call if they have additional information. Periodically check to ensure that your teaching has been effective.

Remember, do not overstep your role as an allied health professional. The teaching you provide should clarify and complement information provided by the physician. A well-planned patient education program helps ensure that patients receive the high-quality health care they deserve.

Critical Thinking Challenges

1. Look at the Maslow's hierarchy pyramid. What level are you on? What steps can you take to reach the self-actualization level? If you are at that level, what steps can you take to ensure that you remain there?
2. Keep track of all of the food that you consume over a 24-hour period. Calculate your total fat and total carbohydrate intake. Do your meals follow the general food pyramid? If not, what do you need to do to improve your nutritional status? Using pictures from magazines, create well-balanced breakfast, lunch, and dinner plates. Hint: your plate should have many colors in the rainbow.
3. Review the list of information that you should teach patients about their medications. Choose two medications, herbal supplements, or vitamins that you have taken. (The medication can be over-the-counter or prescribed.) Using all available resources, write the information for these two medications or supplements.
4. Review the material on fall prevention and preventing childhood injuries. Make a checklist of at least 10 safety tips for both groups. Take your list and visit your neighbor's home. Review these tips with your neighbor. What safety improvements or recommendations were you able to provide?
5. Make a list of preprinted educational materials that every office should have. What professional organizations (e.g., American Heart Association, American Cancer Society) could help provide these materials?

Answers to Checkpoint Questions

1. The purpose of the assessment step in teaching patients is to allow you to gather information about the patient's health care needs and abilities.
2. The purpose of the evaluation step in teaching patients is to allow you to determine how well patients are adapting or applying the new information to their lives.
3. The basic physiologic needs are for air, food, water, rest, and comfort.
4. Six types of conditions or illnesses that may hinder patients' ability to learn effectively are illnesses with moderate to severe pain; illnesses with a poor prognosis or limited rehabilitation; illnesses resulting in weakness or general malaise as a primary symptom; illnesses that impair the patient's mental health or cognitive ability; more than one chronic illness; illnesses that result in respiratory distress or difficulty in breathing.
5. The primary teaching focus for small children and their parents is safety and injury prevention.
6. Any patient who has trouble maintaining balance or uses an ambulation device should be taught fall prevention tips.
7. The five major food groups are bread, cereals, grains, pasta; vegetables; fruits; meat, poultry, fish; and milk, yogurt, cheese.
8. It is important to teach ROM exercises to patients to prevent further loss of motion or disfigurement to their joints.
9. A placebo is the power in believing that a substance or action will help you when there is no chemical reaction that warrants such improvement.
10. The most commonly abused drug is alcohol. Detoxification is the process of clearing drugs out of the patient's body system and treating the withdrawal symptoms.

WWW.GO Websites

Here are some websites that you can search for additional information:

Alcoholics Anonymous
   www.alcoholics-anonymous.org
American Academy of Pediatrics
   www.aap.org
American Cancer Society
   www.cancer.org
American Heart Association
   www.americanheart.org
American Lung Association
   www.lungusa.org
Food and Drug Administration
   www.fda.gov
Food and Nutrition Information Center
   www.nal.usda.gov/fnic
National Center for Complementary and Alternative Medicine
   www.nccam.nih.gov
National Institute of Drug Abuse
   www.nida.nih.gov

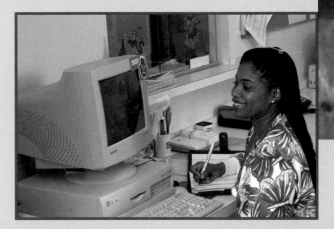

Medical Emergencies: First Aid and CPR

Medical Office Emergencies

CHAPTER OBJECTIVES

In this chapter, you'll learn:

1. To spell and define the key terms.
2. To describe the role of the medical assistant in an emergency before the ambulance arrives.
3. To identify the five types of shock and the management of each.
4. To describe how burns are classified and managed.
5. To explain the management of allergic reactions.

6. To describe the management of poisoning and the role of the poison control center.
7. To list the three types of hyperthermic emergencies and the treatment for each type.
8. To discuss the treatment of hypothermia.
9. To describe the role of the medical assistant in managing psychiatric emergencies.

KEY TERMS

allergen
anaphylactic shock
cardiogenic shock
contusion
ecchymosis
full-thickness burn

heat cramps
heat stroke
hematoma
hyperthermia
hypothermia
hypovolemic shock

infarction
ischemia
melena
neurogenic shock
partial-thickness burn
seizure

septic shock
shock
splint
superficial burn

MEDICAL OFFICE EMERGENCY PROCEDURES

Emergency medical care is the immediate care given to sick or injured persons. When properly performed, it can mean the difference between life and death, rapid recovery and long hospitalization, temporary disability and permanent disability. Emergency medical care in the medical office entails identifying the emergency, delivering basic first aid, and furnishing temporary assistance or basic life support until a rescue squad and advanced life support can be obtained.

An emergency can occur anywhere and to anyone. For example, a patient who is being seen for a routine examination may have a heart attack, collapse, and require immediate cardiopulmonary resuscitation (CPR). A diabetic patient or coworker may lapse into a diabetic coma. A patient may fall down a flight of stairs and receive trauma to the head or limbs. In a life-threatening situation, the well-prepared medical assistant can obtain important information and perform lifesaving procedures before the ambulance or rescue squad arrives, increasing the patient's chance for survival. Medical assistants should be certified in CPR and removing foreign body airway obstructions. Effective January 1, 2005, the American Association of Medical Assistants requires certified medical assistants who are renewing their credentials to demonstrate proof of current CPR certification. This training may be provided by the American Red Cross, American Heart Association, American Safety and Health Institute, or National Safety Council. You should contact one of these agencies for specific information regarding training and certification. This chapter is not meant to provide a comprehensive study of all aspects of emergency care; it briefly reviews the information in such a training course.

Emergency Action Plan

Every medical office should have an emergency action plan, including the following:

- The local emergency rescue service telephone number (usually 911)
- Location of the nearest hospital emergency department
- Telephone number of the local or regional poison control center
- Procedures for various emergencies
- List of office personnel who are trained in CPR
- Location and list of contents of the emergency medical kit or crash cart

Whether confronted with a cardiac emergency or psychiatric crisis, medical assistants must be able to coordinate multiple ongoing events while rendering patient care. Contributing to the complexity of a medical emergency are such factors as panicky family members, the arrival of emergency personnel, and possibly language barriers. You must be able to remain calm in these situations while reacting competently and professionally.

Emergency Medical Kit

Proper equipment and supplies should be readily available in a medical emergency. Although the office's equipment and supplies vary with the medical specialty, emergency equipment and supplies are fairly standard. This equipment should be kept in a designated location that is accessible to all staff. Standard supplies for a medical emergency kit are listed in Box 14-1. Although items used

---

Box 14-1

EMERGENCY MEDICAL KIT AND EQUIPMENT

These are standard supplies that can be used to make up an emergency medical kit:

- Activated charcoal
- Adhesive strip bandages, assorted sizes
- Adhesive tape, 1- and 2-inch rolls
- Alcohol (70%)
- Alcohol wipes
- Antimicrobial skin ointment
- Chemical ice pack
- Cotton balls
- Cotton swabs
- Disposable gloves, latex
- Elastic bandages, 2- and 3-inch widths
- Gauze pads, 2 × 2 and 4 × 4 inch widths
- Roller, self-adhesive gauze, 2- and 4-inch widths
- Safety pins, various sizes
- Scissors
- Syrup of ipecac
- Thermometer
- Triangular bandage
- Tweezers

In addition to these contents, the following equipment should be available:

- Blood pressure cuff (pediatric and adult)
- Stethoscope
- Bag-valve mask device with assorted size masks
- Flashlight or penlight
- Portable oxygen tank with regulator
- Oxygen masks
- Suction unit and catheters

Additional equipment if available:

- Various sizes of endotracheal tubes
- Laryngoscope handle and various sizes of blades
- Automatic external defibrillator
- Intravenous supplies (catheters, administration set tubing, assorted solutions)
- Emergency drugs including atropine, epinephrine, and sodium bicarbonate

during an emergency should be replaced as soon as possible, a medical assistant or other staff member, such as a nurse, should check the contents of the emergency kit or crash cart regularly, perhaps weekly, to verify that contents are available and that no item has gone beyond the expiration date. If so, the expired items should be replaced immediately.

The Emergency Medical Services System

The initial element of any emergency medical services (EMS) system is citizen access. The availability of rapid, systematic intervention by personnel specifically trained in providing emergency care is an integral part of the EMS system. Most communities have a 911 system to report emergencies and summon help by telephone. The communications operator at the local EMS station will answer the call, take the information, and alert the EMS, fire, or police department as needed. In communities without a 911 system, emergency calls are usually made directly to the local ambulance, fire, or police department. You should know the emergency system used in your community. Emergency phone numbers should be prominently displayed by all telephones in the medical office.

Some communities have an enhanced 911 system that automatically identifies the caller's telephone number and location. If the telephone is disconnected or the caller loses consciousness, the communications operator can still send emergency personnel to the scene. In the medical office, an emergency requiring notification of the EMS includes situations that are life threatening or have the potential to become life threatening, such as the symptoms of a heart attack, **shock**, or severe breathing difficulties. In each of these cases, the medical assistant provides immediate care to the patient, including CPR if necessary, while directing another staff member to notify the physician. During assessment of the emergency by the physician, the medical assistant should continue to provide first aid or be prepared to assist the physician in administering first aid while another staff member notifies the EMS. The staff member who calls EMS should be able to describe the emergency to the communications operator. The operator will then know what level of emergency personnel and rescue equipment to send. Excellent communication skills and cooperation between health care team members is essential during a medical office emergency.

Documentation in the medical record is an important responsibility in all patient care, including emergency care. EMS personnel depend on accurate and complete information regarding the patient's symptoms, the nature of the emergency, and any treatment performed prior to their arrival. This information should be placed in the patient's record in chronological order as events occurred or treatments were performed. Any vital signs taken during the emergency should also be recorded. Emergencies that involve visitors or staff must also be documented, and in this case, a blank paper or progress note page will be sufficient to record the details and outline the care provided. Information should include but not be limited to the following:

1. Basic identification, including name, age, address, and location of the patient's emergency contact if known.
2. The chief complaint if known.
3. Times of events, beginning with recognition of the emergency, management techniques, and changes in patient's condition.
4. The patient's vital signs.
5. Specific emergency management rendered in the office, such as CPR, bandaging, splinting, and medications administered before and after the emergency.
6. Observations of the patient's condition, including any slurred speech, lethargy, confusion, and so on.
7. Any medical history, allergies, or current medications if known.

When the EMS personnel arrive, assist them as necessary. Let them examine the patient and take over the emergency care. You can also help by removing any obstacles to removal of the patient by stretcher and keeping family members in the reception area or a private room.

Checkpoint Question

1. What should you attempt to document before the ambulance arrives in an emergency?

PATIENT ASSESSMENT

The two primary objectives in assessment of the patient are to identify and correct any life-threatening problems and provide necessary care. Each step of the assessment must be managed effectively before proceeding to the next. For example, airway, breathing, and circulation must be intact before you take a history. In addition, survey the scene quickly to identify hazards or clues to the patient's condition. For example, an elderly person found at the bottom of a stairway will likely have head or neck injuries and should be treated in such a way as to avoid moving the head, neck, or spinal column. Emesis found near a person that resembles coffee grounds may be a clue to bleeding in the gastrointestinal system that may result from peptic ulcer disease and hemorrhage.

Recognizing the Emergency

When providing emergency care, do not assume that the obvious injuries are the only ones. Less noticeable or internal injuries may also have occurred during an accident. You should look for the causes of the injury, which may provide a clue to the extent of physical damage. For example, the elderly patient who fell down the stairs may have a noticeable bump on

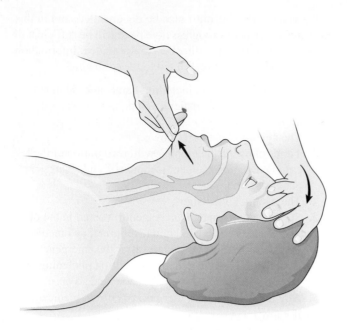

FIGURE 14-1. The head tilt–chin lift technique for opening the airway. The head is tilted backward with one hand (*down arrow*) while the fingers of the other hand lift the chin forward (*up arrow*).

the forehead; this is obvious, but perhaps the patient has an injury in the cervical spine that is not as readily noticeable. In the case of an injury to the head or back when spinal fracture is possible, be especially careful not to move the victim any more than necessary and avoid rough handling.

The Primary Assessment

Once you are at the victim's side, an initial survey of the patient is the first step in emergency care. This is a rapid evaluation, usually done in less than 45 seconds. The purpose of the primary assessment is to identify and correct any life-threatening problems. Quickly assess the following aspects of the patient:

- Responsiveness
- Airway
- Breathing
- Circulation

Checking for responsiveness means noting whether the patient is conscious or unconscious. If the patient is unconscious, attempt to awaken the patient by speaking and touching the shoulder. If no response occurs, assess the patient's airway by using the head tilt–chin lift method. Patients who may have neck injuries should have the airway opened using the jaw thrust method to avoid further injury to the spinal cord (Figs. 14-1 and 14-2). An unconscious patient who is supine is likely to have a partial or total airway obstruction caused by the tongue falling back into the oropharynx, producing snoring respirations or total airway obstruction. Opening the patient's airway may be necessary to allow adequate respiration.

Once the airway is open, evaluate the patient's breathing by watching for movement of the chest up or down while listening and feeling over the mouth and nose for signs of adequate ventilation. If the patient is not breathing, artificial respiration must be started immediately. A face mask with a one-way valve or a bag–valve–mask device is recommended when performing rescue breathing and should be used if available (Fig. 14-3). Respirations that are too fast, too slow, or irregular also require medical intervention. Immediate intervention for these conditions may include breathing into a mask or paper bag for respirations that are too fast (hyperventilation) or administering oxygen as directed by the physician. Any obvious noises, such as stridor or wheezes, are noted and reported to the physician.

Evaluate circulation in adults and children by checking the carotid pulse (Fig. 14-4). The brachial pulse is used to evaluate circulation in infants. If no pulse is found, begin cardiopulmonary resuscitation immediately (Fig. 14-5). Some medical offices may have an automatic external defibrillator (AED) as part of the emergency medical kit (Fig. 14-6). Although these devices should not be used on infants, adults and children with life-threatening heart rhythms have an increased chance of survival if defibrillated quickly and appropriately. Training to use the AED is included in most CPR classes today.

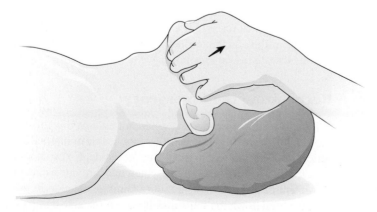

FIGURE 14-2. The jaw thrust technique for opening the airway. The hands are placed on either side of the head. The fingers of both hands grasp behind the angle of the jaw, bringing it up (*arrow*).

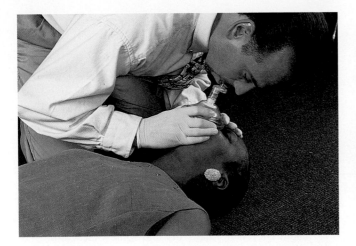

FIGURE 14-3. Using the bag–valve–mask, begin rescue breathing if no breathing is noted in the primary survey.

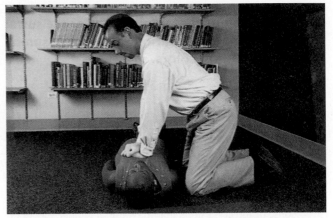

FIGURE 14-5. Chest compressions should be started if no signs of circulation, including a pulse, are present.

Also check for any hemorrhage, and if it is found, control the bleeding quickly. If a pulse is present or becomes palpable during CPR, note the rate and quality frequently. Evaluate perfusion, or blood flow through the tissues, by checking the temperature and moisture of the skin.

Checkpoint Question

2. What is the purpose of the primary assessment?

The Secondary Assessment

After conducting a primary assessment and assessing that the patient's airway, breathing, and circulation are adequate, a secondary assessment can be performed. The secondary assessment includes asking the patient questions to obtain additional information and performing a more thorough physical evaluation to find less obvious problems than those noted in the primary assessment. To gain an accurate impression during the secondary assessment, the following four areas are assessed:

1. General appearance. The patient's skin color and moisture, facial expression, posture, motor activity, speech, and state of alertness provide important clues about the mental and physical condition. Check for a medical bracelet or necklace. Medicine bottles in a pocket or purse can also be helpful.

   Level of consciousness. By the time you have completed the primary survey and noted the patient's general appearance, the level of consciousness may be apparent. A decrease in oxygen to the cells of the brain, neurological damage from a cerebrovascular accident (stroke), and intracranial swelling are just

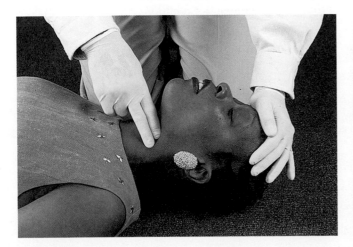

FIGURE 14-4. Check for circulation by palpating the carotid pulse.

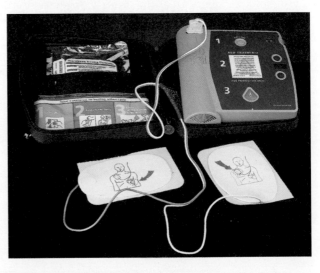

FIGURE 14-6. The automatic external defibrillator can be used to defibrillate a life-threatening heart rhythm.

Ñ Spanish Terminology

Tiene dolor?	Do you have pain?
Tiene dificultad para respirar?	Are you having any problem breathing?
Cuando ocurrio el accidente?	When did the accident happen?
Calmese, por favor. La ambulancia esta en camino.	Calm down. The ambulance is on the way.

some of the conditions that may alter a patient's level of consciousness. The AVPU system uses a common language to describe the patient's level of consciousness:

- A, *A*wake and alert
- V, responds to *v*oice
- P, responds only to *p*ain
- U, *U*nresponsive or unconscious

2. Vital signs. After noting the general appearance and determining the level of consciousness, assess the vital signs, including the pulse and respiratory rates and blood pressure. Assessment of temperature is important for patients who have altered skin temperature or have been exposed to environmental temperature extremes. Patients with a history of infection, chills, or fever and children with **seizures** should always have their temperature taken.

3. Skin. An initial evaluation of the temperature and moisture of skin should have been noted during the primary survey. A more thorough look should now be

taken. Skin is normally dry and somewhat warm. Moist, cool skin may indicate poor blood flow to the tissues and possibly shock. The color of the skin should be noted as an indication of the circulation near the surface of the body and oxygenation of the tissues. Table 14-1 summarizes abnormal skin colors and the possible causes or conditions.

The Physical Examination

A head-to-toe survey that includes examination of the head and neck, chest and back, abdomen, and extremities in this sequence should be done only after completing the primary and secondary surveys. Although the physician usually performs this examination, you must be prepared to assist as needed while continuing to reassure the patient.

Head and neck. If a cervical spine injury is suspected, immediately immobilize the spine and avoid manipulating the neck during examination of the head. Inspect the face for

Table 14-1	ABNORMAL SKIN COLORS AND THEIR CAUSES	
Color	**Possible Cause**	**Possible Conditions**
Pink	Vasodilation Increased blood flow	Heat illness Hot environment Exertion Fever Alcohol consumption
White, pale	Decreased blood flow Decreased red blood cells Vasoconstriction	Shock, fainting Anemia Cold exposure
Blue	Inadequate oxygenation	Airway obstruction Congestive heart failure Chronic bronchitis
Yellow	Increased bilirubin Retention of urinary elements	Liver disease Renal disease

Reprinted with permission from Jones SA, Weigel A, White RD, et al. *Advanced Emergency Care for Paramedic Practice.* Philadelphia: Lippincott, 1992:116.

edema, bruising, bleeding, and drainage from the nose or ears. Examine the mouth for loose teeth and dentures. The condition and severity of a neurological injury or patient with altered consciousness can be assessed by checking the pupils with a flashlight or penlight. The pupils should be checked for several characteristics:

- Equality in size
- Dilation bilaterally in darkness or dim light
- Rapid constriction to light in both eyes
- Equal reaction to light

To evaluate the pupils for these qualities, shade both eyes from the light and use a flashlight or small penlight at an angle 6 to 8 inches from each eye. The conscious patient should not look directly into the light. Report the findings to the physician.

Chest and back. The anterior chest is evaluated to some degree when the patient's respiratory status is evaluated. A further inspection of the chest should be done after removing clothing from a patient with trauma or abnormal vital signs. Patients with cardiac or respiratory complaints should also have their chest more thoroughly evaluated. Palpation of the chest and back may reveal the possibility of rib fractures.

Abdomen. The abdomen of all patients is evaluated, but it is particularly important for those with GI symptoms or suspicion of blood or fluid loss as seen in vaginal bleeding, vomiting, or **melena** (blood in the stool). The abdomen is inspected for scars, bruises, and masses. A distended abdomen may indicate hemorrhage in the abdominal cavity.

Arms and legs. An examination of the arms and legs is the last step of the head-to-toe survey. Inspect the arms and legs for swelling, deformity, and tenderness. Also note any tremors in the hands. To determine the neurological status of the arms and legs, assess strength, movement, range of motion, and sensation, including comparing one side of the body with the other. Muscle strength in the upper extremities is checked by having the patient squeeze both of your hands at the same time. Leg strength may be determined by having the patient push each foot against your hand, again at the same time, while noting any weakness in one side or the other. Assess sensation by using a safety pin or other tool to determine the patient's response to pain. Throughout the examination, you must note the comparison of both sides, including any weakness or decreased sensation in one side or the other. Again, the physician will most likely be performing this examination, but you must be prepared to assist as needed.

Checkpoint Question

3. What diagnostic signs are evaluated in the secondary assessment?

TYPES OF EMERGENCIES

Shock

Shock is lack of oxygen to the individual cells of the body, including the brain, as a result of a decrease in blood pressure. Although the cause of the low blood pressure varies, the body initially adjusts for any type of shock by increasing the strength of the heart contractions and the heart rate while constricting the blood vessels throughout the body. As shock progresses, the body has more difficulty trying to adjust, and eventually tissues and body organs have such severe damage that the shock becomes irreversible and death ensues. Box 14-2 describes the signs and symptoms of shock.

Types of Shock

Hypovolemic shock is caused by loss of blood or other body fluids. If the cause is blood loss, it is hemorrhagic shock. Dehydration caused by diarrhea, vomiting, or profuse sweating can also lead to hypovolemic shock.

Cardiogenic shock is an extreme form of heart failure that occurs when the function of the left ventricle is so compromised that the heart can no longer adequately pump blood to body tissues. This type of shock may follow death of cardiac tissue during a myocardial infarction (heart attack).

TRIAGE

While working in a medical office setting, the following three patients arrive at the same time:

A. A 4-month-old child arrives with his mother. Mother says the child has had vomiting and diarrhea for 2 days and adds, "He is so sleepy and hard to arouse."

B. A 76-year-old man arrives in the office and says, "I was bitten by a spider on my right hand yesterday. My hand is now swollen and hot."

C. A 48-year-old man comes in and says, "I burned my hand on a cup of coffee about 1 hour ago." He is complaining of pain. You notice the hand is red and has two small blisters on the palm.

How do you sort these patients? Whom do you see first? Second? Third?

See patient A first. Anytime there is change in anyone's mental status, it should be treated as a priority. This child may be dehydrated and headed for hypovolemic shock. Patient C should be seen next. Last, see the man with a spider bite.

Box 14-2

SIGNS AND SYMPTOMS OF SHOCK

- Low blood pressure
- Restlessness or signs of fear
- Thirst
- Nausea
- Cool, clammy skin
- Pale skin with cyanosis (bluish color) at the lips and earlobes
- Rapid and weak pulse

Neurogenic shock is caused by a dysfunction of the nervous system following a spinal cord injury. Normally, the diameter of all blood vessels is controlled by the involuntary nervous system and smooth muscles surrounding the vessels. After a spinal cord injury, the nervous system loses control of the diameter of the blood vessels, and vasodilation ensues. Once the blood vessels are dilated, there is not enough blood in the general circulation, so that blood pressure falls and shock ensues.

Anaphylactic shock is an acute general allergic reaction within minutes to hours after the body has been exposed to an offending foreign substance. You must carefully observe patients for this type of shock after giving medications and during allergy testing (see later section on anaphylaxis).

Septic shock is caused by a general infection of the bloodstream in which the patient appears seriously ill. It may be associated with an infection such as pneumonia or meningitis or it may occur without an apparent source of infection, especially in infants and children. Initially, a fever is present, but the body temperature falls, a clinical sign suggestive of sepsis.

Management of the Patient in Shock

Shock can be the result of many types of medical crisis or trauma. After performing the primary and secondary assessments, observe the following list of general guidelines for managing a patient in shock:

1. Observe the patient for and maintain an open airway and adequate breathing.
2. Control bleeding.
3. Administer oxygen as directed by the physician.
4. Immobilize the patient if spinal injuries may be present.
5. Splint fractures.
6. Prevent loss of body heat by covering the patient with a blanket, especially if the patient is cold.
7. Assist the physician with starting an intravenous line as ordered.
8. Elevate the feet and legs of a patient with low systemic blood pressure.

9. Transport the patient to the closest hospital as soon as possible by notifying the EMS.

Checkpoint Question

4. What does *shock* mean?

Bleeding

Soft tissue injuries involve the skin and/or underlying musculature. An open injury to these tissues is a wound. Box 14-3 describes common soft-tissue injuries and wounds.

When a blunt object strikes the body, it may crush the tissue beneath the skin. Although the skin does not always break, severe damage to tissue and blood vessels may cause

Box 14-3

TYPES OF SOFT TISSUE INJURIES

- **Abrasion**, the least serious type of open wound, is little more than a scratch on the surface of the skin. All abrasions, regardless of size, are painful because of the nerve endings involved.
- **Laceration** results from snagging or tearing of tissues that leaves a freely bleeding jagged wound. Skin may be partly or completely torn away, and the laceration may contain foreign matter that can lead to infection. A wound caused by a broken bottle or a piece of jagged metal is a laceration.
- **Major arterial laceration** can cause significant bleeding if the sharp or jagged instrument cuts the wall of a blood vessel, especially an artery. Uncontrolled major arterial bleeding can result in shock and death.
- **Puncture wounds** can result from sharp, narrow objects like knives, nails, and ice picks. Punctures also can be caused by high-velocity penetrating objects, such as bullets. A special case of the puncture wound is the *impaled object wound*, in which the instrument that caused the injury remains in the wound. The object can be anything—a stick, arrow, piece of glass, knife, steel rod—that penetrates any part of the body.
- **Avulsion** is a flap of skin torn loose; it may either remain hanging or tear off altogether. Avulsions usually bleed profusely. Most patients who present with an avulsion work with machinery. Home accidents with lawn mowers and power tools are common causes of avulsion.
- **Amputation** is caused by the ripping, tearing force of industrial and automobile accidents, often great enough to tear away or crush limbs from the body.

WHAT IF

You encounter a person bleeding on the street and you do not have any personal protective equipment with you?

If the person is conscious, instruct him or her to cover the wound and apply pressure with a hand or piece of cloth. You can also make a large, bulky dressing with a piece of clothing and hold it on the area that is bleeding, avoiding direct contact with the victim's blood. In many cases it is up to you to decide whether or not to participate in a street emergency. However, some states have specific laws that require health care professionals to render emergency care.

bleeding within a confined area. This is called a closed wound. Types of closed wounds include **contusions**, **hematomas**, and crush injuries. A contusion is a bruise or collection of blood under the skin or in damaged tissue. The site may swell immediately or 24 to 48 hours later. As blood accumulates in the area, a characteristic black and blue mark, called **ecchymosis**, is seen.

A blood clot that forms at the injury site, generally when large areas of tissue are damaged, is a hematoma. As much as a liter of blood can be lost in the soft tissue when a large bone is fractured. Crush injuries are usually caused by extreme external forces that crush both tissue and bone. Even though the skin remains intact, underlying organs may be severely damaged. Regardless of the type of swelling in a closed wound, the treatment includes the application of ice to reduce and prevent additional swelling to the area.

In an open wound, the skin is broken and the patient is susceptible to external hemorrhage and wound contamination. An open wound may be the only surface evidence of a more serious injury, such as a fracture. Open wounds include abrasions, lacerations, major arterial lacerations, puncture wounds, avulsions, amputations, and impalements. When managing any patient with an open wound, follow standard precautions to protect yourself against disease transmission and to protect the patient from further contamination.

Management of Bleeding and Soft Tissue Injuries

Management of open soft tissue injuries includes controlling bleeding by applying direct pressure and elevating the wound above the level of the heart if possible. Sterile gauze should be used to cover the wound. Management of an am-

putated body part includes controlling the bleeding but also preserving the severed part for possible reattachment later. To preserve the severed body part:

- Place the severed part in a plastic bag.
- Place this bag in a second plastic bag. This second bag will provide added protection against moisture loss.
- Place both sealed bags in a container of ice or ice water, but do not use dry ice.

An impaled object should not be removed but requires careful immobilization of the patient and the injured area of the body. Because any motion of the impaled object can cause additional damage to the surface wound and underlying tissue, you must stabilize the object without removing it by placing gauze pads around the object and securing with tape. The immobilized impaled object can be carefully removed after transportation to the hospital.

Burns

The four major sources of burn injury are thermal, electrical, chemical, and radiation. *Thermal burns*, also called heat burns, result from contact with hot liquids, solids, superheated gases, or flame. *Electrical burns* are caused by contact with low- or high-voltage electricity. Lightning injuries are also considered electrical burns. *Chemical burns* result when wet or dry corrosive substances come into contact with the skin or mucous membranes. The amount of injury with a chemical burn depends on the concentration and quantity of the chemical agent and the length of time it is in contact with the skin. *Radiation burns* are similar to thermal burns and can occur from overexposure to ultraviolet light or from any extreme exposure to radiation.

Classification of Burn Injuries

Classification of burn injuries depends on the depth, or tissue layers involved. Factors that determine the depth of the burn include the agent causing the burn, the temperature, and the length of time exposed. Burns are classified according to the depth of injury: **superficial** (first degree), **partial-thickness** (second degree), or **full-thickness** (third degree). Table 14-2 describes the characteristics of burns according to depth.

Calculation of Body Surface Area

The extent of body surface area (BSA) injured by the burn is most commonly estimated by a method called the rule of nines. This method calculates the percentage of total body surface of individual sections of the body. With the rule of nines for an adult, 9% of the skin is estimated to cover the head and another 9% for each arm, including front and back (Fig. 14-7). Twice as much, or 18%, of the total skin area covers the front of the trunk, another 18% for the back

Table 14-2   CHARACTERISTICS OF BURNS ACCORDING TO DEPTH

Depth, Causes	Skin Involvement	Symptoms	Wound Appearance	Recuperative Course
Superficial (first degree) Sunburn, low intensity, flash	Epidermis	Tingling, hyperesthesia, pain soothed by cooling	Reddened; blanches with pressure; little or no edema	Complete recovery within a week; some peeling
Partial thickness (second degree) Scalds, flash flame	Epidermis, dermis	Pain, hyperesthesia, sensitivity to cold air	Blistered, mottled red base; broken epidermis; weeping surface; edema	Recovery in 2–3 weeks; some scarring, depigmentation; infection may convert to third degree
Full thickness (third degree) Flame, long exposure to hot liquids, electric current	Epidermis, dermis, sometimes subcutaneous tissue	Pain free; shock; hematuria, possible entrance, exit wounds if electrical	Dry, pale white, leathery, or charred; broken skin with fat exposed; edema	Eschar sloughs; grafting needed, scarring, loss of contour function; loss of digits or extremity possible

Reprinted with permission from Smeltzer SC, Bare BG. Brunner and Suddarth's Textbook of Medical–Surgical Nursing, ed 8. Philadelphia: Lippincott-Raven, 1996; 1550.

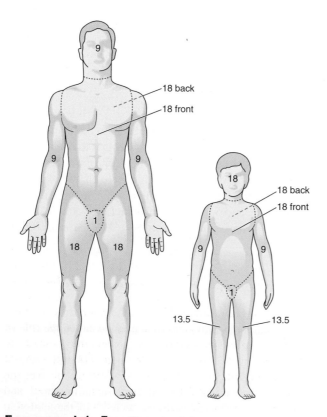

FIGURE 14-7. The rule of nines.

of the trunk, and 18% for each lower extremity. The area around the genitals is the additional 1% of the BSA. In infants and children, the percentages are the same except that the head is 18% and each lower extremity is 13.5% of the total BSA.

Management of the Burn Victim

Follow these guidelines for managing burn patients in the medical office:

1. If necessary, eliminate the source of the burn.
2. Have someone notify the physician and call EMS.
3. Assess the patient's airway, breathing, and circulation. Begin CPR if necessary.
4. Remove all jewelry and clothing as necessary to evaluate the extent of the burn.
5. Wrap the patient in a clean, dry sheet.
6. Administer oxygen as instructed by the physician.
7. Treat the patient for shock and accompanying low blood pressure.
8. Assist with the necessary procedures for transporting the patient to the hospital.

Checkpoint Question

5. What are the four major sources of burn injuries?

Musculoskeletal Injuries

Injuries to muscles, bones, and joints are some of the most common problems encountered in providing emergency care. The seriousness varies widely, from simple injuries, such as a fractured finger, to major or life-threatening conditions, such as open fracture to the femur, which can cause severe bleeding. Injuries to muscles, tendons, and ligaments occur when a joint or muscle is torn or stretched beyond its normal limits. Fractures and dislocations are usually associated with external forces, although some arise from disease, such as bone degeneration.

Management of Musculoskeletal Injuries

It is often difficult to distinguish between strains, sprains, fractures, and dislocations in an emergency. Therefore, in most cases assume the area is fractured and immobilize it accordingly. Proper splinting includes immobilizing the joint above and below the fracture site. Splinting helps prevent further injury to soft tissues, blood vessels, and nerves from sharp bone fragments and relieves pain by stopping motion at the fracture site. As soon as possible, apply ice to the injured area to reduce the swelling that commonly occurs with this type of injury, but never attempt to reduce, or put back into place, a dislocated area.

Types of Splints

Any device used to immobilize a sprain, strain, fracture, or dislocated limb is a **splint**. Splinting material may be soft or rigid and can be improvised from almost any object that can provide stability. Commercial types include traction, air, wire ladder, and padded board splints. Regardless of the type of splint, you must examine the extremity for signs of impaired circulation. To check the circulation of an extremity:

- Observe the skin color and nail beds of the affected extremity. A pale or cyanotic color indicates that the circulation is impeded.
- Locate a pulse in the artery distal to the affected extremity. A weak or absent pulse also indicates that circulation is decreased to the area.
- Watch for increased swelling of the extremity. While this may not indicate that the circulation is impaired, the swelling itself can reduce circulation.

If the circulation is impaired with the splint in place, it must be removed or loosened immediately to provide for adequate blood flow or tissue **ischemia** (decrease in oxygen) and **infarction** (death) may occur.

Cardiovascular Emergencies

Cardiovascular disease accounts for nearly 1 million deaths each year in the United States. The most common problem is coronary artery disease. Approximately two-thirds of sudden deaths from coronary artery disease occur out of the hospi-tal, and most occur within 2 hours of the onset of symptoms. As coronary artery disease progresses, less and less oxygen can get to the cardiac muscle, which leads to tissue ischemia and eventual infarction of the cardiac tissue. The early symptoms of a myocardial infarction (heart attack) include the following:

- Chest pain not relieved by rest
- A complaint of pressure in the chest or upper back
- Nausea or indigestion
- Chest pain that radiates up into the neck and jaw or down one arm
- Anxiety

Early treatment, including basic life support, early defibrillation, and advanced life support can prevent many of these deaths. If cardiopulmonary resuscitation is initiated promptly and the patient is rapidly and successfully defibrillated, the patient's survival chances improve. As noted earlier, an automatic external defibrillator, or AED, may be available in your medical office and should be used as soon as possible after it is determined that the victim does not have a pulse. When applied to the patient's chest, the AED will analyze the rhythm and advise the operator to shock, or defibrillate, the patient by simply pressing a button.

Neurological Emergencies

A seizure is caused by an abnormal discharge of electrical activity in the brain. During a seizure, erratic muscle movements, strange sensations, and a complete loss of consciousness can occur. A seizure is not a disease but a manifestation or symptom of an underlying disorder. Epilepsy, head injury, and drug toxicity can cause seizures. A thorough patient history is important when assessing these patients. It should include the following:

- Information about previous seizure disorders
- Frequency of seizures if recurrent
- Prescribed medications
- Any history of head trauma
- Alcohol or drug abuse
- Recent fever
- Stiff neck (as seen in meningitis)
- A history of heart disease, diabetes, or stroke.

When managing a patient having a seizure, you must give priority to assessing the patient's responsiveness, airway, breathing, and circulation. In certain types of seizures, the patient loses consciousness and therefore cannot protect the airway. During the seizure the muscles of the body, including those of the face, will contract tightly. If you attempt to force an object between the teeth to prevent the patient from biting the tongue, the result will most likely be injury to you or the patient. Frequently, patients vomit during the seizure and lose bowel or bladder control. Particular attention and care are necessary to clear and maintain the airway without causing injury to yourself or the patient. Assisting the patient into the recovery position (on one side) will help secretions such as blood or vomit drain from the mouth. Secretions may be removed from the mouth using a suction machine if available.

After gaining control of the airway, perhaps the most important thing you can do for a patient during a seizure is protect the patient from injury. If the patient lost consciousness and fell at the beginning of the seizure, care will be necessary to protect the neck and cervical spine until immobilization can occur.

Allergic and Anaphylactic Reactions

A severe allergic reaction called anaphylaxis causes most emergency department visits related to allergies. An allergic reaction is a generalized reaction that can occur within minutes to hours after the body has been exposed to a substance recognized by the immune system as foreign and to which it is oversensitive. The systemic signs and symptoms of anaphylaxis are more severe than for a simple allergic reaction, but repeated exposure to a substance that produces allergic reactions may ultimately lead to an anaphylactic reaction and should be avoided.

PATIENT EDUCATION

Choking

A common misconception is that only children choke. The reality is that each year many adults choke to death. Here are some important teaching tips for people aged 20 to 70:

- Chew your food. Focus on eating. Do not eat and drive a car at the same time.
- Avoid excessive alcohol consumption, especially while eating.
- Laugher and talking increase your chance of choking. Do not talk with food in your mouth.

Here are some important teaching points for older people:

- Be sure dentures fit snugly. Go for an annual dental evaluation.
- As we age, our saliva glands produce less saliva. Saliva is needed to dissolve food into small pieces and also helps with swallowing. Therefore, pay special attention while you eat. Older patients need to chew food longer and take smaller bites.

Common Allergens

An **allergen** is a substance that gives rise to hypersensitivity or allergy. The allergen may be a drug, insect venom, food, or pollen and may be injected, ingested, inhaled, or absorbed through the skin or mucous membranes. A person may have symptoms within seconds after exposure to an allergen, or the reaction may be delayed for several hours. You must ask every patient about allergies at every visit and indicate them on the front of the patient's chart and the medication record. Check the patient's medical record and ask about allergies *before* administering any medications in the office; this is essential to prevent allergic reactions or anaphylaxis in patients with known hypersensitivity.

Although the exact incidence of anaphylactic reactions is difficult to pinpoint, it is estimated that 1% to 2% of patients who receive penicillin in the United States have some form of allergy to the drug and that 1 in 50,000 injections of penicillin results in death from anaphylaxis. However, you must be alert to the signs and symptoms of allergic reactions after administering any medication, not just penicillin. Patients with moderate to severe allergy symptoms often receive frequent injections of specific allergens to reduce the symptoms associated with allergies. These patients should be monitored especially closely for anaphylaxis, and they should not be permitted to leave the office for a prescribed amount of time, often 20 to 30 minutes after the injection. When documenting that an injection was given, you should also note the condition of the patient upon discharge.

Signs and Symptoms

The initial signs and symptoms of an allergic reaction may include severe itching, a feeling of warmth, tightness in the throat or chest, or a rash. The primary rule for any exposure is that the sooner the symptoms occur after the exposure, the more severe the reaction is likely to be. Be observant and ready to treat any patient who has these symptoms, since airway obstruction, cardiovascular collapse, and shock can occur if the situation worsens. Since the primary cause of death in an anaphylactic reaction is swelling of the tissues in the airway, leading to airway obstruction, observe the patient closely for signs of airway involvement, including wheezing, shortness of breath, and coughing. Choking or tightness in the neck and throat may signal this danger. Tachycardia, hypotension, pale skin, dryness of the mouth, diaphoresis (profuse sweating), and other signs of shock may also be present.

Management of Allergic and Anaphylactic Reactions

The patient having a severe allergic reaction will often be anxious. Some allergic reactions are mild, without respiratory problems or signs of shock. These simple reactions can be managed by administering oxygen or medications such as antihistamines to relieve symptoms as directed by the physician. If respiratory involvement occurs without signs of shock, the physician may order that epinephrine (1:1000) be given subcutaneously. The patient with a severe anaphylactic reaction who is in shock needs more aggressive therapy, including additional medications, an intravenous line, and monitoring of the cardiac rhythm. The primary goal when treating a patient having an anaphylactic reaction is restoring respiratory and circulatory function. The following steps are required for managing allergic reactions, including anaphylaxis:

- Do not leave the patient, but have another staff member request that the physician immediately evaluate the patient and bring the emergency kit or cart, including oxygen.
- Assist the patient to a supine position.
- Assess the patient's respiratory and circulatory status by obtaining the blood pressure, pulse, and respiratory rates.
- Observe the skin color and warmth.
- If the patient complains of being cold or is shivering, cover with a blanket.
- Upon the direction of the physician, start an intravenous line and administer oxygen and other medications as ordered.
- Document vital signs and any medications and treatments.
- Communicate relevant information to the EMS personnel, including copies of the progress notes or medication record as needed.

 Checkpoint Question

6. What is the primary cause of death in anaphylaxis?

Poisoning

The likelihood that one will be exposed to toxins in the home or workplace is increasing. Over-the-counter and prescription medications are common in homes. Household chemicals are an additional hazard and are often designed to have a pleasant odor and color. Industrial chemicals offer another possibility of poisoning. These chemicals may affect a single victim or many victims in the event of a hazardous materials incident. Most toxic exposures occur in the home, and almost 50% occur in children aged 1 to 3 years. While about 90% of reported poisonings are accidental, intentional exposures usually affect adolescents and adults, and they tend to have a higher death rate. Fortunately, deaths from drug overdoses and poisoning are rare, but you must know how to respond if a patient comes to the office or telephones with a possible poisoning.

Poison Control Center

The American Association of Poison Control Centers (AAPCC) has established standards and regional poison control centers throughout the country. These centers are staffed by physicians, nurses, and pharmacists. When information about a poisoning or drug overdose is not readily available, the poison control center is a valuable resource, and the phone number should be posted near all phones in the medical office. The professionals at the poison control center can usually evaluate a potential or known toxic exposure, instruct the caller in the use of syrup of ipecac to induce vomiting if indicated, and check on the patient's progress by follow-up telephone calls.

Management of Poisoning Emergencies

Exactly how and when a poison control center is consulted should be part of the medical office's protocol. Few toxic substances have specific antidotes, so the management of the poisoning is aimed at treating the signs and symptoms and assessing the involved organ systems. The patient may go to the medical office after the poisoning, or more commonly, the patient or caregiver telephones the office requesting information. In either situation, you must obtain the following information *before* making the call to poison control:

- The nature of the poisoning (ingested, inhaled, skin exposure)
- The age and weight of the victim
- The name of the substance
- An estimate of the amount of poison
- When the exposure occurred
- The patient's present signs and symptoms

Once the poison control center has been notified and instructions given, you must be prepared to treat the patient as directed and notify the EMS to transport the patient to the hospital. Never give a patient syrup of ipecac or otherwise induce vomiting unless directed to do so by the professionals at the poison control center.

Heat- and Cold-Related Emergencies

Environmental temperature is one of the many variables to which the body normally adjusts, maintaining equilibrium. Human beings depend on the ability to control core body temperature within a range of several degrees. Measured rectally, this core temperature is 37.6°C (99.6°F). The peripheral temperature is usually lower (98.6°F orally). Several conditions can disrupt the normal heat-regulating mechanisms of the body. These are divided into two main categories: **hyperthermia** and **hypothermia**.

Hyperthermia

Hyperthermia is the general condition of excessive body heat. Correct management depends on assessment of the underlying cause. The first type of hyperthermia includes **heat cramps**: muscle cramping that follows a period of heavy exertion and profuse sweating in a hot environment. While sweat is primarily water, it also contains the electrolyte sodium, which is needed for muscle function. Heavy sweating, which is a normal compensatory mechanism to cool the body, will result in a sodium deficit, which compromises muscle function and produces muscle cramps. A patient with heat cramps often complains of cramping in the calves of the legs and in the abdomen. Cramping may also occur in the hands, arms, and feet. Mental status and blood pressure usually remain normal, although an increased pulse rate is common.

Heat cramps signal the need for cooling and rest. In uncomplicated cases, the patient is encouraged to take fluids by mouth, but nausea may make intravenous infusion necessary. If the patient is able to take fluids by mouth, give a commercial electrolyte solution such as Gatorade, or salt can be added to water or fruit juice at 1 teaspoon per pint. Cramps can sometimes be prevented entirely with similar oral intake before physical exertion and every 20 minutes during exercise. Salt tablets are not recommended because they may cause nausea.

Heat exhaustion results most often from physical exertion in a hot environment without adequate fluid replacement. Body temperature usually remains normal or slightly above normal. Patients have central nervous system symptoms such as headache, fatigue, dizziness, or syncope (fainting). Although the skin is typically moist and the pulse rate is high, skin color, blood pressure, and respiratory rate vary with the degree to which the body is able to hold off the distress. Patients in late stages of heat exhaustion have pale skin, low blood pressure, and rapid respiration.

Heat stroke is a true emergency. The body is no longer able to compensate for the rapid rise in body temperature (past 105°F) and may undergo brain damage or death. Heat stroke victims can deteriorate quickly to coma, and many patients have seizures. The skin is classically hot, flushed, and dry. Vital signs are elevated initially but may drop, with ensuing cardiopulmonary arrest. Heat stroke demands rapid cooling of the body. After alerting the physician, follow office policy for the management of hyperthermia and heat stroke, which will include these steps:

- Move the patient to a cool area.
- Remove clothing that may be holding in the heat.
- Place cool, wet cloths or a wet sheet on the core surface areas of the body where the ability to cool the central blood is the greatest: the scalp, neck, axilla, and groin.
- Administer oxygen as directed by the physician and apply a cardiac monitor.
- Notify the EMS for transportation to the hospital.

Hypothermia

The body's core temperature can drop several degrees without loss of normal body function. The body usually tolerates a 3° to 4°F drop in temperature without symptoms; hypothermia is an abnormally low body temperature, below 35°C (95°F). Internal metabolic factors and significant heat loss to the external environment can lead to hypothermia. Very cold air and immersion in cold water can cause a rapid drop in core temperature. These are the signs and symptoms of hypothermia:

- Cool, pale skin
- Lethargy and mental confusion
- Shallow, slow respirations
- Slow, faint pulse rate

Basic management of hypothermia includes handling the patient gently, removing wet clothing, and covering the patient to prevent further cooling. If there is evidence of rewarming (skin warm, respirations approaching normal, no shivering) and the patient is alert and able to swallow, give warm fluids by mouth. Avoid drinks that constrict peripheral blood vessels, such as those that contain caffeine (coffee and tea). Fluids that cause dilation of the blood vessels, such as alcohol, should also be avoided. Warm beverages with sugar, such as hot chocolate, can be given to begin replacement of the fuel that the body needs to restore normal heat production. No fluids should be given by mouth to patients who have a diminished or changing level of consciousness.

Frostbite

Windy subfreezing weather creates the greatest risk for **frostbite**. Small body parts with a high ratio of surface area to tissue mass (fingers, toes, ears, and nose) are most vulnerable to frostbite, although larger areas of the extremities are also vulnerable during profound cooling. Exposure to cold can cause tissues to freeze, and the frozen cells die.

The type and duration of contact are the two most important factors in determining the extent of frostbite injury. Touching cold fabric, for example, is not nearly as dangerous as coming into direct contact with cold metal, particularly if the skin is wet or even damp. The combination of wind and cold is dangerous. *Superficial frostbite* appears as firm and waxy gray or yellow skin in an area that loses sensation after hurting or tingling. Prolonged exposure can lead to blistering and eventually *deep frostbite*, which most often affects the hands and feet. No warning symptoms appear after the initial loss of feeling. Freezing progresses painlessly once the nerve endings are numb. Skin becomes inelastic and the entire area feels hard to the touch. Deep frostbite results in tissue death, and the affected tissue must be removed surgically or amputated.

Superficial frostbite can be managed by warming the affected part with another body surface, for example placing an ungloved hand over the nose or ears. Management for more than superficial frostbite is rapid rewarming after any systemwide hypothermia has been corrected. Deep frostbite should be managed only in the hospital to prevent further damage to the tissue. After notifying the EMS, you may be asked to do the following as directed by the physician:

- Immerse the frozen tissue in lukewarm water (41°C, 105°F) until the area becomes pliable and the color and sensation return.
- Do not apply dry heat.
- Do not massage the area; massage may cause further tissue damage.
- Avoid breaking any blisters that may form.

If rewarming is not attempted, bandage the frostbitten part with dry sterile dressings while waiting for the EMS to transport the patient to the hospital. Frostbitten tissue is similar to burned tissue in that it is vulnerable to infection. Take care to keep the affected part as clean as possible. All frostbite victims should be assessed for hypothermia. Clothing offers good protection against weather only if it is loose enough to avoid restricting circulation. Tight gloves, cuffs, boots, and straps add to the danger.

Behavioral and Psychiatric Emergencies

Psychological distress may be mild, moderate, or severe. The degree of intensity determines the type and amount of intervention necessary. A psychiatric emergency is different from an emotional crisis, and you must know how to differentiate between the two. A psychiatric emergency is any situation in which the patient's moods, thoughts, or actions are so disordered or disturbed that harm or death may result for the patient or others if no intervention occurs. An emotional crisis, on the other hand, is a situation with much less intensity. While it may be distressing to the patient, in most cases it is not likely to end in danger, harm, or death without immediate intervention. However, if neglected entirely, an emotional crisis may escalate to a full psychiatric emergency.

A true behavioral emergency, like a medical emergency, carries a serious threat. Urgent behavioral situations usually require some form of professional psychological evaluation and intervention and require transportation to the hospital. The following guidelines are useful for handling a psychiatric emergency:

- Notify the physician and the EMS as directed.
- Offer reassurance and general support to the patient and any caregivers or family members who may be present.
- Accurately document information, including vital signs and the patient's behavior.

SUMMARY

Medical assisting requires interpersonal skills and the ability to communicate clearly, but it is equally important for you to recognize the need for immediate medical intervention when faced with an emergency. If you are prepared with the appropriate knowledge and training to deal with emergencies, you can provide first aid and life support measures that can mean the difference between life and death. In addition, being prepared will lend you confidence in administering first aid and life support, which will reassure your patient, family members, and other members of the health care team.

Critical Thinking Challenges

1. When an emergency occurs, the patient's family members may become anxious and emotionally distraught. How can you help to calm an anxious family member?
2. Reread the "What If" question in this chapter. Analyze how you would respond to such a situation.
3. Investigate the Good Samaritan law in your state.

Answers to Checkpoint Questions

1. Before the ambulance arrives, you should document basic identification, the chief complaint, times that specific events occurred, vital signs, techniques used to treat the patient, and any observations.
2. The purpose of the primary assessment is to identify and correct any life-threatening problems.
3. The diagnostic signs of the secondary assessment are general appearance, level of consciousness, vital signs, and skin appearance.
4. Shock is defined as lack of oxygen to individual cells resulting from low blood pressure.
5. The four major types of burn injuries are thermal, electrical, chemical, and radiation.
6. The primary cause of death from anaphylaxis is airway obstruction.

 ### Websites

American Association of Poison Control Centers
    www.aapcc.org
American Heart Association www.americanheart.org
American Red Cross www.redcross.org
American Safety and Health Institute
    www.ashinstitute.com
National Safety Council www.nsc.org

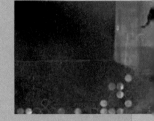

Appendices

APPENDIX A

GLOSSARY OF PREFIXES, SUFFIXES, AND COMBINING FORMS

Term Component to English

a-.............................without
ab-...........................away from
abdomin/o...............abdomen
-ac............................pertaining to
acous/o.................hearing
acr/o.....................extremity or topmost
-acusis.....................hearing condition
ad-...........................to, toward, or near
aden/o...................gland
adip/o....................fat
adren/o..................adrenal gland
aer/o......................air or gas
-al...........................pertaining to
albumin/o..............protein
-algia......................pain
allo-.......................other
alveol/o.................alveolus (air sac)
ambi-......................both
an-...........................without
ana-.......................up, apart
an/o.......................anus
andr/o....................male
angi/o....................vessel
ankyl/o..................crooked or stiff
ante-......................before
anti-.......................against or opposed to
aort/o....................aorta
appendic/o............appendix
aque/o...................water
-ar..........................pertaining to
-arche.....................beginning
arteri/o..................artery
arthr/o...................joint, articulation
articul/o................joint
-ary........................pertaining to
-ase........................enzyme
-asthenia..............weakness
ather/o...................fatty paste
-ation.....................process
atri/o......................atrium
audi/o....................hearing
aur/i.......................ear
auto-......................self
bacteri/o...............bacteria
balan/o..................glans penis
bi-...........................two or both
bil/i........................bile

-blast......................germ or bud
blast/o...................germ or bud
blephar/o...............eyelid
brachi/o.................arm
brady-....................slow
bronch/o................bronchus (airway)
bronchi/o...............bronchus (airway)
bronchiol/o...........bronchiole (little airway)
bucc/o....................cheek
capn/o....................carbon dioxide
carb/o....................carbon dioxide
carcin/o.................cancer
cardi/o...................heart
cata-......................down
-cele.......................pouching or hernia
celi/o......................abdomen
-centesis................puncture for aspiration
cephal/o................head
cerebell/o..............cerebellum (little brain)
cerebr/o.................cerebrum (largest part of brain)
cerumin/o..............wax
cervic/o.................neck or cervix
cheil/o...................lip
chir/o.....................hand
chol/e....................bile
chondr/o................cartilage (gristle)
chrom/o.................color
chromat/o..............color
chyl/o....................juice
circum-..................around
cis/o......................cut
col/o......................colon
colon/o..................colon
colp/o....................vagina (sheath)
con-.......................together or with
conjunctiv/o..........conjunctiva (to join together)
contra-..................against or opposed to
corne/o..................cornea
coron/o..................circle or crown
cost/o.....................rib
crani/o...................skull
crin/o.....................to secrete
cutane/o................skin

cyan/o....................blue
cyst/o....................bladder or sac
cyt/o......................cell
dacry/o..................tear
dactyl/o.................digit (finger or toe)
de-.........................from, down, or not
dent/i.....................teeth
derm/o...................skin
dermat/o................skin
-desis.....................binding
dextr/o...................right, or on the right side
dia-........................across or through
diaphor/o..............profuse sweat
dips/o....................thirst
dis-........................separate from or apart
doch/o....................duct
duoden/o...............duodenum
-dynia....................pain
dys-.......................painful, difficult, or faulty
-e...........................noun marker
e-...........................out or away
-eal........................pertaining to
ec-.........................out or away
-ectasis..................expansion or dilation
ecto-......................outside
-ectomy..................excision (removal)
-emesis..................vomiting
-emia.....................blood condition
en-.........................within
encephal/o.............entire brain
endo-.....................within
enter/o...................small intestine
epi-........................upon
epididym/o............epididymis
episi/o....................vulva (covering)
erythr/o..................red
esophag/o..............esophagus
esthesi/o................sensation
eu-.........................good or normal
ex-.........................out or away
exo-.......................outside
extra-.....................outside
fasci/o...................fascia (a band)
femor/o..................femur

fibr/o	fiber	immun/o	safe	melan/o	black
gangli/o	ganglion (knot)	infra-	below or under	men/o	menstruation
gastr/o	stomach	inguin/o	groin	mening/o	meninges (membrane)
-gen	origin or production	inter-	between		
		intra-	within	meningi/o	meninges (membrane)
-genesis	origin or production	ir/o	iris (colored circle)		
gen/o	origin or production	irid/o	iris (colored circle)	meso-	middle
				meta-	beyond, after, or change
ger/o	old age	-ism	condition of		
gingiv/o	gums	iso-	equal, like	-meter	instrument for measuring
gli/o	glue	-ist	one who specializes in		
glomerul/o	glomerulus (little ball)			metr/o	uterus
		-itis	inflammation	-metry	process of measuring
gloss/o	tongue	-ium	structure or tissue		
glott/o	opening	jejun/o	jejunum (empty)	micro-	small
gluc/o	sugar	kerat/o	hard or cornea	mono-	one
glyc/o	sugar	ket/o	ketone bodies	morph/o	form
glycos/o	sugar	keton/o	ketone bodies	multi-	many
gnos/o	knowing	kinesi/o	movement	muscul/o	muscle
-gram	record	kyph/o	humpback	my/o	muscle
-graph	instrument for recording	lacrim/o	tear	myc/o	fungus
		lact/o	milk	myel/o	bone marrow or spinal cord
-graphy	process of recording	lapar/o	abdomen		
		laryng/o	larynx (voice box)	myos/o	muscle
gynec/o	woman	lei/o	smooth	myring/o	eardrum
hem/o	blood	-lepsy	seizure	narc/o	stupor, sleep
hemat/o	blood	leuc/o	white	nas/o	nose
hemi-	half	leuk/o	white	nat/i	birth
hepat/o	liver	lex/o	word or phrase	necr/o	death
hepatic/o	liver	lingu/o	tongue	neo-	new
herni/o	hernia	lip/o	fat	nephr/o	kidney
hetero-	different	lith/o	stone or calculus	neur/o	nerve
hidr/o	sweat	lob/o	lobe (a portion)	obstetr/o	midwife
hist/o	tissue	-logist	one who specialized in the study or treatment of	ocul/o	eye
histi/o	tissue			-oid	resembling
homo-	same			-ole	small
hormon/o	hormone (an urging on)	-logy	study of	olig/o	few or deficient
		lord/o	bent	-oma	tumor
hydr/o	water	lumb/o	loin (lower back)	onych/o	nail
hyper-	above or excessive	lymph/o	clear fluid	oophor/o	ovary
hypn/o	sleep	-lysis	breaking down or dissolution	ophthalm/o	eye
hypo-	below or deficient			-opia	condition of vision
hyster/o	uterus	macro-	large or long	opt/o	eye
-ia	condition of	-malacia	softening	or/o	mouth
-iasis	formation of or presence of	mamm/o	breast	orch/o	testis (testicle)
		-mania	abnormal impulse (attraction) toward	orchi/o	testis (testicle)
iatr/o	treatment			orchid/o	testis (testicle)
-iatrics	treatment	mast/o	breast	orth/o	straight, normal, or correct
-iatry	treatment	meat/o	opening		
-ic	pertaining to	mega-	large	-osis	condition or increase
-icle	small	megal/o	large		
ile/o	ileum	-megaly	enlargement	oste/o	bone
				ot/o	ear

-ous .... pertaining to
ov/i .... egg
ov/o .... egg
ovari/o .... ovary
ox/o .... oxygen
pachy- .... thick
palat/o .... palate
pan- .... all
pancreat/o .... pancreas
para- .... alongside of or abnormal
-paresis .... slight paralysis
patell/o .... knee cap
path/o .... disease
pector/o .... chest
ped/o .... child or foot
pelv/i, pelv/o .... hip bone
-penia .... abnormal reduction
per- .... through
peri- .... around
perine/o .... perineum
peritone/o .... peritoneum
-pexy .... suspension or fixation
phac/o .... lens (lentil)
phag/o .... eat or swallow
phak/o .... lens (lentil)
pharyng/o .... pharynx (throat)
phas/o .... speech
-phil .... attraction for
-philia .... attraction for
phleb/o .... vein
phob/o .... exaggerated fear or sensitivity
phon/o .... voice or sound
phor/o .... to carry or bear
phot/o .... light
phren/o .... diaphragm (also mind)
physi/o .... physical, nature
plas/o .... formation
-plasia .... formation
-plasty .... surgical repair or reconstruction
-plegia .... paralysis
pleur/o .... pleura
-pnea .... breathing
pneum/o .... air or lung
pneumon/o .... air or lung
pod/o .... foot
-poiesis .... formation
poly- .... many

post- .... after or behind
pre- .... before
presby/o .... old age
pro- .... before
proct/o .... anus and rectum
prostat/o .... prostate
psych/o .... mind
-ptosis .... falling or downward displacement
pulmon/o .... lung
purpur/o .... purple
py/o .... pus
pyel/o .... basin
pylor/o .... pylorus (gate-keeper)
quadr/i .... four
radi/o .... radius (a bone of the forearm); radiation (especially x-ray)
re- .... again or back
rect/o .... rectum
ren/o .... kidney
reticul/o .... a net
rctin/o .... rctina
retro- .... backward or behind
rhabd/o .... rod shaped or striated (skeletal)
rhin/o .... nose
-rrhage .... to burst forth
-rrhagia .... to burst forth
-rrhaphy .... suture
-rrhea .... discharge
-rrhexis .... rupture
salping/o .... uterine (fallopian) tube; also eustachian tube
sarc/o .... flesh
schiz/o .... split, division
scler/o .... hard or sclera
scoli/o .... twisted
-scope .... instrument for examination
-scopy .... examination
seb/o .... sebum (oil)
semi- .... half
sial/o .... saliva
sigmoid/o .... sigmoid colon
sinistr/o .... left, or on the left side
sinus/o .... hollow (cavity)
somat/o .... body

somn/i .... sleep
somn/o .... sleep
son/o .... sound
-spasm .... involuntary contraction
sperm/o .... sperm (seed)
spermat/o .... sperm (seed)
sphygm/o .... pulse
spin/o .... spine (thorn)
spir/o .... breathing
splen/o .... spleen
spondyl/o .... vertebra
squam/o .... scale
-stasis .... stop or stand
steat/o .... fat
sten/o .... narrow
stere/o .... three-dimensional or solid
stern/o .... sternum (breastbone)
steth/o .... chest
stomat/o .... mouth
-stomy .... creation of an opening
sub- .... below or under
super- .... above or excessive
supra- .... above or excessive
sym- .... together or with
syn- .... together or with
tachy- .... fast
tax/o .... order or coordination
ten/o .... tendon (to stretch)
tend/o .... tendon (to stretch)
tendin/o .... tendon (to stretch)
test/o .... testis (testicle)
thalam/o .... thalamus (a room)
therm/o .... heat
thorac/o .... chest
thromb/o .... clot
thym/o .... thymus gland
thyr/o, thyroid/o .... thyroid gland (shield)
-tic .... pertaining to
toc/o .... labor or birth
tom/o .... to cut
-tomy .... incision
ton/o .... tone or tension
tonsill/o .... tonsil (almond)
top/o .... place
tox/o .... poison
toxic/o .... poison
trache/o .... trachea (windpipe)

trans-................across or through
tri-.....................three
trich/o ....hair
-tripsy ....crushing
troph/o ....nourishment or development
tympan/o..............eardrum
-ula, -ule ....small
uln/o ....ulna (a bone of the forearm)
ultra-.................beyond or excessive
uni-....................one
ur/o ....urine
ureter/o ....ureter
urethr/o ....urethra
urin/o ....urine
uter/o ....uterus
vagin/o ....vagina (sheath)
varic/o................swollen or twisted vein
vas/o ....vessel
vascul/o ....vessel
ven/o...................vein
ventricul/o ....ventricle (belly or pouch)
vertebr/o ....vertebra
vesic/o ....bladder or sac
vesicul/o ....bladder or sac
vitre/o ....glassy
vulv/o ....vulva (covering)
xanth/o ....yellow
xeno-...................strange
xer/o ....dry
-y ....condition or process of

English to Term Component

abdomen...............abdomin/o, celi/o, lapar/o
abnormal...............para-
abnormal impulse (attraction) toward...............-mania
abnormal reduction............-penia
above ....hyper-, super-, supra-
across ....dia-, trans-
adrenal gland ....adren/o, adrenal/o
after ....meta-, post-

again ....re-
against ....anti-, contra-
air ....aer/o, pneum/o, pneumon/o
air sac ....alveol/o
airway..................bronch/o, bronchi/o
all ....pan-
alongside of ....para-
alveolus ....alveol/o
anus ....an/o
anus and rectum...............proct/o
aorta ....aort/o
apart ....ana-, dis-
appendix ....appendic/o
arm ....brachi/o
around................circum-, peri-
artery ....arteri/o
articulation ....arthr/o
atrium ....atri/o
attraction for.........-phil, -philia
away ....e-, ec-, ex-
away from ....ab-
back ....re-
backward ....retro-
bacteria..............bacteri/o
basin ....pyel/o
bear...................phor/o
before ....ante-, pre-, pro-
beginning ....-arche
behind................post-, retro-
below ....hypo-, infra-, sub-
bent..................lord/o
between ....inter-
beyond ....meta-, ultra-
bile ....bil/i, chol/e
bile duct ....choledoch/o
binding ....-desis
birth ....nat/i, toc/o
black ....melan/o
bladder ....cyst/o, vesic/o, vesicul/o
blood..................hem/o, hemat/o
blood condition ....-emia
blue ....cyan/o
body ....somat/o
bone ....oste/o
bone marrow ....myel/o
both..................ambi-, bi-
brain ....cerebr/o (largest part), encephal/o (entire brain)

breaking down ....-lysis
breast ....mamm/o, mast/o
breathing................-pnea, spir/o
bronchus ....bronch/o, bronchi/o
bud ....-blast, blast/o
burst forth ....-rrhage, -rrhagia
calculus ....lith/o
cancer ....carcin/o
carbon dioxide ......capn/o, carb/o
carry ....phor/o
cartilage ....chondr/o
cavity (sinus) ....atri/o, sin/o
cell ....cyt/o
cerebellum ....cerebell/o
cerebrum...............cerebr/o
cervix ....cervic/o
change ....meta-
cheek ....bucc/o
chest ....pectoro, steth/o, thorac/o
child ....ped/o
circle...................coron/o
clear fluid ....lymph/o
clot ....thromb/o
colon...................col/o, colon/o
colon, sigmoid .....sigmoid/o
color ....chrom/o, chromat/o
colored circle ....ir/o, irid/o
condition...............-osis
condition of ....-ia, -ism, ium, -y
contraction, involuntary ....-spasm
coordination...........tax/o
cornea ....corne/o, kerat/o
correct..................ortho-
creation of an opening..............-stomy
crooked................ankyl/o
crown ....coron/o
crushing ....-tripsy
cut......................cis/o, tom/o
death ....necr/o
deficient ....hypo-, olig/o
development.........troph/o
diaphragm............phren/o
different ....hetero-
difficult.................dys-
digit (finger or toe) ....dactyl/o
dilation or expansion ....-ectasis

discharge	-rrhea
disease	path/o
dissolution	-lysis
division	schiz/o
down	cata-, de-
downward displacement	-ptosis
dry	xer/o
duct	doch/o
duodenum	duoden/o
ear	aur/i, ot/o
eardrum	myring/o, tympan/o
eat, swallow	phag/o
egg	ov/i, ov/o
enlargement	-megaly
enzyme	-ase
epididymis	epididym/o
equal	iso-
esophagus	esophag/o
eustachian tube	salping/o
examination	-scopy
excessive	hyper-, super-, supra-, ultra-
excision (removal)	-ectomy
expansion or dilation	-ectasis
extremity	acr/o
eye	ocul/o, ophthalm/o, opt/o
eyelid	blephar/o
falling	-ptosis
fallopian tube	salping/o
fascia	fasci/o
fast	tachy-
fat	adip/o, lip/o, steat/o
fatty paste	ather/o,
faulty	dys-
fear, exaggerated	phob/o
femur	femor/o
few	olig/o
fiber	fibr/o
fixation	-pexy
flesh	sarc/o
foot	ped/o, pod/o
form	morph/o
formation	plas/o, -plasia, -poiesis
formation of	-iasis
four	quadri-
from	de-

fungus	myc/o
ganglion	gangli/o
gas	aer/o
germ or bud	-blast, blast/o
gland	aden/o
glans penis	balan/o
glassy	vitre/o
glomerulus	glomerul/o
glue	gli/o
good	eu-
groin	inguin/o
gums	gingiv/o
hair	trich/o
half	hemi-, semi-
hand	chir/o
hard	kerat/o, scler/o
head	cephal/o
hearing	acous/o, audi/o
hearing condition	-acusis
heart	cardio/o
heat	therm/o
hernia	-cele, herni/o
hip bone	pelv/i, pelv/o
hormone	hormon/o
humpback	kyph/o
ileum	ile/o
incision	-tomy
increase	-osis
inflammation	-itis
instrument for examination	-scope
instrument for measuring	-meter
instrument for recording	-graph
jejunum (empty)	jejun/o
joint	arthr/o, articul/o
juice	chyl/o
ketone bodies	ket/o, keton/o
kidney	nephr/o, ren/o
kneecap	patell/o
knowing	gnos/o
labor	toc/o
large	macro-, mega-, megal/o
larynx	laryng/o
left, or on the left side	sinistr/o
lens	phac/o, phak/o
light	phot/o
like	iso-

lip	cheil/o
liver	hepat/o, hepatic/o
lobe	lob/o
loin (lower back)	lumb/o
long	macro-
lung	pneum/o, pneumon/o, pulmon/o
male	andr/o
many	multi-, poly-
measuring, instrument for	-meter
measuring, process of	-metry
meninges	mening/o, meningi/o
menstruation	men/o
milk	lact/o
mind	phren/o, psych/o, thym/o
mouth	or/o, stomat/o
movement	kinesi/o
muscle	muscul/o, my/o, myos/o
nail	onych/o
narrow	sten/o
nature	physi/o
near	ad-
neck	cervic/o
nerve	neur/o
net	reticul/o
new	neo-
normal	eu-, ortho-
nose	nas/o, rhin/o
not	de-
nourishment	troph/o
oil	seb/o
old age	ger/o, geront/o, presby/o
one	mono-, uni-
one who specializes in	-ist
one who specializes in the study or treatment of	-logist
opening	glott/o, meat/o
opening, creation of	-stomy
opposed to	anti-, contra-
order	tax/o
origin	-gen, -genesis, gen/o

other	allo-	saliva	sial/o	suspension	-pexy
out	e-, ec-, ex-	scale	squam/o	suture	-rrhaphy
outside	ecto-, exo-, extra-	sclera	scler/o	swallow	phag/o
ovary	oophor/o, ovari/o	sebum	seb/o	sweat	hidr/o
oxygen	ox/o	secrete	crin/o	sweat, profuse	diaphor/o
pain	-algia, -dynia	seizure	-lepsy	tear	dacry/o, lacrim/o
painful	dys-	self	auto-	teeth	dent/i
palate	palat/o	sensation	esthesi/o	tendon	ten/o, tend/o, tendin/o
pancreas	pancreat/o	sensitivity, exaggerated	phob/o	tension	ton/o
paralysis	-plegia	separate from	dis-	testis (testicle)	orch/o, orchi/o, orchid/o, test/o
paralysis, slight	-paresis	sheath	vagin/o		
perineum	perine/o	sigmoid colon	sigmoid/o	thalamus	thalam/o
peritoneum	peritone/o	sinus	sinus/o	thick	pachy-
pertaining to	-ac, -al, -ar, -ary, -eal, -ic, -ous, -tic	skeletal	rhabd/o	thirst	dips/o
		skin	cutane/o, derm/o, dermat/o	three	tri-
pharynx	pharyng/o	skull	crani/o	three-dimensional or solid	stere/o
phrase	lex/o	sleep	hypn/o, narc/o, somn/i, somn/o		
physical	physi/o			throat	pharyng/o
place	top/o	slow	brady-	through	dia-, per-, trans-
pleura	pleur/o	small	-icle, micro-, -ole, -ula, -ule	thymus gland	thym/o
poison	tox/o, toxic/o			thyroid gland	thyr/o, thyroid/o
portion	lob/o	small intestine	enter/o	tissue	hist/o, -ium
pouching	-cele	smooth	lei/o	to or toward	ad-
presence of	-iasis	softening	-malacia	together	con-, sym-, syn-
process	-ation	sound	phon/o, son/o	tone	ton/o
process of	-y	specializes, one who	-ist	tongue	gloss/o, lingu/o
production	-gen, gen/o, -genesis	speech	phas/o	tonsil	tonsill/o
		sperm	sperm/o, spermat/o	topmost	acr/o
prostate	prostat/o	spinal cord	myel/o	trachea	trache/o
protein	albumin/o	spine	spin/o	treatment	iatr/o, -iatrics, -iatry
pulse	sphygm/o	spleen	splen/o		
puncture for aspiration	-centesis	split	schiz/o	treatment, one who specializes in	-logist
		sternum	stern/o		
purple	purpur/o	stiff	ankyl/o	trop/o	to turn
pus	py/o	stomach	gastr/o	tumor	-oma
pylorus	pylor/o	stone	lith/o	turn	trop/o
radius	radi/o	stop or stand	-stasis	twisted	scoli/o
record	-gram	straight	orth/o	two	bi-
recording, process of	-graphy	strange	xeno-	ulna	uln/o
		striated	rhabd/o	under	infra-, sub-
rectum	rect/o	structure	-ium	up	ana-
red	erythr/o	study of	-logy	upon	epi-
resembling	-oid	study of, one who specializes in	-logist	ureter	ureter/o
reticulum	reticul/o			urethra	urethr/o
retina	retin/o	stupor	narc/o	urine	ur/o, urin/o
rib	cost/o	sugar	gluc/o, glyc/o, glycos/o	uterine tube	salping/o
right, or on the right side	dextr/o			uterus	hyster/o, metr/o, uter/o
		surgical repair or reconstruction	-plasty		
rod shaped	rhabd/o				
rupture	-rrhexis				
sac	cyst/o, vesic/o, vesicul/o				
safe	immun/o				

vagina ....colp/o, vagin/o

vein........................phleb/o, ven/o

vein, swollen
   or twisted ....varic/o

ventricle ....ventricul/o

vertebra..................vertebr/o,
                      spondyl/o

vessel ....angi/o, vas/o,
                      vascul/o

vision,
   condition of ......-opia

voice ....phon/o

voice box ....laryng/o

vomiting ....-emesis

vulva......................episi/o, vulv/o

water......................aque/o, hydr/o

wax ....cerumin/o

weakness ....-asthenia

white.....................leuc/o, leuk/o

windpipe................trache/o

with........................con-, sym-, syn-

within ....en-, endo-,
                    intra-

without ....a-, an-

woman ....gynec/o

word ....lex/o

yellow....................xanth/o

APPENDIX B

ABBREVIATIONS AND SYMBOLS

Abbreviations deemed error prone are printed in red.

ā.....................before
A ....anterior; assessment
A&P ....auscultation and percussion
A&W..............alive and well
AB ....abortion
ABG ....arterial blood gas
a.c. ....before meals
ACE................angiotensin-converting enzyme
ACP...............American College of Physicians
ACS...............American College of Surgeons
ACTH ....adrenocorticotrophic hormone
AD.................right ear
ADH ....antidiuretic hormone
ADHD...........attention-deficit/hyperactivity disorder
ad lib..............as desired
AIDS ....acquired immuno-deficiency syndrome
AKA ....above-knee amputation
alb ....albumin
ALS ....amyotrophic lateral sclerosis
ALT...............alanine aminotrans-ferase (enzyme)
a.m. ....morning
AMBS ....American Board of Medical Specialties
amt.................amount
ANS...............autonomic nervous system
AOA ....American Osteopathic Association
AP ....anterior posterior
APKD ....adult polycystic kidney disease
aq...................water
AS ....left ear
ASD...............atrial septal defect
ASHD ....arteriosclerotic heart disease
AST...............aspartate aminotrans-ferase (enzyme)
AU.................both ears
AV..................atrioventricular

Ⓑ ....bilateral
BAEP ....brainstem auditory evoked potentials
BCC ....basal cell carcinoma
BD.................bipolar disorder
b.i.d. ....twice a day
BKA ....below-knee amputation
BM ....black male; bowel movement
BP ....blood pressure
BPH...............benign prostatic hyperplasia/hypertrophy
BRP...............bathroom privileges
BS ....blood sugar
BUN ....blood urea nitrogen
Bx ....biopsy
c̄.....................with
C ....Celsius; centigrade
C&S ....culture and sensitivity
CABG ....coronary artery bypass graft
CAD ....coronary artery disease
cap.................capsule
CAT...............computed axial tomography
CBC ....complete blood count
cc...................cubic centimeter
CC ....chief complaint; car-diac catheterization
CCU ....coronary (cardiac) care unit; critical care unit
CHF...............congestive heart failure
CIN ....cervical intraepithelial neoplasia
CIS ....carcinoma in situ
cm ....centimeter
CNS...............central nervous system
CO.................cardiac output
CO$_2$ ....carbon dioxide
c/o ....complains of
COPD ....chronic obstructive pulmonary disease
CP ....chest pain; cerebral palsy
CPAP ....continuous positive airway pressure

CPD...............cephalopelvic disproportion
CPR...............cardiopulmonary resuscitation
CSF ....cerebrospinal fluid
C-section ....cesarean section
CSII...............continuous subcutaneous insulin infusion
CT ....computed tomography
cu mm ....cubic millimeter
CVA ....cerebrovascular accident
CVS...............chorionic villus sampling
CXR ....chest x-ray
d.....................day
D&C ....dilation and curettage
DC.................Doctor of Chiropractic Medicine
DC, D/C ....discharge; discontinue
DDS...............Doctor of Dental Surgery
DEXA ....dual-energy x-ray absorptiometry
DJD ....degenerative joint disease
DKA ....diabetic ketoacidosis
DM ....diabetes mellitus
DO.................Doctor of Osteopathic Medicine
DPM ....Doctor of Podiatric Medicine
dr ....dram
DRE...............digital rectal examination
DTR...............deep tendon reflex
DVT ....deep vein thrombosis
Dx ....diagnosis
ECG...............electrocardiogram
ECHO ....echocardiogram
ECT...............electroconvulsive therapy
ECU...............emergency care unit
ED ....erectile dysfunction
EDC...............estimated date of confinement
EDD ....estimated date of delivery

EEG...............electroencephalogram
EGD ....esophagogastro-
          duodenoscopy
EIA ....enzyme immunoassay
EKG ....electrocardiogram
EMG ....electromyogram
ENT...............ear, nose, throat
EPS ....electrophysiological
          study
ER ....emergency room
ERCP ....endoscopic retrograde
          cholangio-
          pancreatography
ESR ....erythrocyte
          sedimentation rate
ESWL ....extracorporeal shock
          wave lithotripsy
ETOH ....ethyl alcohol
F ....Fahrenheit
FACP ....Fellow of the
          American College of
          Physicians
FACS ....Fellow of the
          American College of
          Surgeons
FBS ....fasting blood sugar
Fe...................iron (ferrous)
FH ....family history
fl oz ....fluid ounce
FS ....frozen section
FSH ....follicle-stimulating
          hormone
Fx ....fracture
g.....................gram
GAD ....generalized anxiety
          disorder
GERD ....gastroesophageal
          reflux disease
GH.................growth hormone
GI ....gastrointestinal
gm ....gram
gr ....grain
gt ....drop
gtt ....drops
GTT...............glucose tolerance test
GYN ....gynecology
h.....................hour
H&H ....hemoglobin and hema-
          tocrit
H&P ....history and physical
HAV ....hepatitis A virus
HBV ....hepatitis B virus
HCT or Hct ....hematocrit

HCV ....hepatitis C virus
HD.................Huntington disease
HEENT ....head, eyes, ears, nose,
          throat
HGB or Hgb ..hemoglobin
HIV ....human immuno-
          deficiency virus
HPI ....history of present
          illness
HPV...............human papilloma virus
HRT...............hormone replacement
          therapy
h.s.................bedtime (hour of
          sleep); half strength
HSV-1 ....herpes simplex virus
          type 1
HSV-2 ....herpes simplex virus
          type 2
Ht....................height
HTN ....hypertension
Hx ....history
I&D ....incision and drainage
ICD ....implantable
          cardioverter
          defibrillator
ICU ....intensive care unit
ID ....intradermal
Ig ....immunoglobulins
IM ....intramuscular
IMP ....impression
IOL ....intraocular lens
          implant
IP....................inpatient
IUD ....intrauterine device
IV ....intravenous
IVP ....intravenous pyelogram
kg...................kilogram
KUB ....kidney, ureter, bladder
L ....left; liter
L&W ....living and well
LASIK...........laser-assisted in situ
          keratomileusis
lb ....pound
LEEP.............loop electrosurgical
          excision procedure
LH ....luteinizing hormone
LLETZ ....large loop excision of
          transformation zone
LLQ...............left lower quadrant
LP ....lumbar puncture
LTB ....laryngotracheo-
          bronchitis
LUQ ....left upper quadrant

m ....meter
m ....murmur
MCH ....mean corpuscular
          (cell) hemoglobin
MCHC...........mean corpuscular
          (cell) hemoglobin con-
          centration
MCV ....mean corpuscular
          (cell) volume
MD ....muscular dystrophy;
          Medical Doctor
mg ....milligram
MI ....myocardial infarction
ml, mL...........milliliter
mm ....millimeter
MRA ....magnetic resonance
          angiography
MRI...............magnetic resonance
          imaging
MS.................multiple sclerosis;
          musculoskeletal
MSH ....melanocyte-
          stimulating
          hormone
MVP ....mitral valve prolapse
NCV ....nerve conduction
          velocity
NG.................nasogastric
NKA ....no known allergy
NKDA...........no known drug allergy
noc. ....night
NPO...............nothing by mouth
NSAID ....nonsteroidal anti-
          inflammatory drug
NSR...............normal sinus rhythm
O ....objective
O_2 ....oxygen
OA.................osteoarthritis
OB ....obstetrics
OB/GYN ....obstetrics and
          gynecology
OCD ....obsessive-compulsive
          disorder
OCP...............oral contraceptive pill
OD................right eye; Doctor of
          Optometry
OH.................occupational history
OP ....outpatient
OR ....operating room
ORIF.............open reduction,
          internal fixation
OS ....left eye
OU.................both eyes

oz...................ounce
p̄.....................after
P ....plan; posterior; pulse
PA ....posterior anterior
PaCO₂ ....arterial partial pressure of carbon dioxide
PACU ....postanesthetic care unit
PaO₂ ....arterial partial pressure of oxygen
PAP ....Papanicolaou test (smear)
PAR...............postanesthetic recovery
p.c..................after meals
PD ....panic disorder
PDA...............patent ductus arteriosus
PE ....physical examination; pulmonary embolism; polyethylene
PEFR.............peak expiratory flow rate
per ....by
PERRLA ....pupils equal, round, and reactive to light and accommodation
PET ....positron emission tomography
PF ....peak flow
PFT ....pulmonary function testing
pH ....potential of hydrogen
PH ....past history
Ph.D. ....Doctor of Philosophy
PI...................present illness
PID ....pelvic inflammatory disease
PIH ....pregnancy-induced hypertension
PLT ....platelet (count)
p.m. ....afternoon
PMH ....past medical history
PMN ....polymorphonuclear leukocyte
PNS ....peripheral nervous system
p.o..................by mouth
post op...........after operation
PPBS ....postprandial blood sugar
PR ....per rectum
pre-op, preop before operation
p.r.n. ....as needed

PSA ....prostate-specific antigen
PSG ....polysomnography
pt ....patient
PT ....physical therapy; prothrombin time
PTCA ....percutaneous transluminal coronary angioplasty
PTH...............parathyroid hormone
PTSD.............posttraumatic stress disorder
PTT ....partial thromboplastin time
PUD...............peptic ulcer disease
PV ....per vagina
PVC...............premature ventricular contraction
Px ....physical examination
q.....................every
q2h.................every 2 hours
qd ....every day
qh...................every hour
q.i.d. ....four times a day
q.n.s. ....quantity not sufficient
q.o.d. ....every other day
q.s..................quantity sufficient
qt ....quart
R ....right; respiration
RA.................rheumatoid arthritis
RBC ....red blood cell; red blood count
RIA ....radioimmunoassay
RLQ...............right lower quadrant
R/O ....rule out
ROM ....range of motion
ROS...............review of symptoms
RP ....retrograde pyelogram
RRR ....regular rate and rhythm
RSD...............reflex sympathetic dystrophy
RTC...............return to clinic
RTO...............return to office
RUQ ....right upper quadrant
Rx ....recipe; take thou
s̄.....................without
S ....subjective
SA ....sinoatrial
SAB...............spontaneous abortion
SAD...............seasonal affective disorder
SC ....subcutaneous

SCC...............squamous cell carcinoma
SH ....social history
Sig: ....instruction to patient
SLE ....systemic lupus erythematosus
SOB...............shortness of breath
SPECT ....single photon emission computed tomography
SpGr ....specific gravity
SQ ....subcutaneous
SR ....systems review
ss ....one-half
STAT.............immediately
STD ....sexually transmitted disease
Sub-Q ....subcutaneous
SUI ....stress urinary incontinence
suppos ....suppository
SV ....stroke volume
Sx ....symptom
T ....temperature
T₃....................triiodothyronine
T₄....................thyroxine
T&A ....tonsillectomy and adenoidectomy
tab ....tablet
TAB...............therapeutic abortion
TB ....tuberculosis
TEDS.............thromboembolic disease stockings
TEE ....transesophageal echocardiogram
TIA ....transient ischemic attack
t.i.d. .... three times a day
TM.................tympanic membrane
TMR ....transmyocardial revascularization
tPA, TPA........tissue plasminogen activator
TPR ....temperature, pulse, respiration
Tr....................treatment
TSH...............thyroid-stimulating hormone
TURP ....transurethral resection of the prostate
TV ....tidal volume
Tx ....treatment; traction

UA.................urinalysis

UCHD ....usual childhood diseases

UFE................uterine fibroid embolization

URI ....upper respiratory infection

UTI ....urinary tract infection

VC.................vital capacity

VCU, ...voiding VCUG cystourethrogram

VS ....vital signs

VSD...............ventricular septal defect

V_T ....tidal volume

w.a. ....while awake

WBC ....white blood cell; white blood count

WDWN ....well developed and well nourished

wk ....week

WNL ....within normal limits

Wt ....weight

x-ray ....radiography

y.o..................year old

yr ....year

♀ ....female

♂ ....male

#.....................number or pound

° ....degree or hour

↑ ....increased; above

↓ ....decreased; below

ø ....none or negative

♀ ....standing

♀ ....sitting

O— ....lying

× ....times or for

> ....greater than

< ....less than

† ....one

†† ....two

††† ....three

†V̄ ....four

I, II, III, IV, V, VI, VII, VIII, IX, X uppercase Roman numerals 1–10

APPENDIX C

COMMONLY PRESCRIBED DRUGS

The following alphabetical list of commonly prescribed drugs (trade and generic) is based on listings of prescriptions dispensed in the United States in 2003. The classification and major therapeutic uses for each are also provided. Trade name drugs begin with a capital letter; their generic names accompany them in parentheses. All generic names are set in lowercase.

Name	Classification	Major Therapeutic Uses
Accupril (quinapril hydrochloride)	angiotensin-converting enzyme (ACE) inhibitor	hypertension, congestive heart failure (CHF)
Accutane (isotretinoin)	retinoid	acne
acetaminophen and codeine	analgesic/antipyretic and opiate (narcotic) combination	moderate to severe pain, fever
Aciphex (rabeprazole)	proton pump inhibitor (PPI) (gastric acid secretion inhibitor)	peptic ulcer disease (PUD), gastroesophageal reflux disease (GERD)
Actonel (risedronate)	bisphosphonate (bone resorption inhibitor)	osteoporosis, Paget disease
Actos (pioglitazone)	oral antidiabetic	type 2 diabetes mellitus
Adderall XR (amphetamine mixed salts)	amphetamine	attention-deficit/hyperactivity disorder (ADHD)
Advair Diskus (salmeterol/fluticasone)	adrenergic agonist (bronchodilator) and glucocorticoid (anti-inflammatory)	asthma
albuterol	adrenergic agonist (bronchodilator)	asthma, bronchitis
Allegra (fexofenadine)	antihistamine	allergy
Allegra D (fexofenadine/pseudoephedrine)	antihistamine and decongestant combination	allergy with nasal congestion
allopurinol	xanthine oxidase inhibitor	gout
Alphagan P (brimonidine) ophthalmic solution	α_2-adrenergic agonist (antihypertensive)	glaucoma
alprazolam	benzodiazepine (anxiolytic, sedative, hypnotic)	anxiety
Altace (ramipril)	angiotensin-converting enzyme (ACE) inhibitor	hypertension, congestive heart failure (CHF)
Amaryl (glimepiride)	oral antidiabetic	type 2 diabetes mellitus
Ambien (zolpidem)	hypnotic	insomnia
amitriptyline	antidepressant	depression
amoxicillin	penicillin (antibiotic)	bacterial infections
amoxicillin/clavulanate	penicillin (antibiotic) and β-lactamase inhibitor combination	bacterial infections
Apri (desogestrel/ ethinyl estradiol)	oral contraceptive	birth control

Name	Classification	Major Therapeutic Uses
Aricept (donepezil)	acetylcholinesterase inhibitor	Alzheimer disease
Atacand (candesartan)	angiotensin receptor blocker (antihypertensive)	hypertension
atenolol	cardioselective β blocker/β$_1$-adrenergic antagonist (antihypertensive, antiarrhythmic, antianginal)	hypertension, angina pectoris, cardiac arrhythmias
Atrovent (ipratropium)	anticholinergic (bronchodilator)	chronic obstructive pulmonary disease (COPD)
Augmentin (amoxicillin/ clavulanate)	penicillin (antibiotic) and β-lactamase inhibitor combination	bacterial infections
Avalide (irbesartan/ hydrochlorothiazide)	angiotensin receptor blocker (antihypertensive) and diuretic combination	hypertension
Avandia (rosiglitazone)	oral antidiabetic	type 2 diabetes mellitus
Avapro (irbesartan)	angiotensin receptor blocker (antihypertensive)	hypertension
Avelox (moxifloxacin)	fluoroquinolone (antibiotic)	bacterial infections
Aviane (levonorgestrel/ ethinyl estradiol)	oral contraceptive	birth control
Bactrim (trimethoprim/ sulfamethoxazole)	antibacterial and sulfonamide (antibiotic) combination	bacterial infections
Bactroban (mupirocin)	topical antibiotic	bacterial skin infections
Bextra (valdecoxib)	cox-2 inhibitor (nonsteroidal anti-inflammatory drug [NSAID])	pain, inflammation, fever, arthritis
Biaxin (clarithromycin)	macrolide (antibiotic)	bacterial infections
carisoprodol	skeletal muscle relaxant	skeletal muscle spasms and spasticity
Cartia XT (diltiazem)	calcium channel blocker	hypertension, angina pectoris, cardiac arrhythmias
Cefzil (cefprozil)	cephalosporin (antibiotic)	bacterial infections
Celebrex (celecoxib)	cox-2 inhibitor (nonsteroidal anti-inflammatory drug [NSAID])	pain, inflammation, fever, arthritis
Celexa (citalopram)	selective serotonin reuptake inhibitor (SSRI) (antidepressant)	depression
cephalexin	cephalosporin (antibiotic)	bacterial infections
Cipro (ciprofloxacin)	fluoroquinolone (antibiotic)	bacterial infections
ciprofloxacin	fluoroquinolone (antibiotic)	bacterial infections
clonazepam	benzodiazepine (sedative/hypnotic, anticonvulsant, anxiolytic)	epilepsy, seizures, anxiety (panic disorder)
clonidine	α$_2$-adrenergic agonist (antihypertensive)	hypertension

Name	Classification	Major Therapeutic Uses
clotrimazole and betamethasone	topical antifungal and anti-inflammatory combination	fungal infections, some parasites
Combivent (ipratropium/albuterol) inhalation aerosol	anticholinergic and adrenergic agonist combination (bronchodilators)	asthma, chronic bronchitis, emphysema
Concerta (methylphenidate) extended release	central nervous system stimulant	attention-deficit/hyperactivity disorder (ADHD)
Coreg (carvedilol)	cardioselective β blocker/ $β_1$-adrenergic antagonist (antihypertensive, antiarrhythmic, antianginal)	hypertension, congestive heart failure (CHF)
Coumadin (warfarin sodium)	anticoagulant	thromboembolic disorders
Cozaar (losartan)	angiotensin receptor blocker (antihypertensive)	hypertension
cyclobenzaprine	skeletal muscle relaxant	skeletal muscle spasms and spasticity
Depakote (divalproex)	anticonvulsant	epilepsy, migraine prophylaxis, bipolar mania
Detrol LA (tolterodine)	anticholinergic	overactive bladder
diazepam	benzodiazepine (sedative/hypnotic, anticonvulsant, anxiolytic)	anxiety, skeletal muscle spasm, epilepsy, seizures
Diflucan (fluconazole)	antifungal	fungal infections
Digitek (digoxin)	cardiac glycoside	congestive heart failure (CHF), cardiac tachyarrhythmias
Dilantin (phenytoin)	hydantoin (anticonvulsant)	epilepsy, seizures
diltiazem hydrochloride	calcium channel blocker	hypertension, angina pectoris, cardiac arrhythmias
Diovan (valsartan)	angiotensin receptor blocker (antihypertensive)	hypertension
Diovan HCT (valsartan/ hydrochlorothiazide)	angiotensin receptor blocker and diuretic combination (antihypertensive)	hypertension
Ditropan XL (oxybutynin)	anticholinergic (urinary antispasmodic)	overactive bladder
doxycycline	tetracycline (antibiotic)	bacterial, rickettsial, and chlamydial infections
Duragesic (fentanyl)	analgesic, opiate (narcotic)	pain, sedation
Effexor XR (venlafaxine)	antidepressant	depression
Elidel (pimecrolimus) topical cream	immunosuppressant agent	atopic dermatitis
enalapril	angiotensin-converting enzyme (ACE) inhibitor	hypertension, congestive heart failure (CHF)
Endocet (oxycodone/ acetaminophen)	opiate (narcotic) and nonsteroidal anti-inflammatory (NSAID) (analgesic/ antipyretic) combination	moderate to severe pain
Evista (raloxifene)	selective estrogen receptor modulator (SERM)	prevention and treatment of osteoporosis

Name	Classification	Major Therapeutic Uses
Flomax (tamsulosin)	α_1-adrenergic antagonist (antihypertensive, vasodilator)	benign prostatic hypertrophy (BPH)
Flonase (fluticasone) nasal spray	glucocorticoid (anti-inflammatory, immunosuppressant)	allergic rhinitis
Flovent (fluticasone) oral inhalation	glucocorticoid (anti-inflammatory, immunosuppressant)	asthma control
fluoxetine	selective serotonin reuptake inhibitor (SSRI) (antidepressant)	depression
folic acid	vitamin	nutritional supplement
Fosamax (alendronate)	bisphosphonate (bone resorption inhibitor)	osteoporosis, Paget disease
furosemide	diuretic	hypertension, edema associated with congestive heart failure (CHF) or renal disease
gemfibrozil	antihyperlipidemic	hypertriglyceridemia, hyperlipidemia
Glucophage XR (metformin)	oral antidiabetic	type 2 diabetes mellitus
Glucotrol XL (glipizide)	oral antidiabetic	type 2 diabetes mellitus
Glucovance (glyburide/metformin)	oral antidiabetic (combination product)	type 2 diabetes mellitus
glyburide	oral antidiabetic	type 2 diabetes mellitus
Humalog (insulin lispro)	insulin; antidiabetic	type 1 and 2 diabetes mellitus
Humulin (insulin preparation)	insulin; antidiabetic	type 1 and 2 diabetes mellitus
hydrochlorothiazide	diuretic	hypertension, edema associated with congestive heart failure (CHF) or renal disease
hydrocodone and acetaminophen	opiate (narcotic) and nonsteroidal anti-inflammatory drug (NSAID) (analgesic/antipyretic) combination	moderate to severe pain
Hyzaar (losartan/hydrochlorothiazide)	angiotensin receptor blocker and diuretic combination (antihypertensive)	hypertension
ibuprofen	analgesic; nonsteroidal anti-inflammatory drug (NSAID)	pain, inflammation, fever
Imitrex (sumatriptan succinate)	triptan (antimigraine agent)	migraine headache
Inderal LA (propranolol)	β blocker (antihypertensive, antiarrhythmic, antianginal)	hypertension, angina pectoris, cardiac arrhythmias, migraine headache prophylaxis
isosorbide mononitrate	coronary vasodilator (antianginal)	angina pectoris
Kariva (desogestrel/ethinyl estradiol)	oral contraceptive	birth control
Klor-Con (potassium chloride)	potassium salt; electrolyte supplement	potassium deficiency
Lanoxin (digoxin)	cardiac glycoside	congestive heart failure (CHF), cardiac tachyarrhythmias
Lantus (insulin glargine)	insulin; antidiabetic	type 1 and 2 diabetes mellitus

Name	Classification	Major Therapeutic Uses
Lescol XL (fluvastatin)	HMG-CoA reductase inhibitor (statin)	hyperlipidemia, hypercholesterolemia
Levaquin (levofloxacin)	fluoroquinolone (antibiotic)	bacterial infections
Levothroid (levothyroxine)	thyroid hormone	hypothyroidism
Levoxyl (levothyroxine sodium)	thyroid hormone	hypothyroidism
Lexapro (escitalopram)	selective serotonin reuptake inhibitor (SSRI) (antidepressant)	depression
Lipitor (atorvastatin)	HMG-CoA reductase inhibitor (statin)	hyperlipidemia, hypercholesterolemia
lisinopril	angiotensin-converting enzyme (ACE) inhibitor	hypertension
lorazepam	benzodiazepine (sedative/hypnotic, anticonvulsant, anxiolytic)	anxiety, preop sedation, epilepsy, seizures
Lotensin (benazepril)	angiotensin-converting enzyme (ACE) inhibitor	hypertension
Lotrel (amlodipine/benazepril)	calcium channel blocker and angiotensin-converting enzyme (ACE) inhibitor combination	hypertension
Low-Ogestrel (norgestrel/ ethinyl estradiol)	oral contraceptive	birth control
Macrobid (nitrofurantoin)	antibiotic	bacterial infections of urinary tract
meclizine	anticholinergic	motion sickness, vertigo
metformin	oral antidiabetic	type 2 diabetes mellitus
methylprednisolone	glucocorticoid (anti-inflammatory, immunosuppressant)	inflammation, immunological disorders, allergies
metoprolol	cardioselective β blocker (β_1-adrenergic antagonist)	hypertension, angina pectoris
Miacalcin (calcitonin)	hormone	osteoporosis, Paget disease
Microgestin Fe (norethindrone ethinyl estradiol)	oral contraceptive	birth control
MiraLax (polyethylene glycol)	laxative	constipation
Mobic (meloxicam)	nonsteroidal anti-inflammatory drug (NSAID)	osteoarthritis
Monopril (fosinopril)	angiotensin-converting enzyme (ACE) inhibitor	hypertension
naproxen	analgesic, nonsteroidal anti-inflammatory drug (NSAID)	pain, fever, arthritis
Nasacort (triamcinolone) AQ topical nasal spray	glucocorticoid (anti-inflammatory, immunosuppressant)	allergic rhinitis
Nasonex (mometasone) topical nasal spray	glucocorticoid (anti-inflammatory, immunosuppressant)	allergic rhinitis

Name	Classification	Major Therapeutic Uses
Necon (ethinyl estradiol/norethindrone)	oral contraceptive	birth control
Neurontin (gabapentin)	anticonvulsant	postherpetic neuralgia, epilepsy (partial seizures)
Nexium (esomeprazole)	proton pump inhibitor (PPI) (gastric acid secretion inhibitor)	peptic ulcer disease (PUD), gastroesophageal reflux disease (GERD)
Niaspan (niacin)	vitamin	dyslipidemia
nifedipine	calcium channel blocker	hypertension, angina pectoris
NitroQuick (nitroglycerin)	antianginal	coronary vasodilator
Norvasc (amlodipine)	calcium channel blocker	hypertension, angina pectoris
omeprazole	proton pump inhibitor (PPI) (gastric acid secretion inhibitor)	peptic ulcer disease (PUD), gastroesophageal reflux disease (GERD)
Omnicef (cefdinir)	cephalosporin (antibiotic)	bacterial infections
Ortho Evra (norelgestromin/ethinyl estradiol)	contraceptive patch	birth control
Ortho Novum (norethindrone/ethyl estradiol)	oral contraceptive	birth control
Ortho Tri-Cyclen (norgestimate/ethyl estradiol)	oral contraceptive	birth control
oxycodone and acetaminophen	opiate (narcotic) and nonsteroidal anti-inflammatory drug (NSAID) (analgesic/antipyretic) combination	moderate to severe pain
OxyContin (oxycodone)	opiate (narcotic) analgesic	moderate to severe pain
Patanol (olopatadine)	ophthalmic antihistamine	allergic conjunctivitis
Paxil (paroxetine)	selective serotonin reuptake inhibitor (SSRI) (antidepressant)	depression
Penicillin VK (penicillin V potassium)	penicillin (antibiotic)	bacterial infections
Percocet (oxycodone and acetaminophen)	opiate (narcotic) and nonsteroidal anti-inflammatory drug (NSAID) (analgesic/antipyretic) combination	moderate to severe pain
phenobarbital	barbiturate (sedative/hypnotic, anticonvulsant, anxiolytic)	insomnia, epilepsy, seizures, anxiety
phenytoin	hydantoin (anticonvulsant)	epilepsy, seizures
Plavix (clopidogrel)	antiplatelet agent	reduction in stroke or myocardial infarction risk by excessive clot prevention
Plendil (felodipine)	calcium channel blocker	hypertension, angina pectoris
potassium chloride	potassium salt; electrolyte supplement	potassium deficiency
Pravachol (pravastatin)	HMG-CoA reductase inhibitor (statin)	hyperlipidemia, hypercholesterolemia

Name	Classification	Major Therapeutic Uses
prednisone	glucocorticoid (anti-inflammatory, immunosuppressant)	inflammation, immunological disorders, allergy
Premarin (conjugated estrogens)	estrogen derivative	hormone replacement
Prempro (estrogen/medroxyprogesterone)	estrogen/progestin	hormone replacement
Prevacid (lansoprazole)	proton pump inhibitor (PPI) (gastric acid secretion inhibitor)	peptic ulcer disease (PUD), gastroesophageal reflux disease (GERD)
Prilosec (omeprazole)	proton pump inhibitor (PPI) (gastric acid secretion inhibitor)	peptic ulcer disease (PUD), gastroesophageal reflux disease (GERD)
promethazine	antihistamine; sedative and antiemetic	allergy; motion sickness, nausea
promethazine and codeine	antihistamine and opiate (narcotic) antitussive combination	cold and cough
propoxyphene and acetaminophen	opiate (narcotic) analgesic and nonsteroidal anti-inflammatory drug (NSAID) (analgesic/antipyretic) combination	mild to moderate pain
propranolol	β blocker (antihypertensive, antiarrhythmic, antianginal)	hypertension, angina pectoris, cardiac arrhythmias, migraine headache prophylaxis
Proscar (finasteride)	5α-reductase inhibitor	benign prostatic hyperplasia (BPH)
Protonix (pantoprazole)	proton pump inhibitor (PPI) (gastric acid secretion inhibitor)	peptic ulcer disease (PUD), gastroesophageal reflux disease (GERD)
Pulmicort (budesonide) inhalant	glucocorticoid (anti-inflammatory, immunosuppressant)	asthma
ranitidine hydrochloride	H_2 receptor antagonist	peptic ulcer disease (PUD), gastroesophageal reflux disease (GERD)
Remeron (mirtazapine)	atypical antidepressant	depression
Rhinocort Aqua (budesonide) nasal spray	glucocorticoid (anti-inflammatory,-immunosuppressant)	allergic rhinitis
Risperdal (risperidone)	atypical antipsychotic (neuroleptic)	psychoses (e.g., schizophrenia)
Roxicet (oxycodone and acetaminophen)	opiate (narcotic) and nonsteroidal anti-inflammatory drug (NSAID) (analgesic/antipyretic) combination	moderate to severe pain
Seroquel (quetiapine)	atypical antipsychotic (neuroleptic)	psychoses (e.g. schizophrenia)
Singulair (montelukast)	leukotriene receptor antagonist	asthma
Skelaxin (metaxalone)	skeletal muscle relaxant	skeletal muscle spasms and spasticity
spironolactone	potassium sparing diuretic	hypertension, edema
Strattera (atomoxetine)	selective norepinephrine reuptake inhibitor (SNRI)	attention-deficit/hyperactivity disorder (ADHD)

Name	Classification	Major Therapeutic Uses
Synthroid (levothyroxine)	thyroid product	hypothyroidism
temazepam	benzodiazepine (hypnotic)	insomnia
terazosin	α_1-adrenergic antagonist (antihypertensive, vasodilator)	hypertension, benign prostatic hypertrophy
timolol	β blocker (antihypertensive, antiarrhythmic, antianginal)	hypertension, angina pectoris, cardiac arrhythmias, glaucoma (ophthalmic solution)
TobraDex (tobramycin and dexamethasone) ophthalmic solution	antibiotic and corticosteroid combination	external ocular bacterial infections
Topamax (topiramate)	anticonvulsant	epilepsy (partial seizures)
Toprol-XL (metoprolol)	cardioselective β blocker (β_1-adrenergic antagonist)	hypertension, angina pectoris, congestive heart failure (CHF)
trazodone	atypical antidepressant	depression
triamcinolone	glucocorticoid (anti-inflammatory, immunosuppressant)	inflammation, immunological disorders, allergy
triamterene and hydrochlorothiazide (HCTZ)	diuretic combination	hypertension, edema in congestive heart failure (CHF)
Tricor (fenofibrate)	fibric acid derivative	hyperlipidemia, hypertriglyceridemia, hypercholesterolemia
trimethoprim/sulfamethoxazole (TMP-SMX or co-trimoxazole)	antibacterial and sulfonamide (antibiotic) combination	bacterial infections
Trimox (amoxicillin)	penicillin (antibiotic)	bacterial infections
Trivora-28 (levonorgestrel/ ethinyl estradiol)	oral contraceptive	birth control
Tussionex (hydrocodone and chlorpheniramine)	narcotic antitussive and antihistamine combination	cough and cold
Ultracet (tramadol/acetaminophen)	opioid analgesic and nonsteroidal anti-inflammatory drug (NSAID) (analgesic/ antipyretic) combination	pain
Valtrex (valacyclovir)	antiviral	herpes viruses
verapamil	calcium channel blocker	hypertension, cardiac arrhythmias, angina pectoris
Viagra (sildenafil)	phosphodiesterase (type 5) enzyme inhibitor	erectile dysfunction (ED)
Vioxx (rofecoxib)	cox-2 inhibitor (nonsteroidal anti-inflammatory drug [NSAID])	pain, inflammation, fever, arthritis
warfarin	anticoagulant	thromboembolic disorders
Wellbutrin SR (bupropion)	atypical antidepressant	depression
Xalatan (latanoprost) ophthalmic solution	prostaglandin	glaucoma
Yasmin 28 (drospirenone/ ethinyl estradiol)	oral contraceptive	birth control

Name	Classification	Major Therapeutic Uses
Zetia (ezetimibe)	cholesterol absorption inhibitor	hypercholesterolemia
Zithromax (azithromycin dihydrate)	macrolide (antibiotic)	bacterial infections
Zocor (simvastatin)	HMG-CoA reductase inhibitor (statin)	hyperlipidemia, hypercholesterolemia
Zoloft (sertraline)	selective serotonin reuptake inhibitor (SSRI) (antidepressant)	depression
Zyprexa (olanzapine)	atypical antipsychotic (neuroleptic)	psychoses (e.g., schizophrenia)
Zyrtec (cetirizine)	antihistamine	allergy

GLOSSARY OF KEY TERMS

A

abdominopelvic pertaining to the abdomen and pelvis.

abduction movement away from the midline.

abortifacient agent that induces an abortion.

abortion loss of an embryo or fetus before the 20th week of pregnancy.

abscess area of tissue breakdown; a localized space in the body containing pus and liquefied tissue.

absorption transfer of digested nutrients from the digestive tract into the circulation.

accommodation coordinated changes in the lens of the eye that enable one to focus on near and far objects.

acetylcholine (ACh) neurotransmitter; released at synapses within the nervous system and at the neuromuscular junction.

acid substance that can donate a hydrogen ion to another substance.

acid-fast stain procedure used to color cells for viewing under the microscope.

acidosis condition that results from a decrease in the pH of body fluids.

acne disease of the sebaceous glands.

acquired immunodeficiency syndrome (AIDS) viral disease that attacks the immune system, specifically the T-helper lymphocytes with CD4 receptors.

acromegaly condition caused by oversecretion of growth hormone in adults; there is overgrowth of some bones and involvement of multiple body systems.

acrosome caplike structure over the head of the sperm cell that helps the sperm to penetrate the ovum.

ACTH see adrenocorticotropic hormone.

actin one of the two contractile proteins in muscle cells, the other being myosin.

action potential sudden change in the electrical charge on a cell membrane, which then spreads along the membrane; nerve impulse.

active transport movement of a substance into or out of a cell in an opposite direction to the way in which it would normally flow by diffusion; active transport requires energy and transporters.

acupuncture ancient Chinese method of inserting thin needles into the body at specific points to relieve pain or promote healing.

acute referring to a severe but short-lived disease or condition.

Addison disease condition caused by hypofunction of the adrenal cortex.

adduction movement toward the midline.

adenosine triphosphate (ATP) energy-storing compound found in all cells.

ADH see antidiuretic hormone.

adhesion holding together of two surfaces or parts; band of connective tissue between parts that are normally separate; molecular attraction between contacting bodies.

adipose referring to a type of connective tissue that stores fat or to fats.

adrenal gland endocrine gland located above the kidney; suprarenal gland.

adrenaline see Epinephrine.

adrenergic an activity or structure that responds to epinephrine (adrenaline).

adrenocorticotropic hormone (ACTH) hormone produced by the pituitary that stimulates the adrenal cortex.

aerobic requiring oxygen.

afferent carrying toward a given point, such as a sensory neuron that carries nerve impulses toward the central nervous system.

agglutination clumping of cells due to an antigen-antibody reaction.

agranulocyte leukocyte without visible granules in the cytoplasm when stained; lymphocyte or monocyte.

AIDS see acquired immunodeficiency syndrome.

albinism a hereditary disorder that affects melanin production.

albumin protein in blood plasma and other body fluids; helps maintain the osmotic pressure of the blood.

albuminuria presence of albumin in the urine, usually as a result of a kidney disorder.

aldosterone hormone released by the adrenal cortex that promotes the reabsorption of sodium and water in the kidneys.

alkali substance that can accept a hydrogen ion (H^+); substance that donates a hydroxide ion (OH^-); a base.

alkalosis condition that results from an increase in the pH of body fluids.

allele one member of the gene pair that controls a given trait.

allergen substance that causes hypersensitivity; substance that induces allergy.

allergy tendency to react unfavorably to a certain substance that is normally harmless to most people; hypersensitivity.

alopecia baldness.

alternative an option or substitute to the standard medical treatment plan, e.g. herbal therapies, acupuncture, hypnosis.

alveolus small sac or pouch; usually a tiny air sac in the lungs through which gases are exchanged between the outside air and the blood; tooth socket; pl., alveoli.

Alzheimer disease unexplained degeneration of the cerebral cortex and hippocampus with intellectual impairment, mood changes and confusion.

amblyopia loss of vision in a healthy eye because it cannot work properly with the other eye.

amino acid building block of protein.

amniocentesis removal of fluid and cells from the amniotic sac for prenatal diagnostic tests.

amniotic pertaining to the sac that surrounds and cushions the developing fetus or to the fluid that fills that sac.

amphiarthrosis slightly movable joint.

amyotrophic lateral sclerosis (ALS) disorder of the nervous system in which motor neurons are destroyed.

anabolism metabolic building of simple compounds into more complex substances needed by the body.

anacusis complete hearing loss.

anaerobic not requiring oxygen.

analgesic relieving pain; a pain-relieving agent that does not cause loss of consciousness.

anaphase the third stage of mitosis in which chromosomes separate to opposite sides of the cell.

anaphylactic shock severe allergic reaction within minutes to hours after exposure to a foreign substance.

anaphylaxis severe, life-threatening allergic response.

anastomosis communication between two structures, such as blood vessels.

anatomy study of body structure.

androgen any male sex hormone.

anemia abnormally low level of hemoglobin or red cells in the blood, resulting in inadequate delivery of oxygen to the tissues.

anesthesia loss of sensation, particularly of pain; drug with this effect is an anesthetic.

aneurysm bulging sac in the wall of a vessel.

angina severe choking pain; disease or condition producing such pain. Angina pectoris is suffocating pain in the chest, usually caused by lack of oxygen supply to the heart muscle.

angioplasty use of a balloon inserted with a catheter to open a blocked vessel.

angiotensin substance formed in the blood by the action of the enzyme renin from the kidneys; it increases blood pressure by causing constriction of the blood vessels and stimulating the release of aldosterone from the adrenal cortex.

anion negatively charged particle (ion).

anorexia chronic loss of appetite. Anorexia nervosa is a psychological condition in which a person may become seriously, even fatally, weakened from lack of food.

anoxia see hypoxia.

ANP see atrial natriuretic peptide.

ANS see autonomic nervous system.

antagonist muscle that has an action opposite that of a given movement; substance that opposes the action of another substance.

anterior toward the front or belly surface; ventral.

anthelmintic agent that acts against worms; vermicide; vermifuge.

antibiotic substance produced by living cells that kills or arrests the growth of bacteria.

antibody (Ab) substance produced in response to a specific antigen; immunoglobulin.

anticipatory grief grief experienced prior to the impending death of a loved one.

antidiuretic hormone (ADH) hormone released from the posterior pituitary gland that increases the reabsorption of water in the kidneys, thus decreasing the volume of urine excreted.

antigen (Ag) foreign substance that produces an immune response.

antineoplastic acting against a neoplasm (tumor).

antioxidant substances in the diet that protect against harmful free radicals.

antipyretic drug that reduces fever.

antiseptic substance that prevents pathogens from multiplying but does not necessarily kill them.

antiserum serum containing antibodies that may be given to provide passive immunity; immune serum.

antitoxin antibody that neutralizes a toxin.

antivenin antibody that neutralizes a snake venom.

anus distal opening of the digestive tract.

aorta the largest artery; carries blood out of the left ventricle of the heart.

apex the pointed region of a cone-shaped structure.

aphasia loss or defect in language communication; loss of the ability to speak or write is expressive aphasia; loss of understanding of written or spoken language is receptive aphasia.

apnea temporary cessation of breathing.

apocrine referring to a gland that releases some cellular material along with its secretions.

aponeurosis broad sheet of fibrous connective tissue that attaches muscle to bone or to other muscle.

appendicular skeleton part of the skeleton that includes the bones of the upper extremities, lower extremities, shoulder girdle, and hips.

appendix fingerlike tube of lymphatic tissue attached to the first portion of the large intestine; vermiform (wormlike) appendix.

aqueous humor watery fluid that fills much of the eyeball anterior to the lens.

aqueous pertaining to water; an aqueous solution is one in which water is the solvent.

arachnoid middle layer of the meninges.

areolar referring to loose connective tissue, any small space, or to an areola, a circular area of marked color.

arrector pili muscle attached to a hair follicle that raises the hair.

arrhythmia abnormal rhythm of the heartbeat; dysrhythmia.

arteriole vessel between a small artery and a capillary.

arteriosclerosis hardening of the arteries.

artery vessel that carries blood away from the heart.

arthritis inflammation of the joints.

arthrocentesis puncture of a joint to withdraw fluid.

arthroscope instrument for examining the interior of the knee and surgically repairing the knee.

articular   pertaining to a joint.

ascites   abnormal collection of fluid in the abdominal cavity.

asepsis   condition in which no pathogens are present; adj., aseptic.

assessment   process of gathering information about the patient and the presenting condition.

assimilation   absorption of newly perceived information into the existing subjective conscious schema structure.

asthma   allergy-induced inflammation and constriction of the air passageways.

astigmatism   visual defect due to an irregularity in the curvature of the cornea or the lens.

ataxia   lack of muscular coordination; irregular muscular action.

atelectasis   incomplete expansion of the lung; collapsed lung.

atherosclerosis   hardening of the arteries due to the deposit of yellowish, fatlike material in the lining of these vessels.

atom   smallest subunit of a chemical element.

atomic number   the number of protons in the nucleus of an element's atoms; a number characteristic of each element.

atopic dermatitis   skin condition that may involve redness, blisters, pimples, scaling, and crusting; eczema.

ATP   see Adenosine triphosphate.

atrial natriuretic peptide (ANP)   hormone produced by the atria of the heart that lowers blood pressure.

atrioventricular (AV) node   part of the conduction system of the heart.

atrium   one of the two upper chambers of the heart; adj., atrial.

atrophy   wasting or decrease in size of a part.

attenuated   weakened.

autoclave   instrument used to sterilize material with steam under pressure.

autoimmunity   abnormal reactivity to one's own tissues.

autologous   related to self, such as blood or tissue taken from one's own body.

autonomic nervous system (ANS)   the part of the nervous system that controls smooth muscle, cardiac muscle, and glands; the visceral or involuntary nervous system.

autosome   a chromosome not involved in sex determination. There are 44 autosomes (22 pairs) in humans.

AV node   see Atrioventricular node.

axial skeleton   the part of the skeleton that includes the skull, spinal column, ribs, and sternum.

axilla   hollow beneath the arm where it joins the body; armpit.

axon   fiber of a neuron that conducts impulses away from the cell body.

B

B cell   agranular white blood cell that gives rise to antibody-producing plasma cells in response to an antigen; B lymphocyte.

bacillus   rod-shaped bacterium; pl., bacilli.

bacteriostasis   condition in which bacterial growth is inhibited but the organisms are not killed.

bacterium   type of microorganism; pl., bacteria.

band cell   immature neutrophil.

basal ganglia   gray masses in the lower part of the forebrain that aid in muscle coordination.

base   substance that can accept a hydrogen ion (H^+); substance that donates a hydroxide ion (OH_-); an alkali.

basophil   granular white blood cell that shows large, dark blue cytoplasmic granules when stained with basic stain.

behaviorism   theory of conduct that regards normal and abnormal behaviors as the result of conditioned reflexes separate from the concept of will or choice.

Bell palsy   facial paralysis caused by damage to the facial nerve (VII), usually on one side of the face.

benign   describing a tumor that does not spread; not recurrent nor becoming worse.

bereavement   expected reactions of grief and sadness after learning of the loss of a loved one.

bias   formation of an opinion without foundation or reason; prejudice.

BiCaps   words or phrases with unusual capitalization.

bile   substance produced in the liver that emulsifies fats.

bilirubin   pigment derived from the breakdown of hemoglobin and found in bile.

biofeedback   a method for controling involuntary responses by means of electronic devices that monitor changes and feed information back to a person.

biopsy   removal of tissue or other material from the living body for examination, usually under the microscope.

block   a type of letter format in which the date, subject line, closing and signatures are to the right margin; all other lines are justified left.

blood urea nitrogen (BUN)   amount of nitrogen from urea in the blood; test to evaluate kidney function.

bolus   a concentrated mass; the portion of food that is moved to the back of the mouth and swallowed.

bone   hard connective tissue that makes up most of the skeleton, or any structure composed of this type of tissue.

Bowman capsule   enlarged portion of the nephron that contains the glomerulus; glomerular capsule.

bradycardia   heart rate of less than 60 beats per minute.

brain   the central controlling area of the central nervous system (CNS).

brain stem   portion of the brain that connects the cerebrum with the spinal cord; contains the midbrain, pons, and medulla oblongata.

Broca area   area of the cerebral cortex concerned with motor control of speech.

bronchiole   microscopic branch of a bronchus.

bronchoscope   endoscope for examination of the bronchi and removal of small objects from the bronchi.

bronchus   large air passageway in the lung; pl., bronchi.

buffer   substance that prevents sharp changes in the pH of a solution.

bulbourethral gland   gland that secretes mucus to lubricate the urethra and tip of penis during sexual stimulation; Cowper gland.

bulimia   eating disorder also known as binge-purge syndrome.

bulk transport   movement of large amounts of material through the plasma membrane of a cell.

Bulla   vesicle.

BUN   see Blood urea nitrogen.

bursa   small, fluid-filled sac found in an area subject to stress around bones and joints; pl., bursae.

bursitis   inflammation of a bursa.

C

calcitonin   hormone from the thyroid gland that lowers blood calcium levels and promotes deposit of calcium in bones; thyrocalcitonin.

calcitriol   the active form of vitamin D; dihydroxycholecalciferol.

calculus   stone, such as a urinary stone; pl calculi.

calyx   cuplike extension of the renal pelvis that collects urine; pl. calyces.

cancellous   referring to spongy bone tissue.

cancer   tumor that spreads to other tissues; a malignant neoplasm.

capillary   microscopic vessel through which exchanges take place between the blood and the tissues.

carbohydrate   simple sugar or compound made from simple sugars linked together, such as starch or glycogen.

carbon dioxide (CO2)   the gaseous waste product of cellular metabolism.

carbon   element that is the basis of organic chemistry.

carcinogen   cancer-causing substance.

carcinoma   malignant growth of epithelial cells; a form of cancer.

cardiac   pertaining to the heart.

cardiogenic shock   type of shock in which the left ventricle fails to pump enough blood for the body to function.

cardiopulmonary resuscitation (CPR)   method to restore heartbeat and breathing by mouth-to-mouth resuscitation and closed chest cardiac massage.

cardiovascular system   the system consisting of the heart and blood vessels that transports blood throughout the body.

caries   tooth decay.

carotenemia   yellowish color of the skin caused by eating excessive amounts of carrots and other deeply colored vegetables.

carrier   individual who has a gene that is not expressed but that can be passed to offspring.

cartilage   type of hard connective tissue found at the ends of bones, the tip of the nose, larynx, trachea and the embryonic skeleton.

CAT   see Computed tomography.

catabolism   metabolic breakdown of substances into simpler substances; includes the digestion of food and the oxidation of nutrient molecules for energy.

catalyst   substance that speeds the rate of a chemical reaction.

cataract   opacity of the eye's lens or lens capsule.

catheter   tube that can be inserted into a vessel or cavity; may be used to remove fluid, such as urine or blood; v., catheterize.

cation   positively charged particle (ion).

caudal   toward or nearer to the sacral region of the spinal column.

cecum   small pouch at the beginning of the large intestine.

cell   basic unit of life.

cell membrane   outer covering of a cell; regulates what enters and leaves cell; plasma membrane.

cellular respiration   series of reactions by which nutrients are oxidized for energy within the cell.

central nervous system (CNS)   part of the nervous system that includes the brain and spinal cord.

centrifuge   an instrument that separates materials in a mixture based on density.

centriole   rod-shaped body near the nucleus of a cell; functions in cell division.

cerebellum   small section of the brain located under the cerebral hemispheres; functions in coordination, balance, and muscle tone.

cerebral cortex   the very thin outer layer of gray matter on the surface of the cerebral hemispheres.

cerebral palsy   disorder caused by brain damage occurring before or during the birth process.

cerebrospinal fluid (CSF)   fluid that circulates in and around the brain and spinal cord.

cerebrovascular accident (CVA)   condition involving obstruction of blood flow to brain tissue or bleeding into brain tissue, usually as a result of hypertension or atherosclerosis; stroke.

cerebrum   largest part of the brain; composed of two cerebral hemispheres.

cerumen   earwax; adj., ceruminous.

cervix   constricted portion of an organ or part, such as the lower portion of the uterus; neck; adj., cervical.

chemistry   study of the composition and properties of matter.

chemoreceptor   receptor that responds to chemicals in body fluids.

chemotherapy   treatment of a disease by administration of a chemical agent.

Cheyne-Stokes respiration   rhythmic variation in the depth of respiratory movements alternating with periods of apnea due to depression of the breathing centers.

chlamydia   a type of very small bacterium that can exist only within a living cell; members of this group cause inclusion conjunctivitis, trachoma, sexually transmitted infections, and respiratory diseases.

cholecystokinin (CCK)   hormone from the duodenum that stimulates release of pancreatic enzymes and bile from the gallbladder.

cholelithiasis   gallstones.

cholesterol an organic fatlike compound found in animal fat, bile, blood, myelin, liver, and other parts of the body.

cholinergic an activity or structure that responds to acetylcholine.

chondrocyte cell that produces cartilage.

chordae tendineae fibrous threads that stabilize the AV valve flaps in the heart.

choriocarcinoma very malignant tumor made of placental tissue.

choroid pigmented middle layer of the eye.

choroid plexus vascular network in the ventricles of the brain that forms cerebrospinal fluid.

chromosome dark-staining, threadlike body in the nucleus of a cell; contains genes that determine hereditary traits.

chronic referring to a disease that develops slowly, persists over a long time, or is recurring.

chyle milky-appearing fluid absorbed into the lymphatic system from the small intestine. It consists of lymph and droplets of digested fat.

chyme mixture of partially digested food, water, and digestive juices that forms in the stomach.

cicatrix scar.

cilia hairs or hairlike processes, such as eyelashes or microscopic extensions from the surface of a cell; sing., cilium.

ciliary muscle eye muscle that controls the shape of the lens.

circumcision surgery to remove the foreskin of the penis.

circumduction circular movement at a joint.

cirrhosis chronic disease, usually of the liver, in which active cells are replaced by inactive scar tissue.

cisterna chyli first part of the thoracic lymph duct, which is enlarged to form a temporary storage area.

clarification explanation; removal of confusion or uncertainty.

clitoris small organ of great sensitivity in the external genitalia of the female.

CNS see Central nervous system.

coagulation clotting, as of blood.

coccus a round bacterium; pl., cocci.

cochlea coiled portion of the inner ear that contains the organ of hearing.

colic spasm of visceral muscle.

collagen flexible white protein that gives strength and resilience to connective tissue, such as bone and cartilage.

colloid mixture in which suspended particles do not dissolve but remain distributed in the solvent because of their small size (*e.g.*, cytoplasm); colloidal suspension.

colon main portion of the large intestine.

colostrum secretion of the mammary glands released prior to secretion of milk.

communicable describing a disease that can be transmitted from one person to another.

complement group of blood proteins that helps antibodies to destroy foreign cells.

compliance the ease with which the lungs and thorax can be expanded.

compound substance composed of two or more chemical elements.

computed tomography (CT) imaging method in which multiple radiographic views taken from different angles are analyzed by computer to show a cross-section of an area; used to detect tumors and other abnormalities; also called computed axial tomography (CAT).

concha shell-like bone in the nasal cavity; pl., conchae.

concrete mental operations stage of cognitive development in Piaget's theory of development, in which the individual engages in mental manipulations of internal images of tangible objects.

concussion injury resulting from a violent blow or shock.

condyle rounded projection, as on a bone.

cone receptor cell in the retina of the eye; used for vision in bright light.

congenital present at birth.

conjunctiva membrane that lines the eyelid and covers the anterior part of the sclera (white of the eye).

conscious being aware and having perception of the environment; having the ability to filter that information through the mind with the awareness of doing so.

constipation infrequency of or difficulty with defecation.

contraception prevention of an ovum's fertilization or implantation of a fertilized ovum; birth control.

contusion collection of blood in tissues after an injury; a bruise.

conventional grief feelings of sadness expected or experienced after a loss.

convergence the centering of both eyes on the same visual field.

convulsion series of muscle spasms; seizure.

cookies tiny files that are left on your computer's hard drive by a website.

coping mechanisms unconscious methods of alleviating intense stressors.

cornea clear portion of the sclera that covers the anterior of the eye.

coronary referring to the heart or to the arteries supplying blood to the heart.

corpus callosum thick bundle of myelinated nerve cell fibers, deep within the brain, that carries nerve impulses from one cerebral hemisphere to the other.

corpus luteum yellow body formed from ovarian follicle after ovulation; produces progesterone.

cortex outer layer of an organ, such as the brain, kidney, or adrenal gland.

coryza nasal discharge; acute coryza is the common cold.

countercurrent mechanism mechanism for concentrating urine as it flows through the distal portions of the nephron.

covalent bond chemical bond formed by the sharing of electrons between atoms.

CPR see Cardiopulmonary resuscitation.

cranial pertaining to the cranium, the part of the skull that encloses the brain; toward the head or nearer to the head.

creatine phosphate compound in muscle tissue that stores energy in high energy bonds.

creatinine nitrogenous waste product in the blood or eliminated in urine.

crenation shrinking of a cell, as when placed in a hypertonic solution.

crista receptor for the sense of dynamic equilibrium; pl. cristae.

croup loud barking cough associated with upper respiratory infection in children.

cryoprecipitate precipitate formed when plasma is frozen and then thawed.

cryptorchidism failure of the testis to descend into the scrotum; undescended testicle.

CSF see cerebrospinal fluid.

CT see computed tomography.

culture a laboratory process whereby microorganisms are grown in a special medium often for the purpose of identifying a causative agent in an infectious disease.

cultures the way of life, including commonly held beliefs, of a group of people.

Cushing syndrome condition caused by overactivity of the adrenal cortex.

cutaneous referring to the skin.

cuticle extension of the stratum corneum that seals the space between the nail plate and the skin above the nail root.

cyanosis bluish discoloration of the skin and mucous membranes resulting from insufficient oxygen in the blood.

cystic duct duct that carries bile into and out of the gallbladder.

cystic fibrosis hereditary disease involving thickened secretions and electrolyte imbalances.

cystitis inflammation of the urinary bladder.

cytology study of cells.

cytoplasm substance that fills the cell, consisting of a liquid cytosol and organelles.

cytosol liquid portion of the cytoplasm, consisting of nutrients, minerals, enzymes and other materials in water.

D

deamination removal of amino groups from proteins in metabolism.

decubitus lying down.

defecation act of eliminating undigested waste from the digestive tract.

defense mechanisms methods for protecting the ego from anxiety associated with conflicting urges and restrictions of the id and superego.

degeneration breakdown, as from age, injury, or disease.

deglutition act of swallowing.

dehydration excessive loss of body fluid.

demeanor the way a person looks, behaves, and conducts himself or herself.

dementia gradual and usually irreversible loss of intellectual function.

denaturation change in structure of a protein, such as an enzyme, so that it can no longer function.

dendrite fiber of a neuron that conducts impulses toward the cell body.

denial saying that something is not true; refusing to acknowledge.

deoxyribonucleic acid (DNA) genetic material of the cell; makes up the chromosomes in the nucleus of the cell.

depolarization a sudden reversal of the charge on a cell membrane.

depression persistent and prolonged mood of sadness that extends beyond two weeks duration.

dermal papillae extensions of the dermis that project up into the epidermis; they contain blood vessels that supply the epidermis.

dermatitis inflammation of the skin.

dermatome a region of the skin supplied by a single spinal nerve.

dermatosis any skin disease.

dermis true skin; deeper part of the skin.

detoxification clearing of drugs from the body and treating the withdrawal symptoms.

dextrose glucose, a simple sugar.

diabetes insipidus condition due to insufficient secretion of ADH from the posterior pituitary; there is excessive loss of water.

diabetes mellitus disease of insufficient insulin in which excess glucose is found in blood and urine; characterized by abnormal metabolism of glucose, protein, and fat.

diagnosis identification of an illness.

dialysis method for separating molecules in solution based on differences in their ability to pass through a semipermeable membrane; method for removing nitrogenous waste products from the body, as by hemodialysis or peritoneal dialysis.

diaphragm dome-shaped muscle under the lungs that flattens during inhalation; separating membrane or structure.

diaphysis shaft of a long bone.

diarrhea abnormally frequent watery bowel movements.

diarthrosis freely movable joint; synovial joint.

diastole relaxation phase of the cardiac cycle; adj., diastolic.

diencephalon region of the brain between the cerebral hemispheres and the midbrain; contains the thalamus, hypothalamus, and pituitary gland.

diffusion movement of molecules from a region where they are in higher concentration to a region where they are in lower concentration.

digestion process of breaking down food into absorbable particles.

digestive system the system involved in taking in nutrients, converting them to a form the body can use and absorbing them into the circulation.

dihydroxycholecalciferol the active form of vitamin D.

dilation   widening of a part, such as the pupil of the eye, a blood vessel, or the uterine cervix; dilatation.

disaccharide   compound formed of two simple sugars linked together, such as sucrose and lactose.

discrimination   making a difference in favor of or against someone.

disease   illness; abnormal state in which part or all of the body does not function properly.

disinfection   killing of pathogens but not necessarily harmless microbes.

dissect   to cut apart or separate tissues for study.

distal   farther from the origin of a structure or from a given reference point.

DNA   see deoxyribonucleic acid.

documentation   the process of recording patient information.

dominant   referring to a gene that is always expressed if present.

dopamine   a neurotranmitter.

dorsal   toward the back; posterior.

dorsiflexion   bending the foot upward at the ankle.

Down syndrome   a congenital disorder usually due to an extra chromosome 21; trisomy 21.

downloading   transferring information from an outside location to your computer.

duct   tube or vessel.

ductus deferens   tube that carries sperm cells from the testis to the urethra; vas deferens.

duodenum   first portion of the small intestine.

dura mater   outermost layer of the meninges.

dysmenorrhea   painful or difficult menstruation.

dyspnea   difficult or labored breathing.

dysphasia   difficulty speaking.

dysphonia   impairment of voice; hoarseness.

E

ecchymosis   characteristic black and blue mark that results from blood as it accumulates under the skin.

eccrine   referring to sweat glands that regulate body temperature and vent directly to the surface of the skin through a pore.

ECG   see electrocardiograph.

echocardiograph   instrument to study the heart by means of ultrasound; the record produced is an echocardiogram.

eclampsia   serious and sometimes fatal condition involving convulsions, liver damage, and kidney failure that can develop from pregnancy-induced hypertension.

ectopic   out of a normal place, as a pregnancy or heartbeat.

eczema   see atopic dermatitis.

edema   accumulation of fluid in the tissue spaces.

EEG   see electroencephalograph.

effector   muscle or gland that responds to a stimulus; effector organ.

efferent   carrying away from a given point, such as a motor neuron that carries nerve impulses away from the central nervous system.

effusion   escape of fluid into a cavity or space; the fluid itself.

ego   in Freudian theory, one of the three major divisions in the model of the psychic apparatus that possesses consciousness and memory, and serves to mediate between the id and the superego or conscience.

ejaculation   expulsion of semen through the urethra.

EKG   see electrocardiograph.

electrocardiograph (ECG, EKG)   instrument to study the electrical activity of the heart; record made is an electrocardiogram.

electroencephalograph (EEG)   instrument used to study electrical activity of the brain; record made is an electroencephalogram.

electrolyte   compound that separates into ions in solution; substance that conducts an electrical current in solution.

electron   negatively charged particle located in an energy level outside the nucleus of an atom.

electrophoresis   separation of components in a mixture by passing an electrical current through it; components separate on the basis of their charge.

element   one of the substances from which all matter is made; substance that cannot be decomposed into a simpler substance.

elephantiasis   enlargement of the extremities due to block age of lymph flow by small filariae worms.

embolism   the condition of having an embolus (obstruction in the circulation).

embolus   blood clot or other obstruction in the circulation.

embryo   developing offspring during the first 2 months of pregnancy.

emesis   vomiting.

emphysema   pulmonary disease characterized by dilation and destruction of the alveoli.

emulsify   to break up fats into small particles; n., emulsification.

enclosure   indication for the reader that an item is accompanying the letter.

encryption   scrambling E-mail messages as they leave one site and unscrambling them when they arrive at the designated address.

endarterectomy   procedure to remove plaque associated with athersclerosis from the lining of a vessel.

endocardium   membrane that lines the heart chambers and covers the valves.

endocrine   referring to a gland that secretes directly into the bloodstream.

endocrine system   the system composed of glands that secrete hormones.

endocytosis   movement of large amounts of material into a cell (e.g., phagocytosis and pinocytosis).

endolymph   fluid that fills the membranous labyrinth of the inner ear.

endometrium   lining of the uterus.

endomysium   connective tissue around an individual muscle fiber.

endoplasmic reticulum (ER) network of membranes in the cytoplasm of a cell; may be smooth or rough based on absence or presence of ribosomes.

end-organ modified ending on a dendrite that functions as a sensory receptor.

endorphin pain-relieving substance released naturally from the brain.

endosteum thin membrane that lines the marrow cavity of a bone.

endothelium epithelium that lines the heart, blood vessels, and lymphatic vessels.

enucleation removal of the eyeball.

enzyme organic catalyst; speeds the rate of a reaction but is not changed in the reaction.

eosinophil granular white blood cell that shows beadlike, bright pink cytoplasmic granules when stained with acid stain; acidophil.

epicardium membrane that forms the outermost layer of the heart wall and is continuous with the lining of the fibrous pericardium; visceral pericardium.

epicondyle small projection on a bone above a condyle.

epidemic occurrence of a disease among many people in a given region at the same time.

epidermis outermost layer of the skin.

epididymis coiled tube on the surface of the testis in which sperm cells are stored and in which they mature.

epigastric pertaining to the region just inferior to the sternum (breastbone).

epiglottis leaf-shaped cartilage that covers the larynx during swallowing.

epilepsy chronic disorder of the nervous system involving abnormal electrical activity of the brain; characterized by seizures of varying severity.

epimysium sheath of fibrous connective tissue that encloses a muscle.

epinephrine neurotransmitter and hormone; released from neurons of the sympathetic nervous system and from the adrenal medulla; adrenaline.

epiphysis end of a long bone; adj epiphyseal.

episiotomy cutting of the perineum between the vaginal opening and the anus to reduce tissue tearing in childbirth.

epistaxis nosebleed.

epithelium one of the four main types of tissue; forms glands, covers surfaces, and lines cavities; adj., epithelial.

EPO see erythropoietin.

equilibration process of cognitive development in which a person seeks to balance between information and experiences encountered in the environment with existing modes of thought and schemas.

equilibrium sense of balance.

ER see endoplasmic reticulum.

eruption raised skin lesion; rash.

erythema redness of the skin.

erythrocyte red blood cell.

erythropoietin (EPO) hormone released from the kidney that stimulates red blood cell production in the red bone marrow.

esophagus tube that carries food from the throat to the stomach.

estrogen group of female sex hormones that promotes development of the uterine lining and maintains secondary sex characteristics.

Ethernet system that allows the computer to be connected to a cable or DSL system.

etiology study of the cause of a disease or the theory of its origin.

eustachian tube tube that connects the middle ear cavity to the throat; auditory tube.

evaluation the process of indicating how well the patient or person is progressing toward a particular goal; to appraise; to determine the worth or quality of something or someone.

eversion turning outward, with reference to movement of the foot.

excitability in cells, the ability to transmit an electrical current along the plasma membrane.

excoriation scratch into the skin.

excretion removal and elimination of metabolic waste products from the blood.

exfoliation loss of cells from the surface of tissue, such as the skin.

exhalation expulsion of air from the lungs; expiration.

exocrine referring to a gland that secretes through a duct.

exocytosis movement of large amounts of material out of the cell using vesicles.

exophthalmos protrusion (bulging) of the eyes, commonly seen in Graves disease.

extension motion that increases the angle at a joint.

extracellular outside the cell.

extremity limb; an arm or leg.

F

facilitated diffusion movement of material across the plasma membrane as it would normally flow by diffusion but using transporters to speed movement.

fallopian tube see oviduct.

fascia band or sheet of fibrous connective tissue.

fascicle small bundle, as of muscle cells or nerve cell fibers.

fat type of lipid composed of glycerol and fatty acids; triglyceride.

febrile pertaining to fever.

fecalith hardened piece of fecal material that may cause obstruction.

feces waste material discharged from the large intestine; excrement; stool.

feedback return of information into a system, so that it can be used to regulate that system.

fertilization union of an ovum and a spermatozoon.

fetus developing offspring from the third month of pregnancy until birth.

fever abnormally high body temperature.

fibrillation   very rapid, uncoordinated beating of the heart.

fibrin   blood protein that forms a blood clot.

fibrinogen   plasma protein that is converted to fibrin in blood clotting.

filtration   movement of material through a semipermeable membrane under mechanical force.

fimbriae   fringelike extensions of the oviducts that sweep a released ovum into the oviduct.

fissure   deep groove.

flaccid   flabby, limp, soft.

flagellum   long whiplike extension from a cell used for locomotion; pl., flagella.

flatus   gas in the digestive tract; condition of having gas is flatulence.

flexion   bending motion that decreases the angle between bones at a joint.

follicle   sac or cavity, such as the ovarian follicle or hair follicle.

follicle-stimulating hormone (FSH)   hormone produced by the anterior pituitary that stimulates development of ova in the ovary and spermatozoa in the testes.

font   a typeface; affects the way written messages look.

fontanel   membranous area in the infant skull where bone has not yet formed; also spelled fontanelle; "soft spot".

formal operations   stage of cognitive development in Piaget's theory in which the individual can engage in mental manipulation of abstract ideas or symbols that may not have a specific concrete basis.

foramen   opening or passageway, as into or through a bone; pl., foramina.

foramen magnum   large opening in the occipital bone of the skull through which the spinal cord passes to join the brain.

formed elements   cells and cell fragments in the blood.

fornix   a recess or archlike structure.

fossa   hollow or depression, as in a bone; pl., fossae.

fovea   small pit or cup-shaped depression in a surface; the fovea centralis near the center of the retina is the point of sharpest vision.

frontal   describing a plane that divides a structure into anterior and posterior parts.

FSH   see follicle-stimulating hormone.

fulcrum   pivot point in a lever system; joint in the skeletal system.

full block   a type of letter format in which all letter components are justified left.

full-thickness burn   burn that has destroyed all skin layers.

fundus   the deepest portion of an organ, such as the eye or the uterus.

fungus   type of plantlike microorganism; yeast or mold; pl., fungi.

G

gamete   reproductive cell; ovum or spermatozoon.

gamma globulin   protein fraction in the blood plasma that contains antibodies.

ganglion   collection of nerve cell bodies located outside the central nervous system.

gangrene   death of tissue accompanied by bacterial invasion and putrefaction.

gastric-inhibitory peptide (GIP)   hormone from the duodenum that inhibits release of gastric juice and stimulates release of insulin from the pancreas.

gastrin   hormone released from the stomach that stimulates stomach activity.

gastrointestinal (GI)   pertaining to the stomach and intestine or the digestive tract as a whole.

gene   hereditary factor; portion of the DNA on a chromosome.

genetic   pertaining to the genes or heredity.

genotype   genetic make-up of an organism.

gestation   period of development from conception to birth.

GH   see growth hormone.

GI   see gastrointestinal.

gigantism   excessive growth due to oversecretion of growth hormone in childhood.

gingiva   tissue around the teeth; gum.

glans   the enlarged distal portion of the penis.

glaucoma   disorder involving increased fluid pressure within the eye.

glial cells   the connective tissue cells of the nervous system; neuroglia.

glioma   tumor of neuroglial tissue.

glomerular   filtrate Fluid and dissolved materials that leave the blood and enter the kidney nephron through the glomerular (Bowman) capsule.

glomerulonephritis   kidney disease often resulting from antibodies to a streptococcal infection.

glomerulus   cluster of capillaries in the glomerular (Bowman) capsule of the nephron.

glottis   space between the vocal cords.

glucagon   hormone from the pancreatic islets that raises blood glucose level.

glucocorticoid   steroid hormone from the adrenal cortex that raises nutrients in the blood during times of stress, e.g., cortisol.

glucose   simple sugar; main energy source for the cells; dextrose.

glycemic effect   measure of how rapidly a food raises the blood glucose level and stimulates release of insulin.

glycogen   compound built from glucose molecules that is stored for energy in liver and muscles.

glycolysis   first, anaerobic phase of the metabolic breakdown of glucose for energy.

glycosuria   presence of glucose in the urine.

goblet cell   a single-celled gland that secretes mucus.

goiter   enlargement of the thyroid gland.

Golgi apparatus   system of membranes in the cell that formulates special substances; also called Golgi complex.

gonad   sex gland; ovary or testis.

gonadotropin   hormone that acts on a reproductive gland (ovary or testis) e.g., FSH, LH.

gout   type of arthritis caused by a metabolic disturbance.

Graafian follicle   see ovarian follicle.

gram (g)   basic unit of weight in the metric system.

gram stain   procedure used to color microorganisms for viewing under the microscope.

granulocyte   leukocyte with visible granules in the cytoplasm when stained.

Graves disease   common form of hyperthyroidism.

gray matter   nervous tissue composed of unmyelinated fibers and cell bodies.

greater vestibular gland   gland that secretes mucus into the vagina; Bartholin gland.

grief   great sadness caused by loss.

growth hormone (GH)   hormone produced by anterior pituitary that promotes growth of tissues; somatotropin.

gustatory   pertaining to the sense of taste (gustation).

gyrus   raised area of the cerebral cortex; pl., gyri.

H

Haversian canal   channel in the center of an osteon (haversian system), a subunit of compact bone.

Haversian system   see Osteon.

hay fever   seasonal allergy often due to pollen.

heart   the organ that pumps blood through the cardiovascular system.

heat cramps   type of hyperthermia that causes muscle cramping resulting from high-sodium heat exhaustion; hyperthermia resulting from physical exertion in heat without adequate fluid replacement.

heat stroke   most serious type of hyperthermia; body is no longer able to compensate for elevated temperature.

helminth   worm.

hemapheresis   return of blood components to a donor following separation and removal of desired components.

hematocrit (Hct)   volume percentage of red blood cells in whole blood; packed cell volume.

hematoma   blood clot that forms at an injury site.

hematuria   blood in the urine.

hemocytometer   device used to count blood cells under the microscope.

hemodialysis   removal of impurities from the blood by their passage through a semipermeable membrane in a fluid bath.

hemoglobin (Hb)   iron-containing protein in red blood cells that binds oxygen.

hemolysis   rupture of red blood cells; v., hemolyze.

hemolytic disease of the newborn (HDN)   condition that results from Rh incompatibility between a mother and her fetus; erythroblastosis fetalis.

hemophilia   hereditary bleeding disorder associated with a lack of clotting factors in the blood.

hemopoiesis   production of blood cells; hematopoiesis.

hemorrhage   loss of blood.

hemorrhoids   varicose veins in the rectum.

hemostasis   stoppage of bleeding.

hemothorax   accumulation of blood in the pleural space.

heparin   substance that prevents blood clotting; anticoagulant.

hepatitis   inflammation of the liver.

hereditary   transmitted or transmissible through the genes; familial.

heredity   transmission of characteristics from parent to offspring by means of the genes; the genetic makeup of the individual.

hernia   protrusion of an organ or tissue through the wall of the cavity in which it is normally enclosed.

heterozygous   having unmatched alleles for a given trait; hybrid.

hierarchy   ordering or classification of anything in descending order of importance or value.

hilum   indented region of an organ where vessels and nerves enter or leave.

hippocampus   sea horse-shaped region of the limbic system that functions in learning and formation of long-term memory.

histamine   substance released from tissues during an antigen-antibody reaction.

histology   study of tissues.

HIV   see human immunodeficiency virus.

Hodgkin disease   chronic malignant disease of lymphoid tissue.

homeostasis   state of balance within the body; maintenance of body conditions within set limits.

homozygous   having identical alleles for a given trait; pure-bred.

hormone   secretion of an endocrine gland; chemical messenger that has specific regulatory effects on certain other cells.

host   an organism in or on which a parasite lives.

human chorionic gonadotropin (hCG)   hormone produced by embryonic cells soon after implantation that maintains the corpus luteum.

human immunodeficiency virus (HIV)   the virus that causes AIDS.

human placental lactogen (hPL)   hormone produced by the placenta that prepares the breasts for lactation and maintains nutrient levels in maternal blood.

humoral   pertaining to body fluids, such as immunity based on antibodies circulating in the blood.

Huntington disease   progressive degenerative disorder carried by a dominant gene.

hyaline   clear, glasslike; referring to a type of cartilage.

hydatidiform   mole Benign overgrowth of placental tissue.

hydrocephalus   abnormal accumulation of CSF within the brain.

hydrolysis   splitting of large molecules by the addition of water, as in digestion.

hydrophilic   mixing with or dissolving in water, such as salts; literally "water-loving".

hydrophobic   repelling and not dissolving in water, such as fats; literally "water-fearing".

hymen   fold of membrane near the opening of the vaginal canal.

hypercapnia increased level of carbon dioxide in the blood.

hyperglycemia abnormal increase in the amount of glucose in the blood.

hyperopia farsightedness.

hyperpnea abnormal increase in the depth and rate of respiration.

hypersensitivity exaggerated reaction of the immune system to a substance that is normally harmless to most people; allergy.

hypertension high blood pressure.

hyperthermia general condition of excessive body heat.

hypertonic describing a solution that is more concentrated than the fluids within a cell.

hypertrophy enlargement or overgrowth of an organ or part.

hyperventilation increased amount of air entering the alveoli of the lungs due to deep and rapid respiration.

hypocapnia decreased level of carbon dioxide in the blood.

hypochondriac pertaining to a region just inferior to the ribs.

hypogastric pertaining to an area inferior to the stomach or the most inferior midline region of the abdomen.

hypoglycemia abnormal decrease in the amount of glucose in the blood.

hypophysis pituitary gland.

hypopnea decrease in the rate and depth of breathing.

hypospadias opening of the urethra on the undersurface of the penis.

hypotension low blood pressure.

hypothalamus region of the brain that controls the pituitary and maintains homeostasis.

hypothermia abnormally low body temperature.

hypotonic describing a solution that is less concentrated than the fluids within a cell.

hypoventilation insufficient amount of air entering the alveoli.

hypovolemic shock shock caused by loss of blood or other body fluids.

hypoxemia lower than normal concentration of oxygen in arterial blood.

hypoxia lower than normal level of oxygen in the tissues.

hysterectomy surgical removal of the uterus.

I

iatrogenic resulting from the adverse effects of treatment.

ICSH see Luteinizing hormone.

idiopathic describing a disease without known cause.

ileum the last portion of the small intestine.

ileus intestinal obstruction caused by lack of peristalsis or by muscle contraction.

iliac pertaining to the ilium, the upper portion of the hipbone.

immunity power of an individual to resist or overcome the effects of a particular disease or other harmful agent.

immunization use of a vaccine to produce immunity; vaccination.

immunodeficiency any failure of the immune system.

immunoglobulin (Ig) see antibody.

immunotherapy stimulation of the immune system to fight disease, such as cancer.

impetigo acute, contagious staphylococcal or streptococcal skin infection.

implantation the embedding of the fertilized egg into the lining of the uterus.

implementation the process of initiating and carrying out an action such as a teaching plan or patient treatment

incidence range of occurrence of a disease.

infarct area of tissue damaged from lack of blood supply caused by a vessel blockage.

infarction death of tissues due to lack of oxygen.

infection invasion by pathogens.

infectious mononucleosis acute viral infection associated with enlargement of the lymph nodes.

inferior below or lower.

inferior vena cava large vein that drains the lower part of the body and empties into the right atrium of the heart.

infertility decreased ability to reproduce.

inflammation response of tissues to injury; characterized by heat, redness, swelling, and pain.

influenza acute contagious viral disease of the upper respiratory tract.

infundibulum stalk that connects the pituitary gland to the hypothalamus of the brain.

ingestion the intake of food.

inguinal pertaining to the groin region or the region of the inguinal canal.

inhalation drawing of air into the lungs; inspiration.

insertion muscle attachment connected to a movable part.

insulin hormone from the pancreatic islets that lowers blood glucose level.

integument skin; adj., integumentary.

integumentary system the skin and all its associated structures.

intercalated disk a modified plasma membrane in cardiac tissue that allows rapid transfer of electrical impulses between cells.

intercaps words or phrases with unusual capitalization.

intercellular between cells.

intercostal between the ribs.

interferon (IFN) group of substances released from virus-infected cells that prevent spread of infection to other cells; also nonspecifically boost the immune system.

interleukin a substance released by a T cell or macrophage that stimulates other cells of the immune system.

Internet global system used to connect one computer to another.

interneuron a nerve cell that transmits impulses within the central nervous system.

interpersonal concerning the relations and interactions between persons.

interphase stage in the life of a cell between one mitosis and the next when a cell is not dividing.

interstitial between; pertaining to spaces or structures in an organ between active tissues.

interstitial cell-stimulating hormone (ICSH) see Luteinizing hormone.

intestine organ of the digestive tract between the stomach and the anus, consisting of the small and large intestine.

intracellular within a cell.

intranet a private network system of computers.

intussusception slipping of a part of the intestine into a part below it.

inversion turning inward, with reference to movement of the foot.

ion charged particle formed when an electrolyte goes into solution.

ionic bond chemical bond formed by the exchange of electrons between atoms.

iris circular colored region of the eye around the pupil.

ischemia decrease in oxygen to tissues.

islets groups of cells in the pancreas that produce hormones; islets of Langerhans.

isometric contraction muscle contraction in which there is no change in muscle length but an increase in muscle tension, as in pushing against an immovable force.

isotonic describing a solution that has the same concentration as the fluid within a cell.

isotonic contraction muscle contraction in which the tone within the muscle remains the same but the muscle shortens to produce movement.

isotope form of an element that has the same atomic number as another form of that element but a different atomic weight; isotopes differ in their numbers of neutrons.

isthmus narrow band, such as the band that connects the two lobes of the thyroid gland.

J

jaundice yellowish discoloration of the skin that is usually due to the presence of bile in the blood.

jejunum second portion of the small intestine.

joint area of junction between two or more bones; articulation.

juxtaglomerular (JG) apparatus structure in the kidney composed of cells of the afferent arteriole and distal convoluted tubule that secretes the enzyme renin when blood pressure decreases below a certain level.

K

karyotype picture of the chromosomes arranged according to size and form.

keloid mass or raised area that results from excess production of scar tissue.

keratin protein that thickens and protects the skin; makes up hair and nails.

ketoacidosis acidosis that results from accumulation of ketone bodies in the blood.

kidney organ of excretion.

kilocalorie a measure of the energy content of food; technically, the amount of heat needed to raise 1 kg of water 1° centigrade.

kinesthesia sense of body movement.

Klinefelter syndrome genetic disorder involving abnormal sex chromosomes, usually an extra X chromosome.

Kupffer cells macrophages in the liver that help to fight infection.

Kussmaul respiration deep, rapid respiration characteristic of acidosis (overly acidic body fluids) as seen in uncontrolled diabetes.

kwashiorkor severe protein and energy malnutrition seen in children after weaning.

kyphosis exaggerated lumbar curve of the spine.

L

labium lip; pl labia.

labyrinth inner ear, named for its complex shape.

laceration rough, jagged wound of the skin.

lacrimal referring to tears or the tear glands.

lactation secretion of milk.

lacteal lymphatic capillary that drains digested fats from the villi of the small intestine.

lactic acid organic acid that accumulates in muscle cells functioning without oxygen.

laryngeal pharynx lowest portion of the pharynx, opening into the larynx and esophpagus.

larynx structure between the pharynx and trachea that contains the vocal cords; voice box.

laser device that produces a very intense beam of light.

lateral farther from the midline; toward the side.

learning objectives steps that needed to be achieved to accomplish the learning goal.

lens biconvex structure of the eye that changes in thickness to accommodate for near and far vision; crystalline lens.

lesion wound or local injury.

leukemia malignant blood disease characterized by abnormal development of white blood cells.

leukocyte white blood cell.

leukocytosis increase in the number of white cells in the blood, such as during infection.

leukopenia deficiency of leukocytes in the blood.

leukoplakia thickened white patches on the oral mucous membranes, often due to smoking.

LH see luteinizing hormone.

ligament band of connective tissue that connects a bone to another bone; thickened portion or fold of the peritoneum that supports an organ or attaches it to another organ.

limbic system area between the brain's cerebrum and diencephalon that is involved in emotional states and behavior.

lipid type of organic compound, one example of which is a fat.

liter (L) basic unit of volume in the metric system; 1000 mL; 1.06 qt.

literary search finding professional journal articles on a given subject.

lithotripsy use of external shock waves to shatter stones (calculi).

loop of Henle hairpin shaped segment of the renal tubule between the proximal and distal convoluted tubules.

lordosis exaggerated lumbar curve of the spine.

lumbar pertaining to the region of the spine between the thoracic vertebrae and the sacrum.

lumen central opening of an organ or vessel.

lung Organ of respiration.

lunula the pale half-moon shaped area at the proximal end of the nail.

lupus erythematosus chronic inflammatory autoimmune disease that involves the skin and sometimes other organs.

luteinizing hormone hormone produced by the anterior pituitary that induces ovulation and formation of the corpus luteum in females; in males, it stimulates cells in the testes to produce testosterone and may be called interstitial cell-stimulating hormone (ICSH).

lymph fluid in the lymphatic system.

lymph node mass of lymphoid tissue along the path of a lymphatic vessel that filters lymph and harbors white blood cells active in immunity.

lymphadenitis inflammation of lymph nodes.

lymphadenopathy any disorder of lymph nodes.

lymphangitis inflammation of lymphatic vessels.

lymphatic duct vessel of the lymphatic system.

lymphatic system system consisting of the lymphatic vessels and lymphoid tissue; involved in immunity, digestion, and fluid balance.

lymphedema edema due to obstruction of lymph flow.

lymphocyte agranular white blood cell that functions in immunity.

lymphoma any tumor, benign or malignant, that occurs in lymphoid tissue.

lysosome cell organelle that contains digestive enzymes.

M

macrophage large phagocytic cell that develops from a monocyte; presents antigen to lymphocytes in immune response.

macula spot; flat, discolored spot on the skin, such as a freckle or measles lesion; also called macule; Small yellow spot in the retina of the eye that contains the fovea, the point of sharpest vision; receptor for the sense of static equilibrium.

magnetic resonance imaging (MRI) method for studying tissue based on nuclear movement after exposure to radio waves in a powerful magnetic field.

major histocompatibility complex (MHC) group of genes that codes for specific proteins (antigens) on the surface of cells; these antigens are important in cross-matching for tissue transplantation; they are also important in immune reactions.

malignant describing a tumor that spreads; describing a disorder that tends to become worse and cause death.

malnutrition state resulting from lack of food, lack of an essential component of the diet, or faulty use of food in the diet.

MALT Mucosal-associated lymphoid tissue; tissue in the mucous membranes that helps fight infection.

mammary gland breast.

mammogram radiographic study of the breast.

marasmus severe malnutrition in infants.

margin the blank space around the edges of a piece of paper, such as a letter or page of a book.

mastectomy removal of the breast; mammectomy.

mastication act of chewing.

mastitis inflammation of the breast.

matrix the nonliving background material in a tissue; the intercellular material.

meatus short channel or passageway, as in a bone.

medial nearer the midline of the body.

mediastinum region between the lungs and the organs and vessels it contains.

medulla inner region of an organ; marrow.

medulla oblongata part of the brain stem that connects the brain to the spinal cord.

medullary cavity channel at the center of a long bone that contains bone marrow.

megakaryocyte very large cell that gives rise to blood platelets.

meibomian gland gland that produces a secretion that lubricates the eyelashes.

meiosis process of cell division that halves the chromosome number in the formation of the reproductive cells.

melanin dark pigment found in skin, hair, parts of the eye, and certain parts of the brain.

melanocyte cell that produces melanin.

melanoma malignant tumor of melanocytes.

melatonin hormone produced by the pineal gland.

melena black, tarry stools caused by digested blood from the gastrointestinal tract.

membrane thin sheet of tissue.

memorandum a type of written documentation used for interoffice communication.

Mendelian laws principles of heredity discovered by an Austrian monk named Gregor Mendel.

meninges three layers of fibrous membranes that cover the brain and spinal cord.

menopause time during which menstruation ceases.

menses monthly flow of blood from the female reproductive tract.

menstruation the period of menstrual flow.

mesentery membranous peritoneal ligament that attaches the small intestine to the dorsal abdominal wall.

mesocolon   peritoneal ligament that attaches the colon to the dorsal abdominal wall.

mesothelium   epithelial tissue found in serous membranes.

messages   words sent from one person to another; information sent through spoken, written, or body language.

metabolic rate   rate at which energy is released from nutrients in the cells.

metabolism   all the physical and chemical processes by which an organism is maintained.

metaphase   second stage of mitosis, during which the chromsomes line up across the equator of the cell.

metarteriole   small vessel that connects the arterial system directly with the venous system in a blood shunt; thoroughfare channel.

metastasis   spread of tumor cells; pl., metastases.

meter (m)   basic unit of length in the metric system; 1.1 yards.

MHC   see Major histocompatibility complex.

microbiology   study of microscopic organisms.

micrometer (mm)   1/1000th of a millimeter; micron; an instrument for measuring through a microscope.

microorganism   microscopic organism.

microscope   magnifying instrument used to examine cells and other structures not visible with the naked eye; examples are the compound light microscope, transmission electron microscope (TEM) and scanning electron microscope (SEM).

microvilli   small projections of the plasma membrane that increase surface area; sing., microvillus.

micturition   act of urination; voiding of the urinary bladder.

midbrain   upper portion of the brainstem.

mineral   inorganic substance; in the diet, an element needed in small amounts for health.

mineralocorticoid   steroid hormone from the adrenal cortex that regulates electrolyte balance, e.g. aldosterone.

mitochondria   cell organelles that manufacture ATP with the energy released from the oxidation of nutrients; sing., mitochondrion.

mitosis   type of cell division that produces two daughter cells exactly like the parent cell.

mitral valve   valve between the left atrium and left ventricle of the heart; left AV valve; bicuspid valve.

mixture   blend of two or more substances.

molecule   particle formed by chemical bonding of two or more atoms; smallest subunit of a compound.

monocyte   phagocytic agranular white blood cell.

monosaccharide   simple sugar; basic unit of carbohydrates.

morbidity rate   proportion of people with a specific disease in a given population per unit of time.

mortality rate   percentage of a population that dies from a given disease within a period of time.

motor   describing structures or activities involved in transmitting impulses away from the central nervous system; efferent.

motor end plate   region of a muscle cell membrane that receives nervous stimulation.

motor unit   group consisting of a single neuron and all the muscle fibers it stimulates.

mourning   to demonstrate signs of grief; grieving.

mouth   proximal opening of the digestive tract where food is ingested, chewed, mixed with saliva and swallowed.

MRI   see magnetic resonance imaging.

mucosa   lining membrane that produces mucus; mucous membrane.

mucus   thick protective fluid secreted by mucous membranes and glands; adj., mucous.

multiple sclerosis   disease that affects the myelin sheath around axons leading to neuron degeneration.

murmur   abnormal heart sound.

muscle   tissue that contracts to produce movement; includes skeletal, smooth and cardiac types; adj., muscular.

muscular system   the system of skeletal muscles that moves the skeleton, supports and protects the organs and maintains posture.

mutagen   agent that causes mutation; adj., mutagenic.

mutation   change in a gene or a chromosome.

myalgia   muscular pain.

mycology   study of fungi (yeasts and molds).

myelin   fatty material that covers and insulates the axons of some neurons.

myocardium   middle layer of the heart wall; heart muscle.

myoglobin   compound that stores oxygen in muscle cells.

myoma   usually benign tumor of the uterus; fibroma; fibroid.

myometrium   the muscular layer of the uterus.

myopia   nearsightedness.

myosin   one of the two contractile proteins in muscle cells, the other being actin.

myxedema   condition that results from hypothyroidism in adults.

N

narcotic   drug that acts on the CNS to alter perception and response to pain.

nasopharynx   upper portion of the pharynx located posterior to the nasal cavity.

natural killer (NK) cell   type of lymphocyte that can nonspecifically destroy abnormal cells.

naturopathy   philosophy of helping people to heal themselves by developing healthy lifestyles.

nausea   unpleasant sensation due to disturbance in the upper GI tract that may precede vomiting.

necrosis   tissue death.

negative feedback   self-regulating system in which the result of an action is the control over that action; a method for keeping body conditions within a normal range and maintaining homeostasis.

neoplasm   abnormal growth of cells; tumor; adj., neoplastic.

nephron microscopic functional unit of the kidney.

nerve bundle of neuron fibers outside the central nervous system.

nerve impulse electrical charge that spreads along the membrane of a neuron; action potential.

nervous system the system that transports information in the body by means of electrical impulses.

neuralgia pain in a nerve.

neurilemma thin sheath that covers certain peripheral axons; aids in axon regeneration.

neurogenic shock shock that results from dysfunction of nervous system following spinal cord injury.

neuroglia supporting and protective cells of the central nervous system; glial cells.

neuromuscular junction point at which a nerve fiber contacts a muscle cell.

neuron conducting cell of the nervous system.

neurotransmitter chemical released from the ending of an axon that enables a nerve impulse to cross a synapse.

neutron noncharged particle in the nucleus of an atom.

neutrophil phagocytic granular white blood cell; polymorph; poly; PMN; seg.

nevus mole or birthmark.

nitrogen chemical element found in all proteins.

node small mass of tissue, such as a lymph node; space between cells in the myelin sheath.

nonlanguage not expressed in spoken language, e.g., laughing, sobbing, grunting, sighing.

noncompliance the patient's inability or refusal to follow prescribed orders.

norepinephrine neurotransmitter similar to epinephrine; noradrenaline.

normal saline isotonic or physiologic salt solution.

nosocomial acquired in a hospital, as an infection.

nucleic acid complex organic substance composed of nucleotides that makes up DNA and RNA.

nucleolus small unit within the nucleus that assembles ribosomes.

nucleotide building block of DNA and RNA.

nucleus largest organelle in the cell, containing the DNA, which directs all cell activities; group of neurons in the central nervous system; in chemistry, the central part of an atom.

nutrition the study of food and how it is used for growth, nourishment, and repair.

O

obstipation extreme constipation.

occlusion closing, as of a vessel.

olfactory pertaining to the sense of smell (olfaction).

omentum portion of the peritoneum; greater omentum extends over the anterior abdomen; lesser omentum extends between the stomach and liver.

oncology study of tumors.

ophthalmic pertaining to the eye.

ophthalmoscope instrument for examining the posterior (fundus) of the eye.

opportunistic describing an infection that takes hold because a host has been compromised (weakened) by disease.

organ body part containing two or more tissues functioning together for specific purposes.

organ of Corti receptor for hearing located in the cochlea of the internal ear.

organelle specialized subdivision within a cell.

organic referring to the complex compounds found in living things that contain carbon, and usually hydrogen, and oxygen.

organism individual plant or animal; any organized living thing.

origin source; beginning; muscle attachment connected to a nonmoving part.

oropharynx middle portion of the pharynx, located behind the mouth.

orthopnea difficulty in breathing that is relieved by sitting in an upright position.

osmosis movement of water through a semipermeable membrane.

osmotic pressure tendency of a solution to draw water into it; is directly related to the concentration of the solution.

osseus pertaining to bone tissue.

ossicle one of three small bones of the middle ear: malleus, incus, or stapes.

ossification process of bone formation.

osteoblast bone-forming cell.

osteoclast cell that breaks down bone.

osteocyte mature bone cell; maintains bone but does not produce new bone tissue.

osteon subunit of compact bone, consisting of concentric rings of bone tissue around a central channel; haversian system.

osteopenia reduction in bone density to below average levels.

osteoporosis abnormal loss of bone tissue with tendency to fracture.

otoliths crystals that add weight to fluids in the inner ear and function in the sense of static equilibrium.

ovarian follicle cluster of cells in which the ovum develops within the ovary; Graafian follicle.

ovary female reproductive gland.

oviduct tube that carries ova from the ovaries to the uterus; fallopian tube, uterine tube.

ovulation release of a mature ovum from a follicle in the ovary.

ovum female reproductive cell or gamete; pl., ova.

oxidation chemical breakdown of nutrients for energy.

oxygen (O_2) the gas needed to break down nutrients completely for energy within the cell.

oxygen debt amount of oxygen needed to reverse the effects produced in muscles functioning without oxygen.

oxytocin   hormone from the posterior pituitary that causes uterine contraction and milk ejection ("letdown") from the breasts.

P

pacemaker   sinoatrial (SA) node of the heart; group of cells or artificial device that sets the rate of heart contractions.

palate   roof of the oral cavity; anterior portion is hard palate, posterior portion is soft palate.

pallor   paleness of the skin.

pancreas   large, elongated gland behind the stomach; produces digestive enzymes and hormones (e.g., insulin).

pandemic   disease that is prevalent throughout an entire country, continent, or the world..

Papanicolaou test   histologic test for cervical cancer; Pap test or smear.

papilla   small nipplelike projection or elevation.

papule   firm, raised lesion of the skin.

paracentesis   puncture of the abdominal cavity, usually to remove a fluid accumulation, such as ascites; abdominocentesis.

paralanguage   factors connected with, but not essentially part of language, e.g., tone of voice, volume, pitch.

paraphrasing   restating what you heard using your own words.

parasite   organism that lives on or within another (the host) at the other's expense.

parasympathetic nervous system   craniosacral division of the autonomic nervous system; generally reverses the fight-or-flight (stress) response.

parathyroid gland   any of four to six small glands embedded in the capsule enclosing the thyroid gland; produces parathyroid hormone, which raises the blood calcium level by causing release of calcium from bones.

parietal   pertaining to the wall of a space or cavity.

Parkinson disease   progressive neuro-logic condition characterized by tremors, rigidity of limbs and joints, slow movement, and impaired balance.

partial-thickness burn   burn that involves epidermis and varying levels of the dermis.

parturition   childbirth; labor.

pathogen   disease-causing organism; adj., pathogenic.

pathology   study of disease.

pathophysiology   study of the physiologic basis of disease.

pedigree   family history; used in the study of heredity; family tree.

pelvic inflammatory disease (PID)   ascending infection that involves the pelvic organs; common causes are gonorrhea and chlamydia.

pelvis   basinlike structure, such as the lower portion of the abdomen or the upper flared portion of the ureter (renal pelvis).

pemphigus   an autoimmune skin disease with blistering of the skin.

penis   male organ of urination and sexual intercourse.

perforating canal   channel across a long bone that contains blood vessels and nerves; Volkmann canal.

pericardium   fibrous sac lined with serous membrane that encloses the heart.

perichondrium   layer of connective tissue that covers cartilage.

perilymph   fluid that fills the inner ear's bony labyrinth.

perimysium   connective tissue around a fascicle of muscle tissue.

perineum   pelvic floor; external region between the anus and genital organs.

periosteum   connective tissue membrane covering a bone.

peripheral   located away from a center or central structure.

peripheral nervous system (PNS)   all the nerves and nervous tissue outside the central nervous system.

peristalsis   wavelike movements in the wall of an organ or duct that propel its contents forward.

peritoneum   serous membrane that lines the abdominal cavity and forms outer layer of abdominal organs; forms supporting ligaments for some organs.

peritonitis   inflammation of the peritoneum.

peroxisome   cell organelle that enzymatically destroys harmful substances produced in metabolism.

personality traits   defining characteristics that are unique to each individual.

Peyer patches   clusters of lymphatic nodules in the mucous membranes lining the distal portion of the small intestine.

pH   symbol indicating hydrogen ion (H1) concentration; scale that measures the relative acidity and alkalinity (basicity) of a solution.

phagocyte   cell capable of engulfing large particles, such as foreign matter or cellular debris, through the plasma membrane.

phagocytosis   engulfing of large particles through the plasma membrane.

pharynx   throat; passageway between the mouth and esophagus.

phenotype   all the characteristics of an organism that can be seen or tested for.

phenylketonuria (PKU)   hereditary metabolic disorder involving inability to metabolize the amino acid phenylalanine.

phimosis   tightness of the foreskin.

phlebitis   inflammation of a vein.

phospholipid   complex lipid containing phosphorus.

phrenic   pertaining to the diaphragm.

physiology   study of the function of living organisms.

pia mater   innermost layer of the meninges.

PID   see pelvic inflammatory disease.

pineal gland   gland in the brain that is regulated by light; involved in sleep-wake cycles.

pinna   outer projecting portion of the ear; auricle.

pinocytosis   intake of small particles and droplets by the plasma membrane of a cell.

pituitary gland endocrine gland located under and controlled by the hypothalamus; releases hormones that control other glands; hypophysis.

placebo the power of believing that something will make you better without any chemical reaction that warrants improvement, e.g., sugar pills.

placenta structure that nourishes and maintains the developing fetus during pregnancy.

planning the process of using information gathered during the assessment phase to organize learning or patient care objectives in order to accomplish the specific learning or treatment goal.

plaque a patch or flat area; fatty material that deposits in vessel linings in atherosclerosis.

plasma liquid portion of the blood.

plasma cell cell derived from a B cell that produces antibodies.

plasma membrane outer covering of a cell; regulates what enters and leaves cell; cell membrane.

plasmapheresis separation and removal of plasma from a blood donation and return of the formed elements to the donor.

platelet cell fragment that forms a plug to stop bleeding and acts in blood clotting; thrombocyte.

pleura serous membrane that lines the chest cavity and covers the lungs.

pleurisy inflammation of the pleura; pleuritis.

plexus network of vessels or nerves.

pneumonia inflammation of the lungs, commonly due to infection; pneumonitis.

pneumothorax accumulation of air in the pleural space.

PNS see peripheral nervous system.

poliomyelitis (polio) viral disease of the nervous system that occurs most commonly in children.

polycythemia increase in the number of red cells in the blood.

polydipsia excessive thirst.

polyp protruding growth, often grapelike, from a mucous membrane.

polysaccharide compound formed from many simple sugars linked together, such as starch and glycogen.

pons area of the brain between the midbrain and medulla; connects the cerebellum with the rest of the central nervous system.

portal system venous system that carries blood to a second capillary bed through which it circulates before returning to the heart.

positive feedback a substance or condition that acts within a system to promote more of the same activity.

positron emission tomography (PET) imaging method that uses a radioactive substance to show activity in an organ.

postconventional phase or moral development in which the individual recognizes the importance of societal rules as a basis for behavior but may also follow internal moral principles that supercede these rules.

posterior toward the back; dorsal.

potential an electrical charge, as on the neuron plasma membrane.

precipitation clumping of small particles as a result of an antigen-antibody reaction; seen as a cloudiness.

preconscious level of the mind not present in consciousness, but able to be recalled at will.

preconventional phase of moral development in which moral reasoning is guided by punishments and rewards with a focus on avoiding punishment and obedience to authority without concern for the interests or feelings of others.

preeclampsia see pregnancy induced hypertension.

pregnancy the period during which an embryo or fetus is developing in the body.

pregnancy-induced hypertension (PIH) hypertension, proteinuria and edema associated with a hormone imbalance in the latter part of pregnancy; if untreated, may lead to eclampsia; preeclampsia, toxemia of pregnancy.

preoperational second stage of cognitive development, according to Piaget, that is characterized by the development of internal mental representations (schema) and verbal communication.

prepuce loose fold of skin that covers the glans penis; foreskin.

presbyacusis loss of hearing associated with aging.

presbyopia loss of visual accommodation that occurs with age, leading to farsightedness.

prime mover muscle that performs a given movement; agonist.

prion an infectious protein particle that causes progressive neurodegenerative disease.

PRL see Prolactin.

progeny offspring, descendent.

progesterone hormone produced by the corpus luteum and placenta; maintains the lining of the uterus for pregnancy.

prognosis prediction of the probable outcome of a disease based on the condition of the patient and knowledge about the disease.

prolactin hormone from the anterior pituitary that stimulates milk production in the breasts; PRL.

prone face down or palm down.

proofread read the written draft for accuracy and clarity and correct errors.

prophase first stage of mitosis, during which the chromosomes become visible and the organelles disappear.

prophylaxis prevention of disease.

proprioceptor sensory receptor that aids in judging body position and changes in position; located in muscles, tendons, and joints.

prostaglandin any of a group of hormones produced by many cells; these hormones have a variety of effects.

prostate gland gland that surrounds the urethra below the bladder and contributes secretions to the semen.

protein organic compound made of amino acids; contains nitrogen in addition to carbon, hydrogen, and oxygen (some contain sulfur or phosphorus).

prothrombin clotting factor; converted to thrombin during blood clotting.

prothrombinase blood clotting factor that converts prothrombin to thrombin.

proton positively charged particle in the nucleus of an atom.

protozoon animal-like microorganism; pl., protozoa.

proximal nearer to point of origin or to a reference point.

pruritis intense itching of the skin.

psoriasis chronic skin disease with red, flat areas covered with silvery scales.

psychomotor describes a physical task.

psychosocial related to both psychological and social factors.

ptosis dropping down of a part.

puerperal related to childbirth.

pulmonary circuit pathway that carries blood from the heart to the lungs for oxygenation and then returns the blood to the heart.

pulse wave of increased pressure in the vessels produced by contraction of the heart.

pupil opening in the center of the eye through which light enters.

Purkinje fibers part of the conduction system of the heart; conduction myofibers.

pus Mixture of bacteria and leukocytes formed in response to infection.

pustule vesicle filled with pus.

pylorus distal region of the stomach that leads to the pyloric sphincter.

pyrogen substance that produces fever.

pyruvic acid intermediate product in the breakdown of glucose for energy.

R

radioactivity emission of atomic particles from an element.

radiography production of an image by passage of x-rays through the body onto sensitized film; record produced is a radiograph.

range-of-motion (ROM) range in degrees of angle through which a joint can be extended and flexed.

rash surface skin lesion.

receptor specialized cell or ending of a sensory neuron that can be excited by a stimulus. A site in the cell membrane to which a special substance (e.g., hormone, antibody) may attach.

recessive referring to a gene that is not expressed if a dominant gene for the same trait is present.

reflecting repeat what one heard using open-ended questions.

reflex simple, rapid, automatic response involving few neurons.

reflex arc a pathway through the nervous system from stimulus to response; commonly involves a receptor, sensory neuron, central neuron(s), motor neuron, and effector.

refraction bending of light rays as they pass from one medium to another of a different density.

reinforcement stimulus used in operant conditioning that increases the probability that a given behavior associated with the stimulus will be repeated.

relaxin placental hormone that softens the cervix and relaxes the pelvic joints.

renin enzyme released from the kidney's juxtaglomerular apparatus that indirectly increases blood pressure by activating angiotensin.

repolarization a sudden return to the original charge on a cell membrane following depolarizaiton.

resorption loss of substance, such as that of bone or a tooth.

respiration process by which oxygen is obtained from the environment and delivered to the cells.

respiratory system the system consisting of the lungs and breathing passages involved in exchange of oxygen and carbon dioxide between the outside air and the blood.

reticular formation network in the limbic system that governs wakefulness and sleep.

reticuloendothelial system protective system consisting of highly phagocytic cells in body fluids and tissues, such as the spleen, lymph nodes, bone marrow, and liver.

retina innermost layer of the eye; contains light-sensitive cells (rods and cones).

retroperitoneal behind the peritoneum, as are the kidneys, pancreas, and abdominal aorta.

Rh factor a red cell antigen; D antigen.

rheumatoid arthritis disease of connective tissue that affects the joints.

rhodopsin light-sensitive pigment in the rods of the eye; visual purple.

rib one of the slender curved bones that make up most of the thorax; costa; adj. costal.

ribonucleic acid (RNA) substance needed for protein manufacture in the cell.

ribosome small body in the cell's cytoplasm that is a site of protein manufacture.

rickets softening of bone (osteomalacia) in children, usually caused by a deficiency of vitamin D.

Rickettsia extremely small oval to rod-shaped bacterium that can grow only within a living cell.

RNA see ribonucleic acid.

rod receptor cell in the retina of the eye; used for vision in dim light.

roentgenogram image produced by means of x-rays; radiograph.

rotation twisting or turning of a bone on its own axis.

rugae folds in the lining of an organ, such as the stomach or urinary bladder; sing., ruga.

rule of nines method for estimating the extent of a burn based on multiples of nine.

S

SA node see Sinoatrial node.

sagittal describing a plane that divides a structure into right and left portions.

saliva secretion of the salivary glands; moistens food and contains an enzyme that digests starch.

salt compound formed by reaction between an acid and a base (e.g. NaCl, table salt).

salutation an introductory phrase that greets the reader of a letter.

sarcoma malignant tumor of connective tissue; a form of cancer.

saturated fat fat that has more hydrogen atoms and fewer double bonds between carbons than do unsaturated fats.

scar fibrous connective tissue that replaces normal tissues destroyed by injury or disease; cicatrix.

Schwann cell cell in the nervous system that produces the myelin sheath around peripheral axons.

sclera outermost layer of the eye; made of tough connective tissue; "white" of the eye.

scleroderma an autoimmune disease associated with overproduction of collagen.

scoliosis lateral curvature of the spine.

scrotum sac in which testes are suspended.

search engine program that allows you to find information on the Internet rapidly and effectively.

sebum oily secretion that lubricates the skin; adj., sebaceous.

secondary traits personality traits that have some bearing on a person's behavior but that are not particularly central to what the person does.

secretin hormone from the duodenum that stimulates pancreatic release of water and bicarbonate.

seizure series of muscle spasms; convulsion.

selectively permeable describing a membrane that regulates what can pass through (e.g., the plasma membrane of a cell).

sella turcica saddlelike depression in the floor of the skull that holds the pituitary gland.

semen mixture of sperm cells and secretions from several glands of the male reproductive tract.

semiblock a type of letter format that is styled the same as block, except the first sentence of each paragraph is indented five spaces.

semicircular canal bony canal in the internal ear that contains receptors for the sense of dynamic equilibrium; there are three semicircular canals in each ear.

semilunar shaped like a half-moon, such as the flaps of the pulmonary and aortic valves.

seminal vesicle gland that contributes secretions to the semen.

seminiferous tubules tubules in which sperm cells develop in the testis.

semipermeable capable of being penetrated by some substances and not others.

sensorimotor first stage of cognitive development in Piaget's theory in which individuals largely develop in terms of sensory input and motor output abilities with reflexive responses and gradually expanding to schema and purposeful actions.

sensory describing cells or activities involved in transmitting impulses toward the central nervous system; afferent.

sensory adaptation gradual loss of sensation when sensory receptors are exposed to continuous stimulation.

sepsis presence of pathogenic microorganisms or their toxins in the bloodstream or other tissues; adj., septic.

septicemia presence of pathogenic organisms or their toxins in the bloodstream; blood poisoning.

septic shock shock that results from general infection in the bloodstream.

septum dividing wall, as between the chambers of the heart or the nasal cavities.

serosa serous membrane; epithelial membrane that secretes a thin, watery fluid.

Sertoli cells see Sustentacular cells.

serum liquid portion of blood without clotting factors; thin, watery fluid; adj., serous.

sex-linked referring to a gene carried on a sex chromosome, usually the X chromosome.

sexually transmitted infection (STI) communicable disease acquired through sexual relations; sexually transmitted disease (STD); venereal disease (VD).

shingles viral infection that follows the nerve pathways; caused by the same virus that causes chicken pox; herpes zoster.

shock pertaining to the circulation: a life-threatening condition in which there is inadequate blood flow to the tissues.

sickle cell disease hereditary disease in which abnormal hemoglobin causes red blood cells to change shape (sickle) when they release oxygen.

sign manifestation of a disease as noted by an observer.

sinoatrial (SA) node tissue in the upper wall of the right atrium that sets the rate of heart contractions; the heart's pacemaker.

sinus cavity or channel, such as the paranasal sinuses in the skull bones.

sinus rhythm a normal heart rhythm originating at the SA node.

sinusoid enlarged capillary that serves as a blood channel.

skeletal system the body system that includes the bones and joints.

skeleton the complete bony framework of the body; adj., skeletal.

skull bony framework of the head.

solute substance that is dissolved in another substance (the solvent).

solution homogeneous mixture of one substance dissolved in another; the components in a mixture are evenly distributed and cannot be distinguished from each other.

solvent substance in which another substance (the solute) is dissolved.

somatic nervous system the division of the nervous system that controls voluntary activities and stimulates skeletal muscle.

somatotropin growth hormone.

spasm sudden and involuntary muscular contraction.

specific gravity the weight of a substance as compared to the weight of an equal volume of pure water.

spermatic cord cord that extends through the inguinal canal and suspends the testis; contains blood vessels nerves and ductus deferens.

spermatozoon male reproductive cell or gamete; pl., spermatozoa; sperm cell.

sphincter muscular ring that regulates the size of an opening.

sphygmomanometer device used to measure blood pressure; blood pressure apparatus or cuff.

spina bifida incomplete closure of the spine.

spinal cord nervous tissue contained in the spinal column; major relay area between the brain and the peripheral nervous system.

spirillum corkscrew or spiral-shaped bacterium; pl., spirilla.

spirochete spiral-shaped microorganism that moves in a waving and twisting motion.

spirometer instrument for recording lung volumes; tracing is a spirogram.

spleen lymphoid organ in the upper left region of the abdomen.

splint device used to immobilize a sprain, strain, fracture, or dislocated limb.

spore resistant form of bacterium; reproductive cell in lower plants.

squamous flat and irregular, as in squamous epithelium.

staging a procedure for evaluating the extent of tumor spread.

stain dye that aids in viewing structures under the microscope.

staphylococcus round bacterium found in a cluster resembling a bunch of grapes; pl., staphylococci.

stasis stoppage in the normal flow of fluids, such as blood, lymph, urine, or contents of the digestive tract.

stem cell cell that has the potential to develop into different types of cells.

stenosis narrowing of a duct or canal.

stent small tube inserted into a vessel to keep it open.

stereotyping to place in a fixed mold, without consideration of differences.

sterility complete inability to reproduce.

sterilization process of killing every living microorganism on or in an object; procedure that makes an individual incapable of reproduction.

steroid category of lipids that includes the hormones of the sex glands and the adrenal cortex.

stethoscope instrument for conveying sounds from the patient's body to the examiner's ears.

STI see Sexually transmitted infection.

stimulus change in the external or internal environment that produces a response.

stomach organ of the digestive tract that stores food, mixes it with digestive juices and moves it into the small intestine.

strabismus deviation of the eye resulting from lack of eyeball muscle coordination.

stratified in multiple layers (strata).

stratum a layer; pl. strata.

stratum basale deepest layer of the epidermis; layer that produces new epidermal cells; stratum germinativum.

stratum corneum the thick uppermost layer of the epidermis.

stress a factor that induces body tension; can be positive or negative.

striations stripes or bands, as seen in skeletal muscle and cardiac muscle.

stricture narrowing of a part.

stroke damage to the brain due to lack of oxygen; usually caused by a blood clot in a vessel (thrombus) or rupture of a vessel; cerebrovascular accidnt (CVA).

subacute not as severe as an acute infection nor a long-lasting as a chronic disorder.

subcutaneous under the skin.

submucosa layer of connective tissue beneath the mucosa.

substrate substance on which an enzyme works.

sudoriferous producing sweat; referring to the sweat glands.

sulcus shallow groove, as between convolutions of the cerebral cortex; pl., sulci.

summarizing briefly review the information discussed to determine the patient's comprehension.

superficial burn burn limited to the epidermis..

superego one of three psychodynamic concepts which includes all internal norms and values of society acquired during early development through interactions with parents as figures of societal authority.

superior above; in a higher position.

superior vena cava large vein that drains the upper part of the body and empties into the right atrium of the heart.

supine face up or palm up.

surfactant substance in the alveoli that prevents their collapse by reducing surface tension of the contained fluids.

surfing navigating the Internet.

suspension heterogeneous mixture that will separate unless shaken.

suspensory ligaments filaments attached to the ciliary muscle of the eye that hold the lens in place.

sustentacular cells cells in the seminiferous tubules that aid in development of spermatozoa; Sertoli cells.

suture type of joint in which bone surfaces are closely united, as in the skull; stitch used in surgery to bring parts together or to stitch parts together in surgery.

sympathetic nervous system thoracolumbar division of the autonomic nervous system; stimulates a fight-or-flight (stress) response.

symptom evidence of disease noted by the patient; such evidence noted by an examiner is called a sign or an objective symptom.

synapse junction between two neurons or between a neuron and an effector.

synarthrosis immovable joint.

syndrome group of symptoms characteristic of a disorder.

synergist a substance or structure that enhances the work of another. A muscle that works with a prime mover to produce a given movement.

synovial pertaining to a thick lubricating fluid found in joints, bursae, and tendon sheaths; pertaining to a freely movable (diarthrotic) joint.

system group of organs functioning together for the same general purposes.

systemic referring to a generalized infection or condition.

systemic circuit pathway that carries blood to all tissues of the body except the lungs.

systole contraction phase of the cardiac cycle; adj., systolic.

T

T cell lymphocyte active in immunity that matures in the thymus gland; destroys foreign cells directly; T lymphocyte.

tachycardia heart rate more than 100 beats per minute.

tachypnea excessive rate of respiration.

tactile pertaining to the sense of touch.

target tissue tissue that is capable of responding to a specific hormone.

Tay-Sachs disease hereditary disease affecting fat metabolism.

tectorial membrane part of the hearing apparatus; generates nerve impulses as cilia move against it in response to sound waves.

telophase final stage of mitosis, during which new nuclei form and the cell contents usually divide.

temperament individual differences in the intensity and duration of emotions including the characteristics of one's disposition.

template a skeleton of a letter or document with preset and prespaced elements.

tendinitis inflammation of a tendon.

tendon cord of fibrous connective tissue that attaches a muscle to a bone.

teniae coli bands of smooth muscle in the wall of the large intestine.

testis male reproductive gland; pl., testes.

testosterone male sex hormone produced in the testes; promotes the development of sperm cells and maintains secondary sex characteristics.

tetanus constant contraction of a muscle; infectious disease caused by a bacterium (Clostridium tetani); lockjaw.

tetany muscle spasms due to low blood calcium, as in parathyroid deficiency.

thalamus region of the brain located in the diencephalon; chief relay center for sensory impulses traveling to the cerebral cortex.

therapy treatment.

therapeutic having to do with treating or curing disease; curative.

thoracentesis puncture of the chest for aspiration of fluid in the pleural space.

thorax chest; adj., thoracic.

thrombocyte blood platelet; cell fragment that participates in clotting.

thrombocytopenia deficiency of platelets in the blood.

thrombolytic dissolving blood clots.

thrombosis condition of having a thrombus (blood clot in a vessel).

thrombus blood clot within a vessel.

thymosin hormone produced by the thymus gland.

thymus endocrine gland in the upper portion of the chest; stimulates development of T cells.

thyroid endocrine gland in the neck.

thyroiditis inflammation of the thyroid gland.

thyroid-stimulating hormone (**TSH**) hormone produced by the anterior pituitary that stimulates the thyroid gland; thyrotropin.

thyroxine hormone produced by the thyroid gland; increases metabolic rate and needed for normal growth; T4.

tinea common term for fungal infection of the skin.

tissue group of similar cells that performs a specialized function.

tonicity the osmotic concentration or osmotic pressure of a solution. The effect that a solution will have on osmosis.

tonsil mass of lymphoid tissue in the region of the pharynx.

tonus partially contracted state of muscle; also, tone.

toxemia general toxic condition in which poisonous bacterial substances are absorbed into the bloodstream; presence of harmful substances in the blood as a result of abnormal metabolism.

toxin poison.

toxoid altered toxin used to produce active immunity.

trachea tube that extends from the larynx to the bronchi; windpipe.

tracheostomy surgical opening into the trachea for the introduction of a tube through which a person may breathe.

trachoma acute eye infection caused by chlamydia.

tract bundle of neuron fibers within the central nervous system.

trait characteristic.

transplantation the grafting to a recipient of an organ or tissue from an animal or other human to replace an injured or incompetent part of the body.

transverse describing a plane that divides a structure into superior and inferior parts.

trauma injury or wound.

tricuspid valve valve between the right atrium and right ventricle of the heart.

trigeminal neuralgia severe spasmodic pain affecting the fifth cranial nerve; tic douloureux.

triglyceride simple fat composed of glycerol and three fatty acids.

trigone triangulaar shaped region in the floor of the bladder that remains stable as the bladder fills.

triiodothyronine thyroid hormone that functions with thyroxine to raise cellular metabolism; T3.

tropomyosin a protein that works with troponin to regulate contraction in skeletal muscle.

troponin a protein that works with tropomyosin to regulate contraction in skeletal muscle.

TSH see thyroid-stimulating hormone.

tuberculosis (TB) infectious disease, often of the lung, caused by the bacillus Mycobacterium tuberculosis.

tumor abnormal growth or neoplasm.

tympanic membrane membrane between the external and middle ear that transmits sound waves to the bones of the middle ear; eardrum.

U

ulcer sore or lesion associated with death and disintegration of tissue.

ultrasound very high frequency sound waves.

umbilical cord structure that connects the fetus with the placenta; contains vessels that carry blood between the fetus and placenta.

umbilicus small scar on the abdomen that marks the former attachment of the umbilical cord to the fetus; navel.

unconscious level of consciousness at which thoughts, wishes, and feelings are not retrievable to conscious awareness.

universal solvent term used for water because it dissolves more substances than any other solvent.

unsaturated fat fat that has fewer hydrogen atoms and more double bonds between carbons than do saturated fats.

urea nitrogenous waste product excreted in the urine; end product of protein metabolism.

uremia accumulation of nitrogenous waste products in the blood.

unresolved grief process of grieving becomes prolonged and may be considered abnormal or maladaptive when symptoms are still present two months after the loss.

ureter tube that carries urine from the kidney to the urinary bladder.

urethra tube that carries urine from the urinary bladder to the outside of the body.

urinalysis laboratory examination of the physical and chemical properties of urine.

urinary bladder hollow organ that stores urine until it is eliminated.

urinary system the system involved in elimination of soluble waste, water balance and regulation of body fluids.

urination voiding of urine; micturition.

urine liquid waste excreted by the kidneys.

urticaria hives; allergic skin reaction with elevated red patches (wheals).

uterus muscular, pear-shaped organ in the female pelvis within which the fetus develops during pregnancy.

uvea middle coat of the eye, including the choroid, iris, and ciliary body; vascular and pigmented structures of the eye.

uvula soft, fleshy, V-shaped mass that hangs from the soft palate.

V

vaccination administration of a vaccine to protect against a specific disease; immunization.

vaccine substance used to produce active immunity; usually, a suspension of attenuated or killed pathogens or some component of a pathogen given by inoculation to prevent a specific disease.

vagina distal part of the birth canal that opens to the outside of the body; female organ of sexual intercourse.

valence the combining power of an atom; the number of electrons lost or gained by atoms of an element in chemical reactions.

valve structure that prevents fluid from flowing backward, as in the heart, veins, and lymphatic vessels.

varicose pertaining to an enlarged and twisted vessel, as in varicose vein.

vas deferens tube that carries sperm cells from the testis to the urethra; ductus deferens.

vasectomy surgical removal of part or all of the ductus (vas) deferens; usually done on both sides to produce sterility.

vasoconstriction decrease in the diameter of a blood vessel.

vasodilation increase in the diameter of a blood vessel.

VD venereal disease; see sexually transmitted infection.

vector an insect or other animal that transmits a disease-causing organism from one host to another.

vein vessel that carries blood toward the heart.

vena cava a large vein that carries blood into the right atrium of the heart; superior vena cava or inferior vena cava.

venereal disease (VD) infectious disease acquired through sexual activity; sexually transmitted infection (STI).

venous sinus large channel that drains deoxygenated blood.

ventilation movement of air into and out of the lungs.

ventral toward the front or belly surface; anterior.

ventricle cavity or chamber; one of the two lower chambers of the heart; one of the four chambers in the brain in which cerebrospinal fluid is produced; adj., ventricular.

venule vessel between a capillary and a vein.

vernix caseosa cheeselike sebaceous secretion that covers a newborn.

verruca wart.

vertebra a bone of the spinal column; pl., vertebrae.

vesicle small sac or blister filled with fluid.

vesicular transport use of vesicles to move large amounts of material through the plasma membrane of a cell.

vestibule part of the internal ear that contains receptors for the sense of static equilibrium; any space at the entrance to a canal or organ.

vibrio slight curved or comma-shaped bacterium; pl., vibrios.

villi small fingerlike projections from the surface of a membrane; projections in the lining of the small intestine through which digested food is absorbed; sing., villus.

viroid infectious agent composed of RNA with no protein. Viroids are intracellular parasites linked so far only to diseases in plants.

virtual a paperless system or chart on your computer.

virulence power of an organism to overcome defenses of a host.

virus extremely small infectious agent that can reproduce only within a living cell.

virus a harmful invader that can damage your computer.

viscera organs in the ventral body cavities, especially the abdominal organs; adj. visceral.

viscosity thickness, as of the blood or other fluid.

vitamin organic compound needed in small amounts for health.

vitreous body soft, jellylike substance that fills the eyeball and holds the shape of the eye; vitreous humor.

vocal cords folds of mucous membrane in the larynx used in producing speech.

Volkmann canal see perforating canal.

volvulus twisting of the intestine.

von Willebrand disease hereditary blood clotting disorder in which there is a shortage of von Willebrand factor.

W

Wernicke area portion of the cerebral cortex concerned with speech recognition and the meaning of words.

white matter nervous tissue composed of myelinated fibers.

X-Z

x-ray ray or radiation of extremely short wavelength that can penetrate opaque substances and affect photographic plates and fluorescent screens.

zygote fertilized ovum; cell formed by the union of a sperm and an egg.

INDEX

Page numbers followed by a "f" indicate figures, those followed by a "t" indicate tables, those followed by a "b" indicate boxes, those followed by a "p" indicate procedures.

1

English Fundamentals and Written Communications

CHAPTER COMPETENCIES

Review the information in your text that supports the following course objectives.

Learning Objectives

In this chapter, you'll learn:

1. To spell and define the key terms.

2. To discuss the basic guidelines for grammar, punctuation, and spelling.

3. To describe six key guidelines for medical writing.

4. To discuss the eleven key components of a business letter.

5. To describe the three steps to writing a business letter.

6. To describe the process of writing a memorandum.

Performance Objectives

In this chapter, you'll learn:

1. To write a business letter.

2. To write a memorandum.

CHAPTER OUTLINE

CHAPTER OUTLINE	NOTES
Professional Writing	
Basic Grammar and Punctuation Guidelines	
Basic Spelling Guidelines	
Forming a Sentence	
What is a Subject?	
Nouns	
Pronouns	
What is a Predicate?	
Composing a Paragraph	
Structuring Paragraphs	
Purpose of Writing	

CHAPTER OUTLINE *continued*	NOTES
Guidelines for Medical Writing	
Accuracy	
Spelling	
Capitalization	
Abbreviations and Symbols	
Plural and Possessive	
Numbers	
Letter Development	
Components of a Letter	
Letter Formats	
Full Block	
Block	
Semiblock	
Writing a Business Letter	
Preparation	
Composition	
Editing	
Types of Business Letters	
Memorandum Development	
Components of a Memorandum	

LEARNING SELF-ASSESSMENT EXERCISES

Key Terms

Define the following key terms:

BiCaps _____

block _____

enclosure _____

font _____

full block _____

intercaps _____

margin _____

memorandum _____

proofread _____

salutation _____

semiblock _____

template _____

Matching

Match the definition in part 1 with the correct term in part 2.

PART I

_____ 1. Greeting of the letter

_____ 2. Something included with a letter

_____ 3. Most formal format and most commonly used for
         professional letters

_____ 4. Same as block except first sentence of each para-
         graph is indented five spaces

_____ 5. Date, subject line, closing, and signature flush
         with the right margin

PART 2

a. Full block

b. Block

c. Enclosure

d. Salutation

e. Semiblock

Multiple Choice

1. In letters to a physician, the salutation should
   a. Always be in capital letters
   b. Begin with "Dr."
   c. Begin with "Doctor"
   d. Never use the first name

2. Which of the following items *can* be abbreviated in an inside address?
   a. City
   b. Town
   c. Business title
   d. State

3. The subject line of a letter is
   a. Placed five spaces below the inside address
   b. Mandatory
   c. Used to highlight the intent of a letter
   d. None of the above

4. Which of the following is *not* a step in writing a professional business letter?
   a. Mailing status
   b. Preparation
   c. Editing
   d. Composition

2
Introduction to the Computer

CHAPTER COMPETENCIES

Review the information in your text that supports the following course objectives.

Learning Objectives

1. To identify the basic computer components.

2. To understand the basics of a computer operating system and how to set your preferences.

3. To understand how to create and manage files and folders.

4. To identify the appropriate office software to use for specific tasks.

5. To understand how to create, format, save, and print Word documents.

6. To understand how to create, format, save, and print PowerPoint presentations.

7. To understand how to create, format, save, and print Excel spreadsheets.

CHAPTER OUTLINE	NOTES
The Computer	
Hardware	
Peripherals	
Care and Maintenance of the System and Equipment	
The Computer Operating System	
Setting Your Preferences	
Managing Files and Folders	
Files	
Folders	
Using Office Software	
Discovering Word	
Creating and Formatting Word Documents	
Saving and Printing Word Documents	

CHAPTER OUTLINE *continued*	NOTES
Discovering PowerPoint	
Creating and Formatting Presentations	
Saving and Printing Presentations	
Discovering Excel	
Creating and Formatting Spreadsheets	
Saving and Printing Spreadsheets	

SELF-ASSESSMENT LEARNING EXERCISES

Multiple Choice

1. An example of a special function key is
   a. Alt
   b. Ctrl
   c. Insert
   d. All of the above

2. A freestanding device that is used to control the cursor on a display screen is called a
   a. Login
   b. Modem
   c. Mouse
   d. Indicator

3. A communication device that connects a computer to the standard telephone system is a
   a. Modem
   b. Monitor
   c. Terminal
   d. Cable

3

Computer Applications in the Health Care Setting

CHAPTER COMPETENCIES

Review the information in your text that supports the following course objectives.

Learning Objectives

1. To spell and define the key words
2. To explain the basics of connecting to the Internet
3. To discuss the safety concerns for online searching
4. To describe how to use a search engine
5. To list sites that can be used by professionals and sites geared for patients
6. To describe the benefits of an intranet and explain how it differs from the Internet
7. To describe the various types of clinical software that might be used in a physician's office
8. To describe the various types of administrative software that might be used in a physician's office
9. To describe the benefits of a handheld computer
10. To describe various training options
11. To discuss the ethics related to computer access

Performance Objectives

1. To search a given topic on the Internet
2. To conduct a basic literary search

CHAPTER OUTLINE	NOTES
Internet Basics	
Getting Started and Connected	
Security	
Viruses	
Downloading Information	
Working Offline	
Electronic Mail	
Access	
Composing Messages	

CHAPTER OUTLINE *continued*	NOTES
Address Books	
Attachments	
Opening Electronic Mail	
Medical Applications of the Internet	
Search Engines	
Professional Medical Sites	
Literary Searches	
Insurance-Related Sites	
Patient Teaching Issues Regarding the Internet	
Buying Medications Online	
Financial Assistance for Medications	
Health Records	
Injury Prevention	
Intranet	
Medical Software Applications	
Clinical Applications	
Administrative Applications	
Meeting Maker	
Handheld Computers	
Training Options	
Computer Ethics	

SELF-ASSESSMENT LEARNING EXERCISES

Key Terms

Define the following key terms:

cookies _____

downloading _____

encryption _____

Ethernet _____

Internet _____

intranet _____

literary search _____

search engine _____

surfing _____

virtual _____

virus _____

5 Organization of the Human Body

OVERVIEW

Anatomy is the study of body structure, whereas **physiology** is the study of how the body functions.

Living things are organized from simple to complex levels. The simplest living form is the **cell**, the basic unit of life. Specialized cells are grouped into **tissues**, which, in turn, are combined to form **organs**; these organs form systems, which work together to maintain the body.

The systems include the integumentary system, the body's covering; the skeletal system, the framework of the body; the muscular system, which moves the bones; the nervous system, the central control system that includes the organs of special sense; the endocrine system, which produces the regulatory hormones; the circulatory system, consisting of the heart, blood vessels, and lymphatic vessels that transport vital substances; the respiratory system, which adds oxygen to the blood and removes carbon dioxide; the digestive system, which converts raw food materials into products usable by cells; the urinary system, which removes wastes and excess water; and the reproductive system, by which new individuals of the species are produced.

All the cellular reactions that sustain life comprise **metabolism**, which can be divided into **catabolism** and **anabolism**. In catabolism, complex substances are broken down into simpler molecules. When the nutrients from food are broken down by catabolism, energy is released. This energy is stored in the compound **ATP** (adenosine triphosphate) for use by the cells. In anabolism, simple compounds are built into substances needed for cell activities.

All the systems work together to maintain a state of balance or **homeostasis**. The main mechanism for maintaining homeostasis is **negative feedback**, by which the state of the body is the signal to keep conditions within set limits.

The human body is composed of large amounts of fluid, the amount and composition of which must be constantly regulated. The **extracellular fluid** consists of the fluid that surrounds the cells as well as the fluid circulated in blood and lymph. The fluid within cells is the **intracellular fluid**.

Study of the body requires knowledge of directional terms to locate parts and to relate various parts to each other. Several planes of division represent different directions in which cuts can be made through the body. Separation of the body into areas and regions, together with the use of the special terminology for directions and locations, makes it possible to describe an area within the human body with great accuracy.

The large internal spaces of the body are cavities in which various organs are located. The **dorsal cavity** is subdivided into the **cranial cavity** and the **spinal cavity (canal)**. The **ventral cavity** is subdivided into the **thoracic** and **abdominopelvic cavities**. Imaginary lines are used to divide the abdomen into regions for study and diagnosis.

The metric system is used for all scientific measurements. This system is easy to use because it is based on multiples of 10.

LEARNING THE LANGUAGE: WORD ANATOMY

Complete the following table by writing the correct word part or meaning in the space provided. For each word part, write a term that contains the word part.

Word Part	Meaning	Example
1. -tomy	_____	_____
2. -stasis	_____	_____
3. _____	nature, physical	_____
4. homeo-	_____	_____
5. _____	apart, away from	_____
6. _____	down	_____
7. _____	upward	_____

ADDRESSING THE LEARNING OUTCOMES

I. Writing Exercise

The learning outcomes for Chapter 5 are listed below. These outcomes provide an overview of the major topics covered in this chapter. On a separate piece of paper, try to write out an answer to each outcome. All of the answers can be found in the pages of the textbook. Learning Outcomes 2, 9, 10, 11, and 12 are also addressed in the Coloring Atlas.

1. Define the terms *anatomy* and *physiology*.
2. Describe the organization of the body from chemicals to the whole organism.
3. List 11 body systems and give the general function of each.
4. Define *metabolism* and name the two phases of metabolism.
5. Briefly explain the role of ATP in the body.
6. Differentiate between extracellular and intracellular fluids.
7. Define and give examples of homeostasis.
8. Compare negative feedback and positive feedback.
9. List and define the main directional terms for the body.
10. List and define the three planes of division of the body.
11. Name the subdivisions of the dorsal and ventral cavities.
12. Name and locate subdivisions of the abdomen.
13. Name the basic units of length, weight, and volume in the metric system.
14. Define the metric prefixes *kilo-, centi-, milli-,* and *micro-*.
15. Show how word parts are used to build words related to the body's organization.

II. Labeling and Coloring Atlas

Exercise 5-1: Levels of Organization (text Fig. 5-1)

Instructions

1. Write the name or names of each labeled part on the numbered lines in different colors.
2. Color the different structures on the diagram with the corresponding color. For instance, if you wrote "cell" in blue, color the cell blue.

1. _____

2. _____

3. _____

4. _____

5. _____

6. _____

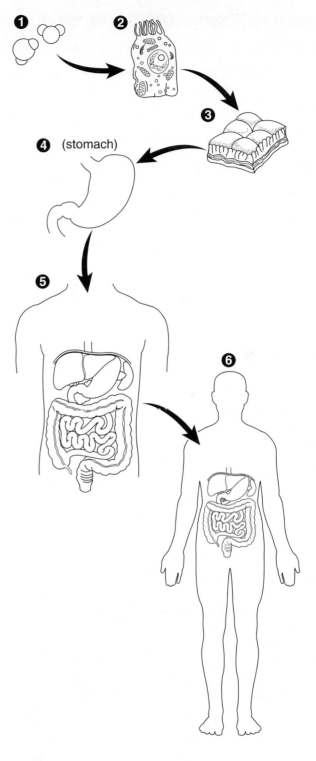

Exercise 5-2: Directional Terms (text Fig. 5-7)

Instructions

1. Write the name of each directional term on the numbered lines in different colors.
2. Color the arrow corresponding to each directional term with appropriate color.

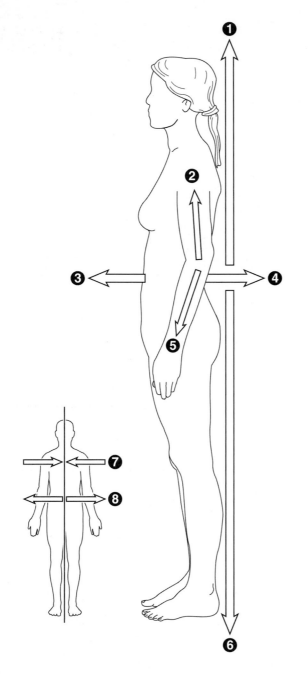
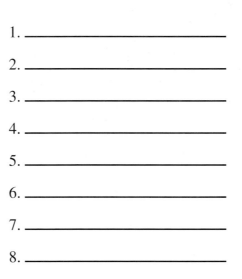

1. _____

2. _____

3. _____

4. _____

5. _____

6. _____

7. _____

8. _____

Exercise 5-3: Planes of Division (text Fig. 5-8)

Instructions

1. Write the names of the three planes of division on the correct numbered lines in different colors.
2. Color each plane in the illustration with its corresponding color.

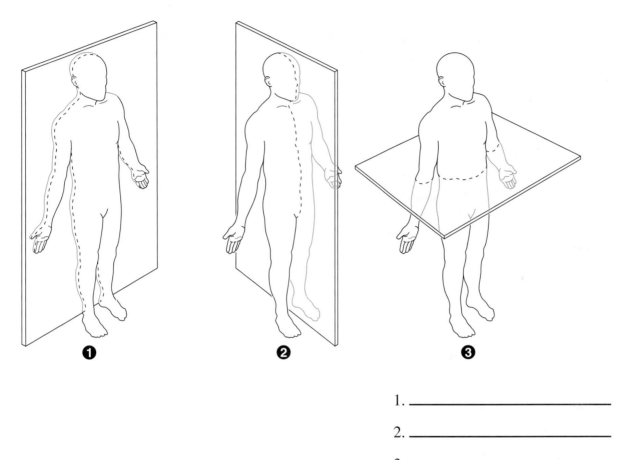

1. _____

2. _____

3. _____

Exercise 5-4: Lateral View of Body Cavities (text Fig. 5-11)

Instructions

1. Write the names of the different body cavities and other structures in the appropriate spaces in different colors. Try to choose related colors for the dorsal cavity subdivisions and for the ventral cavity subdivisions.
2. Color each part with the corresponding color.

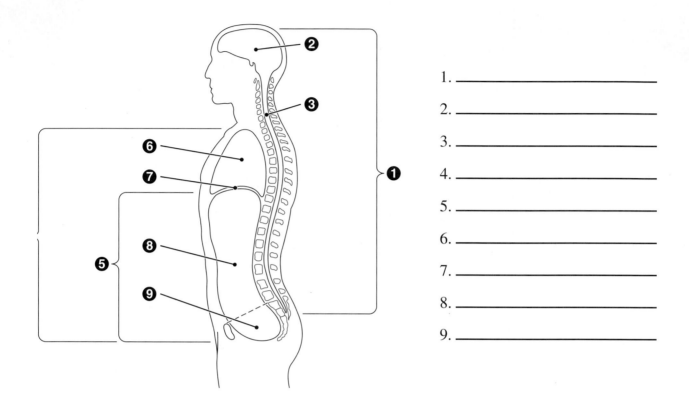

1. _____

2. _____

3. _____

4. _____

5. _____

6. _____

7. _____

8. _____

9. _____

Exercise 5-5: Regions of the Abdomen (text Fig. 5-13)

Instructions

1. Write the names of the nine regions of the abdomen on the appropriate numbered lines in different colors.
2. Color the corresponding region with the appropriate color.

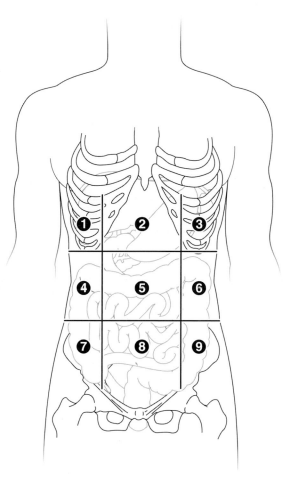

1. _____

2. _____

3. _____

4. _____

5. _____

6. _____

7. _____

8. _____

9. _____

Exercise 5-6: Quadrants of the Abdomen (text Fig. 5-14)

Instructions

1. Write the names of the four quadrants of the abdomen on the appropriate numbered lines in different colors.
2. Color the corresponding quadrant in the appropriate color.

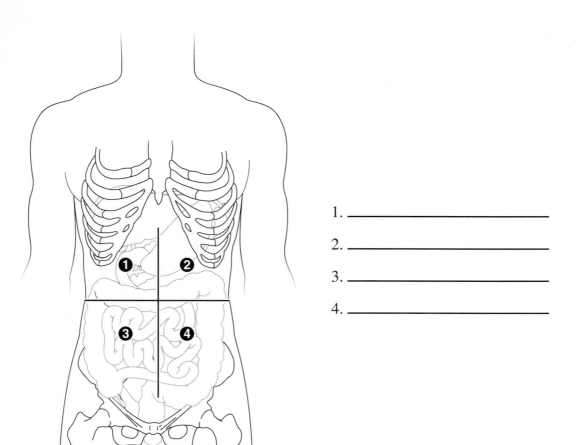

1. _____

2. _____

3. _____

4. _____

MAKING THE CONNECTIONS

The following concept map deals with the body's cavities and their divisions. Complete the concept map by filling in the blanks with the appropriate word or term for the cavity, division, subdivision, or region.

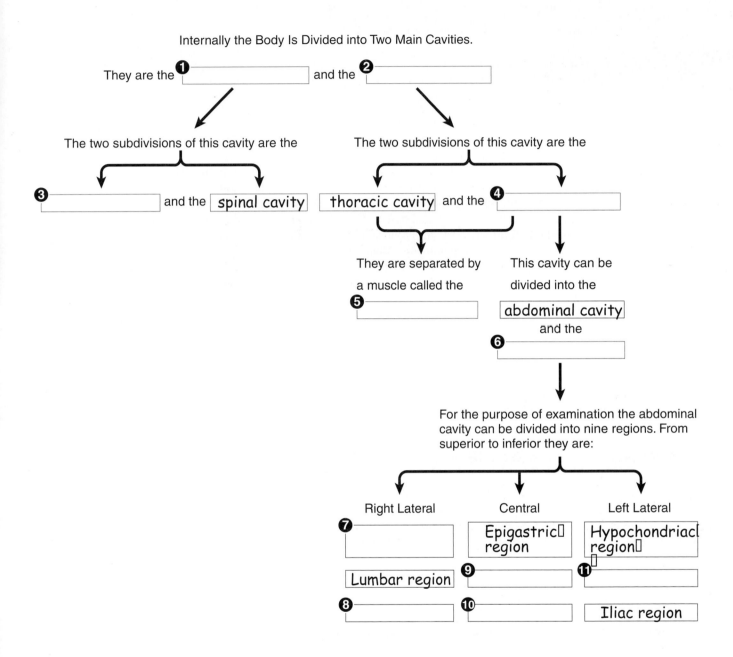

Internally the Body Is Divided into Two Main Cavities.

They are the **1** [   ] and the **2** [   ]

The two subdivisions of this cavity are the

The two subdivisions of this cavity are the

3 [   ] and the | spinal cavity |

| thoracic cavity | and the **4** [   ]

They are separated by a muscle called the

5 [   ]

This cavity can be divided into the

| abdominal cavity |

and the

6 [   ]

For the purpose of examination the abdominal cavity can be divided into nine regions. From superior to inferior they are:

Right Lateral   Central   Left Lateral

7 [   ]

| Epigastric region | | Hypochondriac region |

| Lumbar region | **9** [   ]   **11** [   ]

8 [   ]   **10** [   ] | Iliac region |

6

Tissues, Glands, and Membranes

OVERVIEW

The cell is the basic unit of life. Individual cells are grouped according to function into **tissues**. The four main groups of tissues include **epithelial tissue**, which forms glands, covers surfaces, and lines cavities; **connective tissue**, which gives support and form to the body; **muscle tissue**, which produces movement; and **nervous tissue**, which conducts nerve impulses.

Glands produce substances used by other cells and tissues. **Exocrine glands** produce secretions that are released through ducts to nearby parts of the body. **Endocrine glands** produce hormones that are carried by the blood to all parts of the body.

The simplest combination of tissues is a **membrane**. Membranes serve several purposes, a few of which are mentioned here. They may serve as dividing partitions, may line hollow organs and cavities, and may anchor various organs. Membranes that have epithelial cells on the surface are referred to as **epithelial membranes**. Two types of epithelial membranes are **serous membranes**, which line body cavities and cover the internal organs, and **mucous membranes**, which line passageways leading to the outside.

Connective tissue membranes cover or enclose organs, providing protection and support. These membranes include the fascia around muscles, the meninges around the brain and spinal cord, and the tissues around the heart, bones, and cartilage.

The study of tissues — **histology** — requires much memorization. In particular, you may be challenged to learn the different types of epithelial and connective tissue, as well as the classification scheme of epithelial and connective membranes. Learning the structure of these different tissues and membranes will help you understand the amazing properties of the body — how we can jump from great heights, swim without becoming waterlogged, and fold our ears over without breaking them.

LEARNING THE LANGUAGE: WORD ANATOMY

Complete the following table by writing the correct word part or meaning in the space provided. For each word part, write a term that contains the word part.

Word Part	Meaning	Example
1. _____	cartilage	_____
2. _____	on, upon	_____
3. oste/o-	_____	_____
4. _____	heart	_____
5. osse/o-	_____	_____
6. blast-	_____	_____
7. peri-	_____	_____
8. _____	muscle	_____

9. _____   false   _____

10. hist/o-   _____   _____

11. neur/o-   _____   _____

12. _____   side, rib   _____

ADDRESSING THE LEARNING OUTCOMES

I. Writing Exercise

The learning outcomes for Chapter 6 are listed below. These learning outcomes provide an overview of the major topics covered in this chapter. On a separate piece of paper, try to write out an answer to each learning outcome. All of the answers can be found in the pages of the textbook. Learning Outcomes 1–3 are also addressed in the Coloring Atlas, and Learning Outcome 6 is addressed in the Word Anatomy exercise above.

1. Name the four main groups of tissues and give the location and general characteristics of each.
2. Describe the difference between exocrine and endocrine glands and give examples of each.
3. Give examples of liquid, soft, fibrous, and hard connective tissues.
4. Describe three types of epithelial membranes.
5. List several types of connective tissue membranes.
6. Show how word parts are used to build words related to tissues, glands, and membranes.

II. Labeling and Coloring Atlas

Exercise 6-1: Three Types of Epithelium (text Fig. 6-1)

Instructions

Label each of the following types of epithelium.

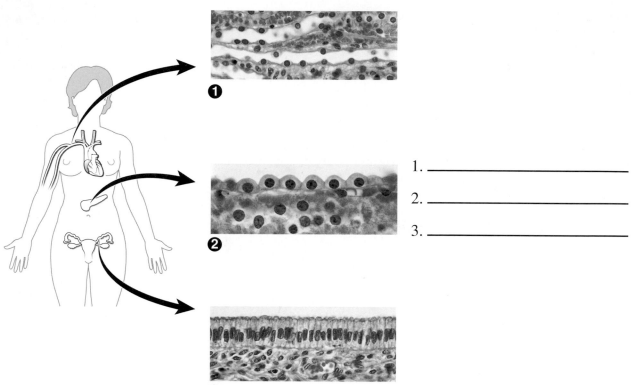

1. _____

2. _____

3. _____

Exercise 6-2: Connective Tissue (text Figs. 6-5 and 6-6)

Instructions

Write the names of the six types of connective tissue in the appropriate blanks in six different colors. Color some of the **cells** of each tissue type with the corresponding color.

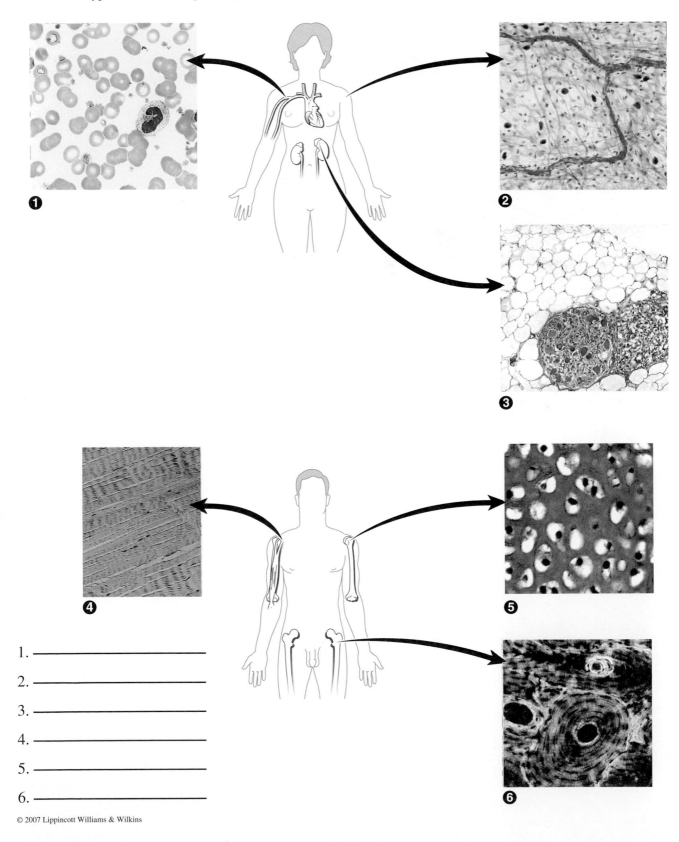

1. _____

2. _____

3. _____

4. _____

5. _____

6. _____

Exercise 6-3: Muscle Tissue (text Fig. 6-7)

Instructions

Write the names of the three types of muscle tissue in the appropriate blanks in different colors. Color some of the muscle cells the appropriate color. Look for the nuclei, and color them a different color.

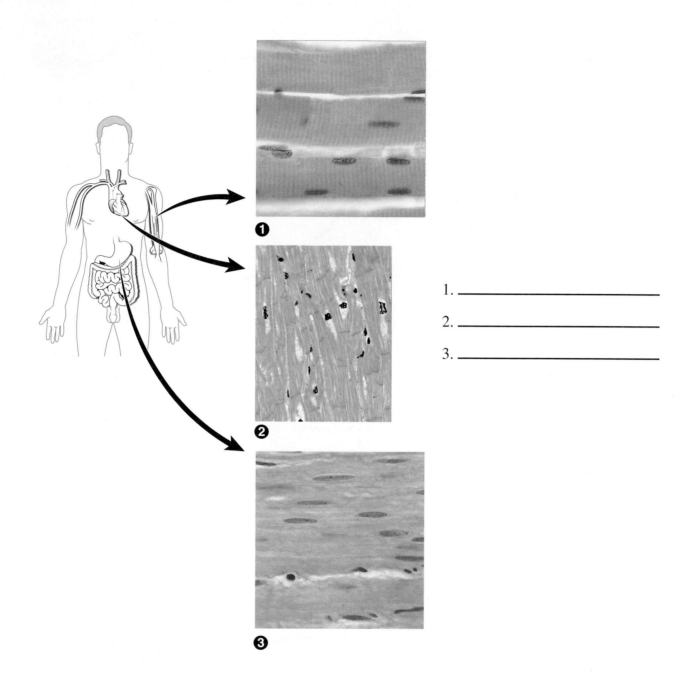

1. _____

2. _____

3. _____

Exercise 6-4: Nervous Tissue (text Fig. 6-8)

Instructions

1. Write the names of each tissue (indicating the plane of the section where appropriate) in boxes 12–9.
2. Label the neural structures and tissues (parts 1–6) using different colors. When possible, color each structure or tissue with the appropriate color.

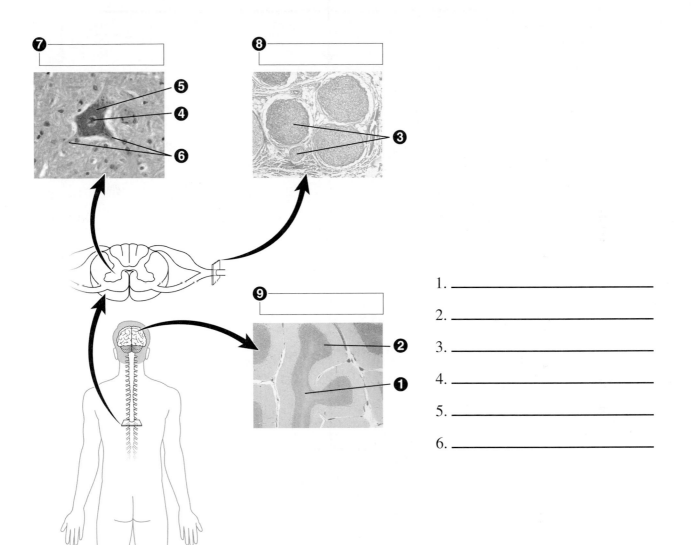

1. _____

2. _____

3. _____

4. _____

5. _____

6. _____

MAKING THE CONNECTIONS

The following concept map deals with the classification of tissues. Complete the concept map by filling in the appropriate word or phrase that classifies or describes the tissue.

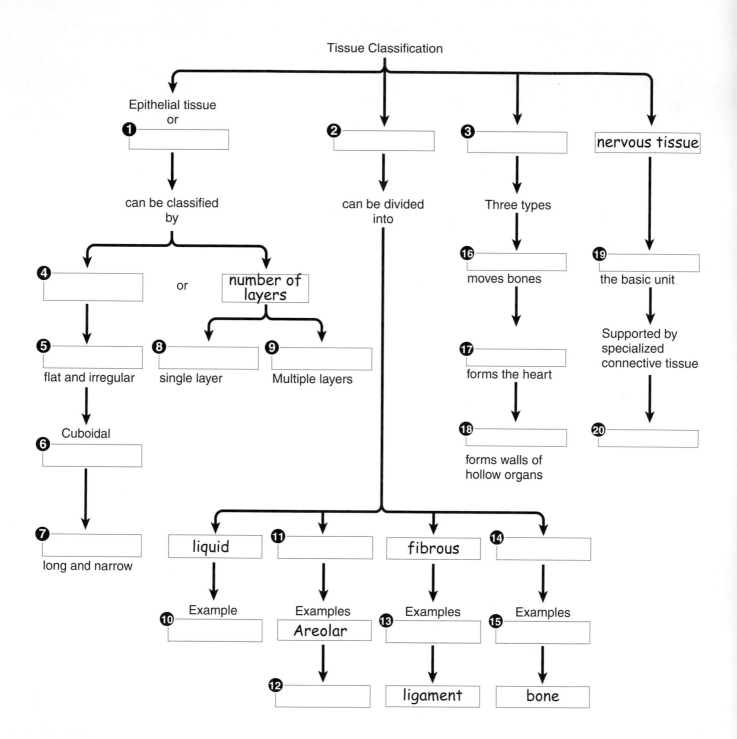

Optional Exercise: Assemble your own concept map summarizing the classification of membranes. Use the following terms: membrane, epithelial tissue membrane, connective tissue membrane, serous, mucous, cutaneous, peritoneum, pleurae, serous pericardium, parietal layer, visceral layer, meninges, fascia, deep, superficial, fibrous pericardium, periosteum, perichondrium. You could also provide some examples of the different membranes, as shown in the concept map provided above.

7

Anatomy and Physiology of the Body Systems

The Integumentary System

LEARNING THE LANGUAGE: WORD ANATOMY

Complete the following table by writing the correct word part or meaning in the space provided. For each word part write a term that contains the word part.

Word Part	Meaning	Example
1. sub-	_____	_____
2. _____	dark, black	_____
3. _____	white	_____
4. _____	hair	_____
5. derm/o	_____	_____
6. _____	horny	_____
7. ap/o-	_____	_____

II. Labeling and Coloring Atlas

Exercise 7-1: The Skin (text Fig. 7-1)

Instructions

1. Write the names of the three skin layers in the numbered boxes 1–3.
2. Write the name of each labeled part on the numbered lines in different colors. Use a light color for structures 4 and 12. Use the same color for structures 15 and 16, for structures 13 and 14, and for structures 8 and 9.
3. Color the different structures on the diagram with the corresponding color. Try to color every structure in the figure with the appropriate color. For instance, structure number 8 is found in three locations.

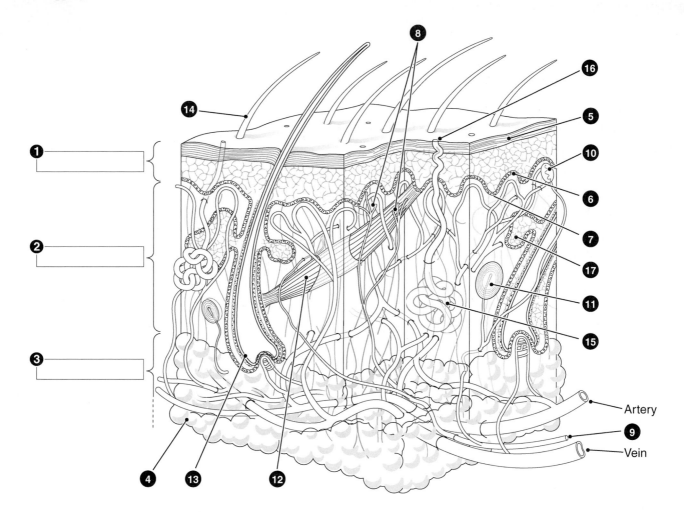

4. _____

5. _____

6. _____

7. _____

8. _____

9. _____

10. _____

11. _____

12. _____

13. _____

14. _____

15. _____

16. _____

17. _____

The Skeleton: Bones and Joints

LEARNING THE LANGUAGE: WORD ANATOMY

Complete the following table by writing the correct word part or meaning in the space provided. For each word part, write a term that contains the word part.

Word Part	Meaning	Example
1. _____	near, beyond	_____
2. -clast	_____	_____
3. _____	rib	_____
4. amphi-	_____	_____
5. arthr/o-	_____	_____
6. _____	away from	_____
7. _____	around	_____
8. _____	toward, added to	_____
9. dia-	_____	_____
10. pariet/o-	_____	_____

II. Labeling and Coloring Atlas

Exercise 7-2: The Skeleton (text Fig. 7-6)

Instructions

1. Write the name of each labeled part on the numbered lines in different colors. Use the same color for structures 24 and 25 and for structures 19 and 20.
2. Color the different structures on the diagram with the corresponding color. Try to color every structure in the figure with the appropriate color. For instance, structure number 3 is found in two locations.

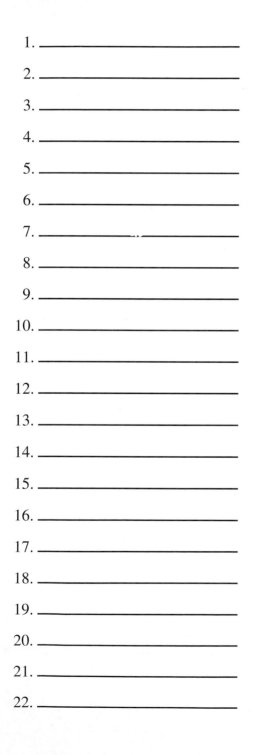

1. _____

2. _____

3. _____

4. _____

5. _____

6. _____

7. _____

8. _____

9. _____

10. _____

11. _____

12. _____

13. _____

14. _____

15. _____

16. _____

17. _____

18. _____

19. _____

20. _____

21. _____

22. _____

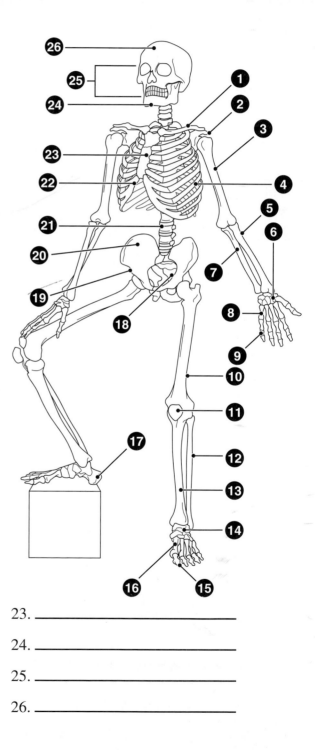

23. _____

24. _____

25. _____

26. _____

The Muscular System

LEARNING THE LANGUAGE: WORD ANATOMY

Word Part	Meaning	Example
1. _____	muscle	_____
2. brachi/o	_____	_____
3. _____	nutrition, nurture	_____
4. erg/o	_____	_____
5. metr/o	_____	_____
6. _____	four	_____
7. _____	tone, tension	_____
8. _____	flesh	_____
9. vas/o	_____	_____
10. iso-	_____	_____

II. Labeling and Coloring Atlas

Exercise 7-3: Structure of a Skeletal Muscle (text Fig. 7-10)

Instructions

Label each of the indicated parts.

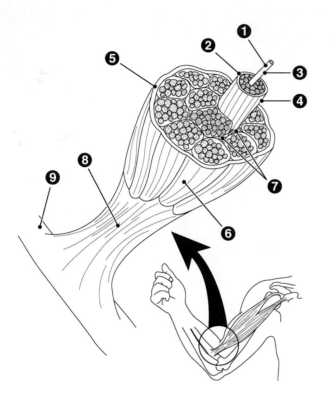
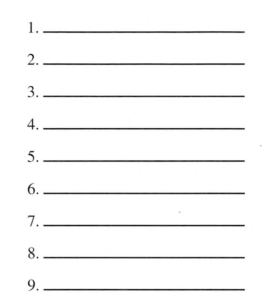

1. _____

2. _____

3. _____

4. _____

5. _____

6. _____

7. _____

8. _____

9. _____

Exercise 7-4: Neuromuscular Junction (text Fig. 7-12)

Instructions

Label each of the indicated parts.

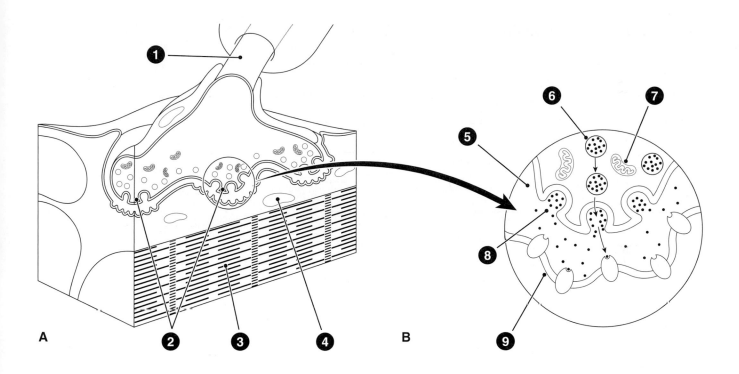

A

B

1. _____

2. _____

3. _____

4. _____

5. _____

6. _____

7. _____

8. _____

9. _____

The Nervous System: The Spinal Cord and Spinal Nerves

LEARNING THE LANGUAGE: WORD ANATOMY

Word Part	Meaning	Example
1. _____	sheath	_____
2. re-	_____	_____
3. soma-	_____	_____
4. _____	nerve, nervous tissue	_____
5. _____	remove	_____
6. aut/o	_____	_____
7. post-	_____	_____

II. Labeling and Coloring Atlas

Exercise 7-5: Anatomic divisions of the nervous system (text Fig. 7-13)

Label the parts and divisions of the nervous system shown below.

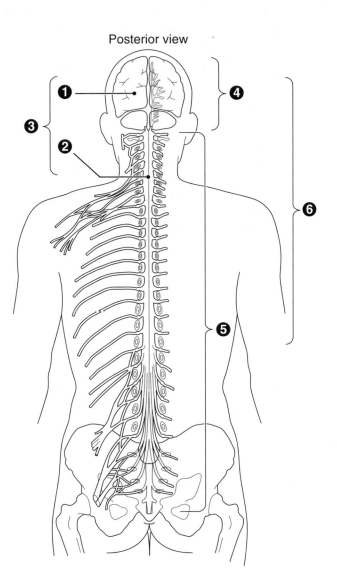

Posterior view

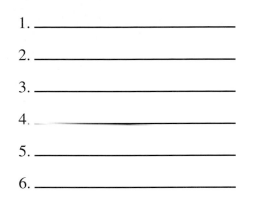

1. _____

2. _____

3. _____

4. _____

5. _____

6. _____

Exercise 7-6: The Motor Neuron (text Fig. 7-14)

Instructions

1. Write the name of each labeled part on the numbered lines in different colors. Structures 4–6 will not be colored, so write their names in black.
2. Color the different structures on the diagram with the corresponding color.
3. Add large arrows showing the direction the nerve impulse will travel, from the dendrites to the muscle.

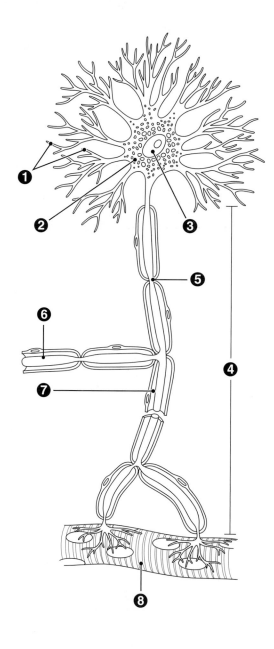

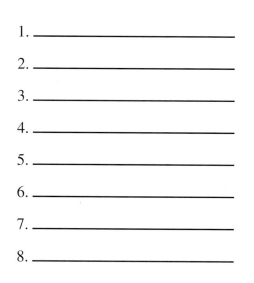

1. _____

2. _____

3. _____

4. _____

5. _____

6. _____

7. _____

8. _____

Exercise 7-7: Formation of a Myelin Sheath (text Fig. 7-16)

Instructions

1. Write the name of each labeled part on the numbered lines in different colors. Structures 4 and 7 to 9 will not be colored, so write their names in black.
2. Color the different structures on the diagram with the corresponding color. Make sure you color the structure in all parts of the diagram. For instance, structure 3 is visible in three locations.

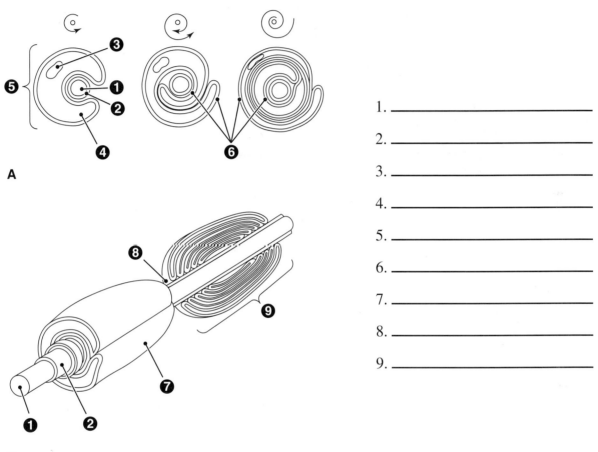

1. _____

2. _____

3. _____

4. _____

5. _____

6. _____

7. _____

8. _____

9. _____

The Nervous System: The Brain and Cranial Nerves

LEARNING THE LANGUAGE: WORD ANATOMY

Word Part	Meaning	Example
1. _____	cut	_____
2. chori/o-	_____	_____
3. _____	tongue	_____
4. encephal/o-	_____	_____
5. cerebr/o-	_____	_____
6. _____	opposed, against	_____
7. _____	lateral, side	_____
8. gyr/o	_____	_____

II. Labeling and Coloring Atlas

Exercise 7-8: Brain: Sagittal Section (text Fig. 7-17)

Instructions

1. Write the names of the four labeled brain divisions in lines 1 to 4, using four different colors. Use red for 2 and blue for 3. DO NOT COLOR THE DIAGRAM YET.
2. Write the name of each labeled structure on the appropriate numbered line in different colors. Use different shades of red for structures 5 and 6 and different shades of blue for structures 8–10.
3. Color each structure on the diagram with the appropriate color.

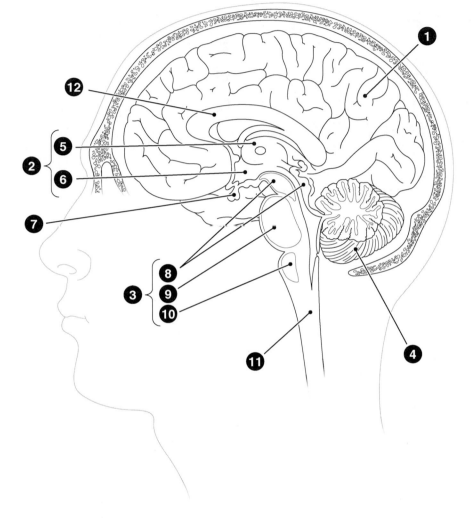

1. _____   7. _____

2. _____   8. _____

3. _____   9. _____

4. _____   10. _____

5. _____   11. _____

6. _____   12. _____

Exercise 7-9: Meninges and Related Parts (text Fig. 7-19)

Instructions

1. Write the name of each labeled part on the numbered lines in different colors. Use the same color for structures 7 and 8. Write the names of structures 4, 10, and 12 in black.
2. Color the structures on the diagram with the corresponding color. Do not color structures 4, 10, and 12.

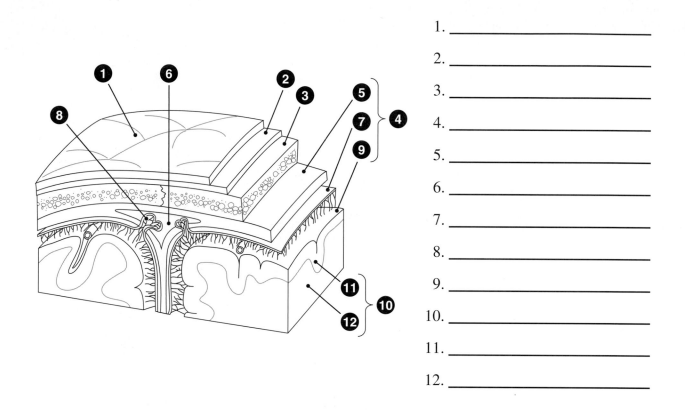

1. _____

2. _____

3. _____

4. _____

5. _____

6. _____

7. _____

8. _____

9. _____

10. _____

11. _____

12. _____

Exercise 7-10: Flow of Cerebrospinal Fluid (text Fig. 7-20)

Instructions

1. Write the name of each labeled part on the numbered lines in different colors. Use light colors for structures 5–12.
2. Color the structures on the diagram with the corresponding color. The boundaries between structures 5–12 (inclusive) are not always well defined. For instance, structure 6 is continuous with structure 7. You can overlap your colors to signify this fact.
3. Draw arrows to indicate the direction of CSF flow.

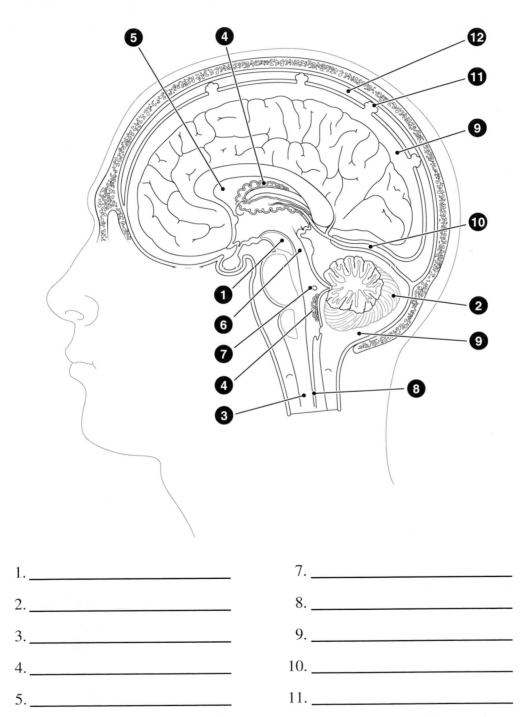

1. _____   7. _____

2. _____   8. _____

3. _____   9. _____

4. _____   10. _____

5. _____   11. _____

6. _____   12. _____

Exercise 7-11: Ventricles of the Brain (text Fig. 7-21)

Instructions

1. Write the name of each labeled part on the numbered lines in different colors. Write the names of structures 5, 6, and 9 in black, because they will not be colored.
2. Color the structures on the diagram with the corresponding color (except for structures 5, 6, and 9). The boundaries between structures are not always well defined. For instance, structure 2 is continuous with structure 4. You can overlap your colors to signify this fact.

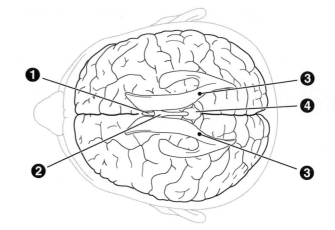

1. _____

2. _____

3. _____

4. _____

5. _____

6. _____

7. _____

8. _____

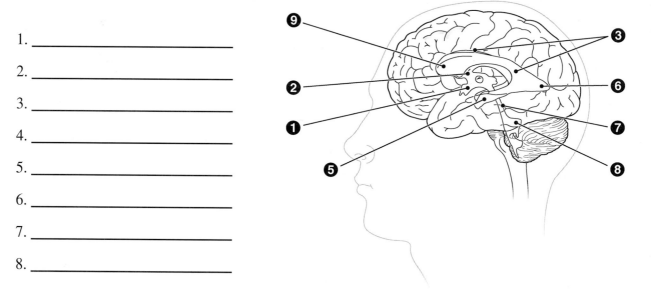

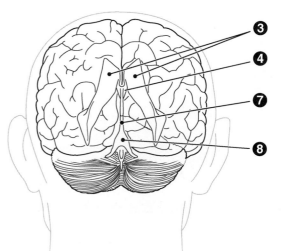

The Sensory System

LEARNING THE LANGUAGE: WORD ANATOMY

Complete the following table by writing the correct word part or meaning in the space provided. For each word part, write a term that contains the word part.

Word Part	Meaning	Example
1. presby-	_____	_____
2. _____	stone	_____
3. _____	drum	_____
4. _____	yellow	_____
5. _____	hearing	_____

II. Labeling and Coloring Atlas

Exercise 7-12: The Lacrimal Apparatus (text Fig. 7-23)

Label the indicated parts.

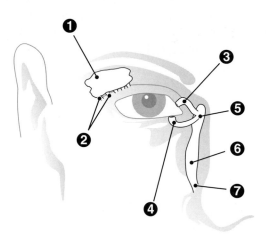

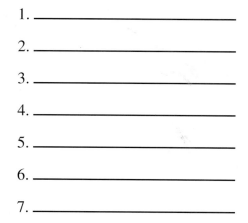

1. _____

2. _____

3. _____

4. _____

5. _____

6. _____

7. _____

Exercise 7-13: The Eye (text Fig. 7-24)

Instructions

1. Write the name of each labeled part on the numbered lines in different colors. Use the same color for structures 3 and 4 and structures 6–9 (inclusive). Write the name of structure 1 in black, because it will not be colored.
2. Color the different structures on the diagram with the corresponding color. Some structures are present in more than one location on the diagram. Try to color all of a particular structure in the appropriate color. For instance, only one of the suspensory ligaments is labeled, but color both suspensory ligaments.

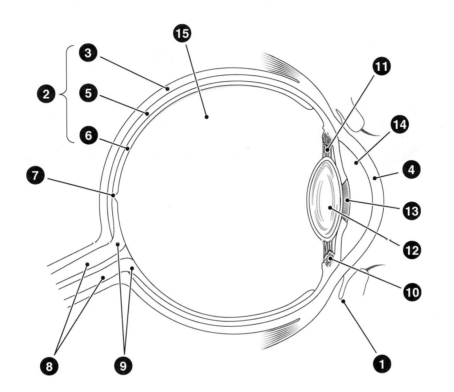
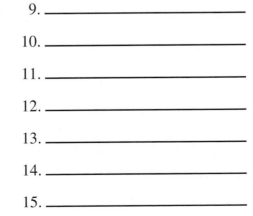
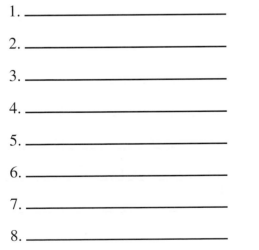

1. _____

2. _____

3. _____

4. _____

5. _____

6. _____

7. _____

8. _____

9. _____

10. _____

11. _____

12. _____

13. _____

14. _____

15. _____

Exercise 7-14: The Ear (text Fig. 7-25)

Instructions

1. Write the names of the three ear divisions on the appropriate lines (1–3).
2. Write the names of the labeled parts on the numbered lines in different colors. Use black for structures 12–14, because they will not be colored.
3. Color each part with the corresponding color (except for parts 12–14).

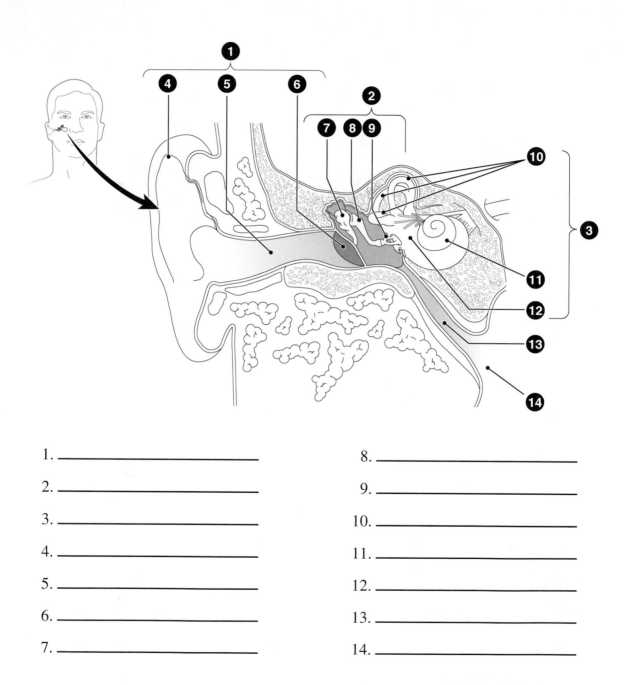

1. _____

2. _____

3. _____

4. _____

5. _____

6. _____

7. _____

8. _____

9. _____

10. _____

11. _____

12. _____

13. _____

14. _____

Exercise 7-15: The Inner Ear (text Fig. 7-27)

Label the indicated parts.

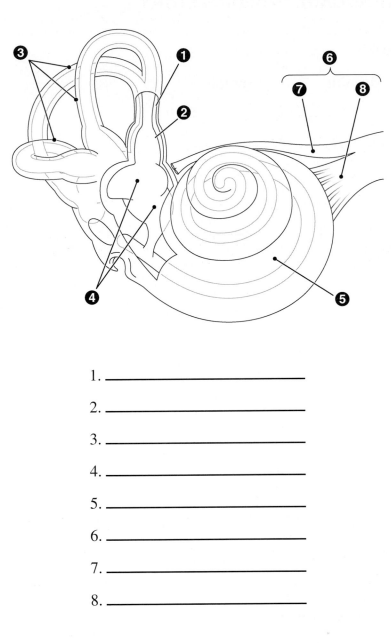

1. _____

2. _____

3. _____

4. _____

5. _____

6. _____

7. _____

8. _____

The Endocrine System

LEARNING THE LANGUAGE: WORD ANATOMY

Complete the following table by writing the correct word part or meaning in the space provided. For each word part, write a term that contains the word part.

Word Part	Meaning	Example
1. trop/o	——————	——————
2. ——————	cortex	——————
3. -poiesis	——————	——————
4. natri-	——————	——————
5. ——————	male	——————
6. ——————	milk	——————
7. ren/o	——————	——————
8. insul/o-	——————	——————
9. oxy	——————	——————
10. nephr/o	——————	——————

II. Labeling and Coloring Atlas

Exercise 7-16: The Endocrine Glands (text Fig. 7-29)

Instructions

1. Write the name of each labeled part on the numbered lines in different colors.
2. Color the different structures on the diagram with the corresponding color. Some structures are present in more than one location on the diagram. Try to color all of a particular structure in the appropriate color. For instance, color both adrenal glands, although only one is indicated by a leader line.

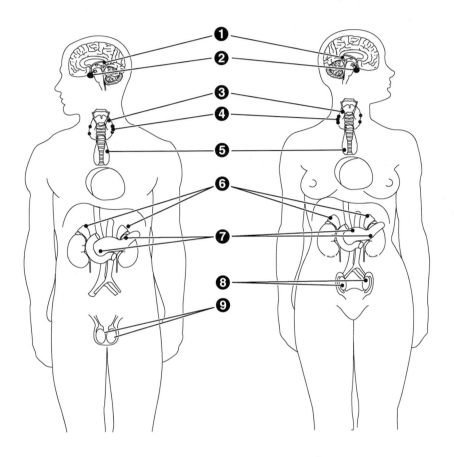

1. _____

2. _____

3. _____

4. _____

5. _____

6. _____

7. _____

8. _____

9. _____

Circulation and the Heart

LEARNING THE LANGUAGE: WORD ANATOMY

Complete the following table by writing the correct word part or meaning in the space provided. For each word part, write a term that contains the word part.

Word Part	Meaning	Example
1. _____	chest	_____
2. sin/o	_____	_____
3. cardi/o	_____	_____
4. _____	lung	_____
5. _____	slow	_____
6. _____	rapid	_____

II. Labeling and Coloring Atlas

Exercise 7-17: Layers of the Heart Wall and Pericardium (text Fig. 7-31)

Instructions

1. Write the terms "heart wall" and "serous pericardium" in the appropriate boxes.
2. Write the names of the different structures on the numbered lines in different colors. Use black for structure 6, because it will not be colored.
3. Color the structures on the diagram (except structure 6) with the appropriate colors.

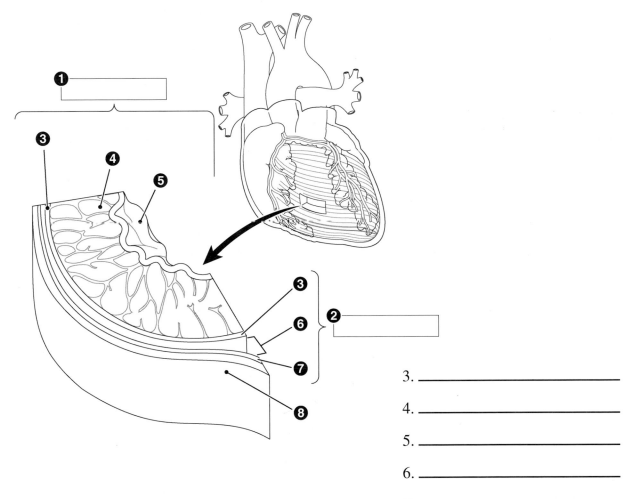

3. _____

4. _____

5. _____

6. _____

7. _____

8. _____

Exercise 7-18: The Heart Is a Double Pump (text Fig. 7-33)

Instructions

1. Label the indicated parts.
2. Color the oxygenated blood red and the deoxygenated blood blue.
3. Use arrows to show the direction of blood flow.

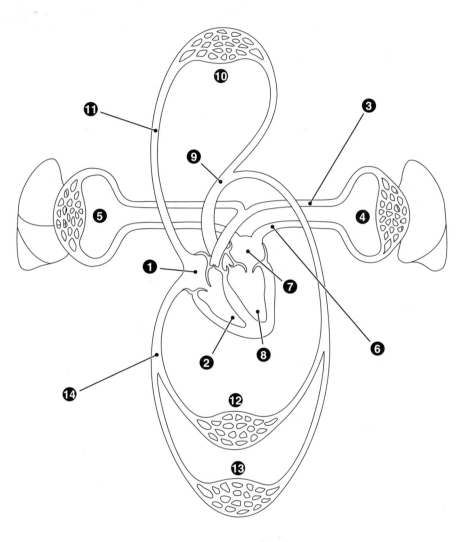

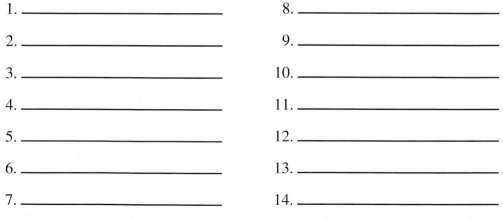

1. _____   8. _____

2. _____   9. _____

3. _____   10. _____

4. _____   11. _____

5. _____   12. _____

6. _____   13. _____

7. _____   14. _____

Exercise 7-19: The Heart and Great Vessels (text Fig. 7-34)

Instructions

1. Label the indicated parts.
2. Color the oxygenated blood red and the deoxygenated blood blue.
3. Use arrows to show the direction of blood flow.

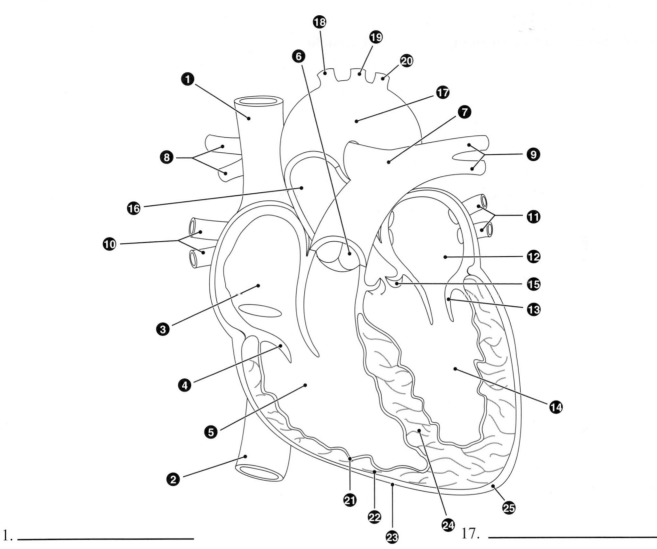

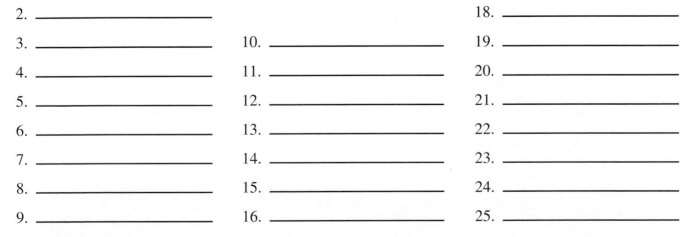

1. _____

2. _____

3. _____   10. _____   17. _____

4. _____   11. _____   18. _____

5. _____   12. _____   19. _____

6. _____   13. _____   20. _____

7. _____   14. _____   21. _____

8. _____   15. _____   22. _____

9. _____   16. _____   23. _____

                                                              24. _____

                                                              25. _____

The Lymphatic System and Lymphoid Tissue

LEARNING THE LANGUAGE: WORD ANATOMY

Complete the following table by writing the correct word part or meaning in the space provided. For each word part, write a term that contains the word part.

Word Part	Meaning	Example
1. _____	gland	_____
2. lingu/o	_____	_____
3. -oid	_____	_____

II. Labeling and Coloring Atlas

Exercise 7-20: Lymphatic System in Relation to the Cardiovascular System (text Fig. 7-35)

Instructions

1. Label the indicated parts.
2. Color the oxygenated blood red, the deoxygenated blood blue, and the lymph yellow.

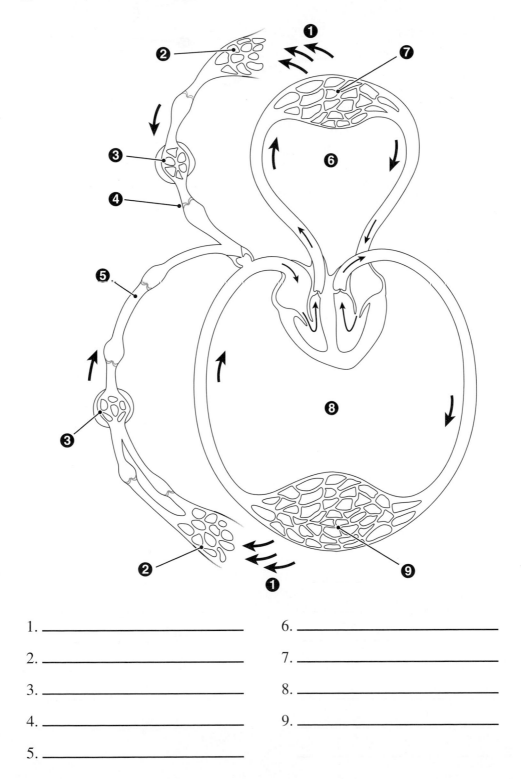

1. _____   6. _____

2. _____   7. _____

3. _____   8. _____

4. _____   9. _____

5. _____

Exercise 7-21: Lymphatic System (text Fig. 7-38)

Label the indicated parts.

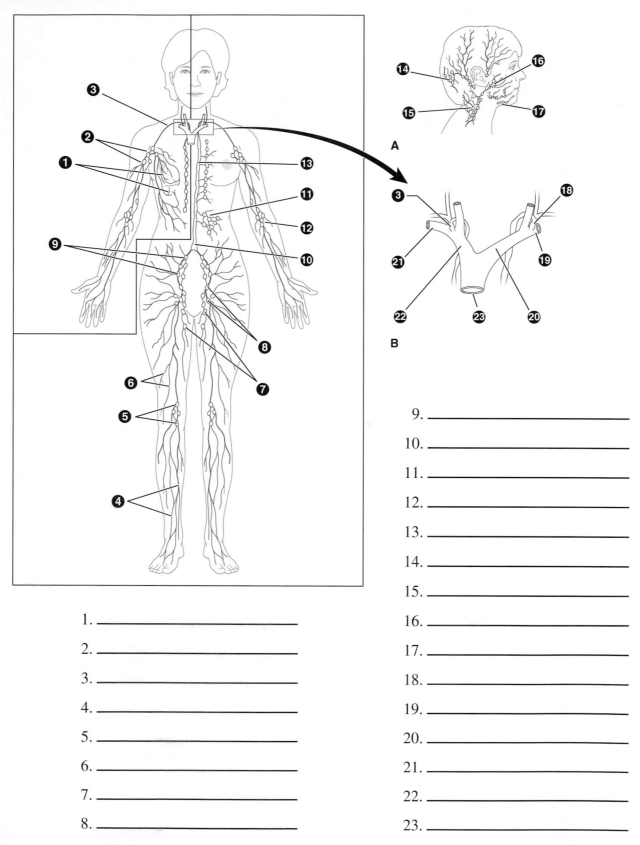

1. _____

2. _____

3. _____

4. _____

5. _____

6. _____

7. _____

8. _____

9. _____

10. _____

11. _____

12. _____

13. _____

14. _____

15. _____

16. _____

17. _____

18. _____

19. _____

20. _____

21. _____

22. _____

23. _____

Exercise 7-22: Lymph Node (text Fig. 7-39)

Label the indicated parts.

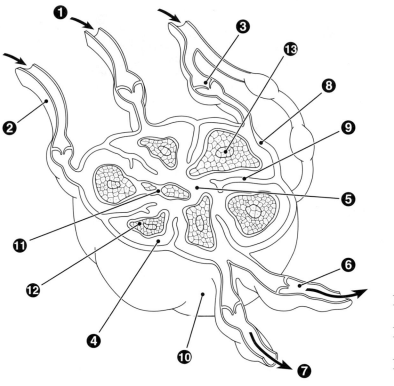
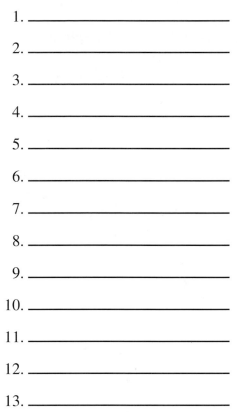

1. _____

2. _____

3. _____

4. _____

5. _____

6. _____

7. _____

8. _____

9. _____

10. _____

11. _____

12. _____

13. _____

The Respiratory System

LEARNING THE LANGUAGE: WORD ANATOMY

Word Part	Meaning	Example
1. spir/o-	_____	_____
2. _____	nose	_____
3. -pnea	_____	_____
4. _____	carbon dioxide	_____
5. _____	lung	_____
6. _____	air, gas	_____
7. orth/o-	_____	_____
8. or/o	_____	_____

II. Labeling and Coloring Atlas

Exercise 7-23: Respiratory System (text Fig. 7-41)

Instructions

1. Label the indicated parts.
2. Color all of the structures that encounter air green.
   Color structures containing oxygenated blood red.
   Color structures containing deoxygenated blood blue.

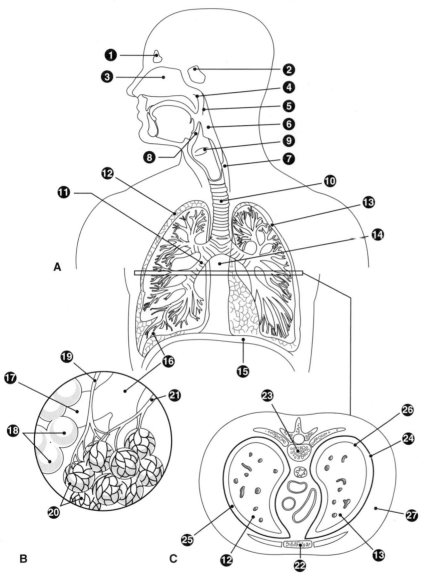

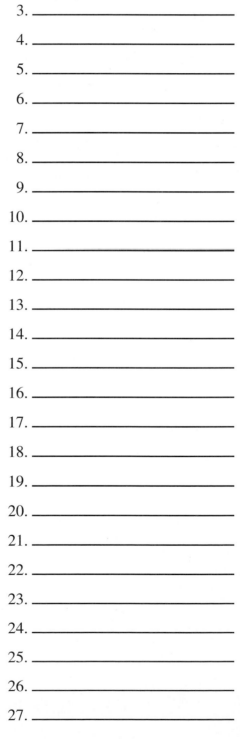

1. _____

2. _____

3. _____

4. _____

5. _____

6. _____

7. _____

8. _____

9. _____

10. _____

11. _____

12. _____

13. _____

14. _____

15. _____

16. _____

17. _____

18. _____

19. _____

20. _____

21. _____

22. _____

23. _____

24. _____

25. _____

26. _____

27. _____

Exercise 7-24: The Larynx (text Fig. 7-42)

Instructions

1. Write the name of each labeled part on the numbered lines in different colors.
2. Color the different parts on the diagram with the corresponding color.

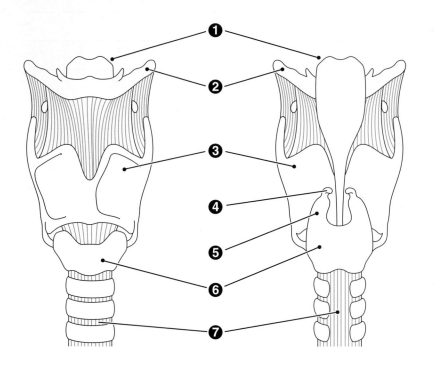

1. _____

2. _____

3. _____

4. _____

5. _____

6. _____

7. _____

The Digestive System

LEARNING THE LANGUAGE: WORD ANATOMY

Word Part	Meaning	Example
1. mes/o-	_____	_____
2. _____	intestine	_____
3. _____	stomach	_____
4. _____	away from	_____

II. Labeling and Coloring Atlas

Exercise 7-25: The Wall of the Small Intestine (text Fig. 7-46)

Instructions

1. Write the names of the intestinal layers and associated structures on the appropriate numbered lines in different colors. Use the same color for parts 6 and 7.
2. Color the layers and structures on the diagram with the appropriate color.

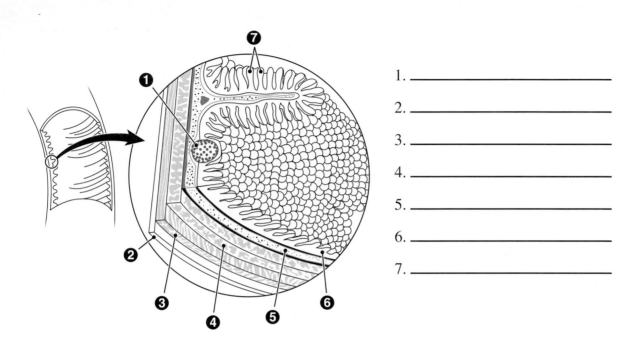

1. _____

2. _____

3. _____

4. _____

5. _____

6. _____

7. _____

Exercise 7-26: Abdominal Cavity Showing Peritoneum (text Fig. 7-48)

Instructions

1. Write the names of the abdominal organs on the appropriate numbered lines 1–9 in different colors. Use the same color for parts 3 and 4.
2. Color the organs on the diagram with the appropriate color.
3. Label the parts of the peritoneum (lines 10–14). Color the greater and lesser peritoneal cavities in contrasting colors.

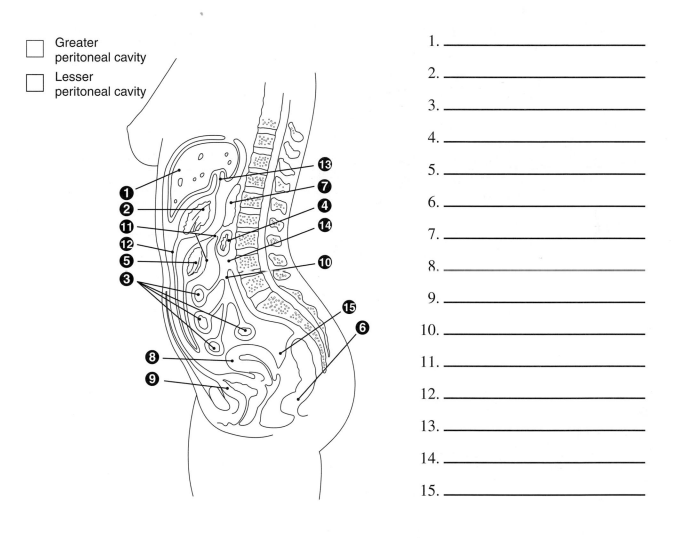

☐ Greater peritoneal cavity

☐ Lesser peritoneal cavity

1. _____

2. _____

3. _____

4. _____

5. _____

6. _____

7. _____

8. _____

9. _____

10. _____

11. _____

12. _____

13. _____

14. _____

15. _____

Exercise 7-27: Digestive System (text Fig. 7-49)

Instructions

1. Trace the path of food through the digestive tract by labeling parts 1–12. You can color all of these structures orange.
2. Write the names of the accessory organs and ducts on the appropriate lines in different colors. Use black for structure 20, because it will not be colored.
3. Color the accessory organs on the diagram with the appropriate colors.

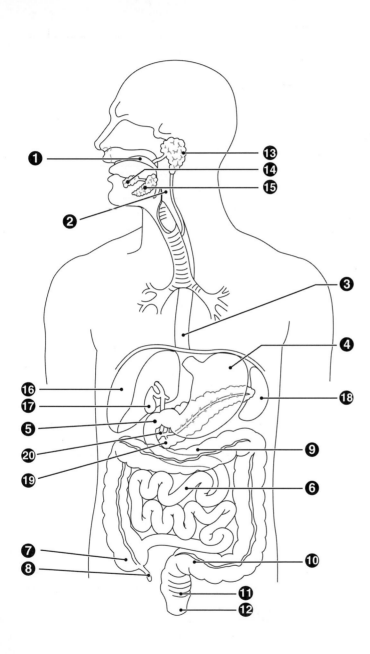

1. _____

2. _____

3. _____

4. _____

5. _____

6. _____

7. _____

8. _____

9. _____

10. _____

11. _____

12. _____

13. _____

14. _____

15. _____

16. _____

17. _____

18. _____

19. _____

20. _____

The Urinary System and Body Fluids

LEARNING THE LANGUAGE: WORD ANATOMY

Word Part	Meaning	Example
1. _____	night	_____
2. intra-	_____	_____
3. _____	partial, half	_____
4. osmo-	_____	_____
5. nephr/o-	_____	_____
6. _____	many	_____
7. _____	backward, behind	_____
8. _____	next to	_____
9. ren/o	_____	_____
10. extra-	_____	_____

II. Labeling and Coloring Atlas

Exercise 7-28: Male Urinary System (text Fig. 7-50)

Instructions

1. Write the names of the arteries on the appropriate numbered lines in red, and color the arteries (except for the small box) on the diagram.
2. Write the names of the veins on the appropriate numbered lines in blue, and color the veins (except for the small box) on the diagram.
3. Write the names of the remaining structures on the appropriate numbered lines in different colors, and color the structures on the diagram.
4. Put arrows in the small boxes to indicate the direction of blood/urine movement.

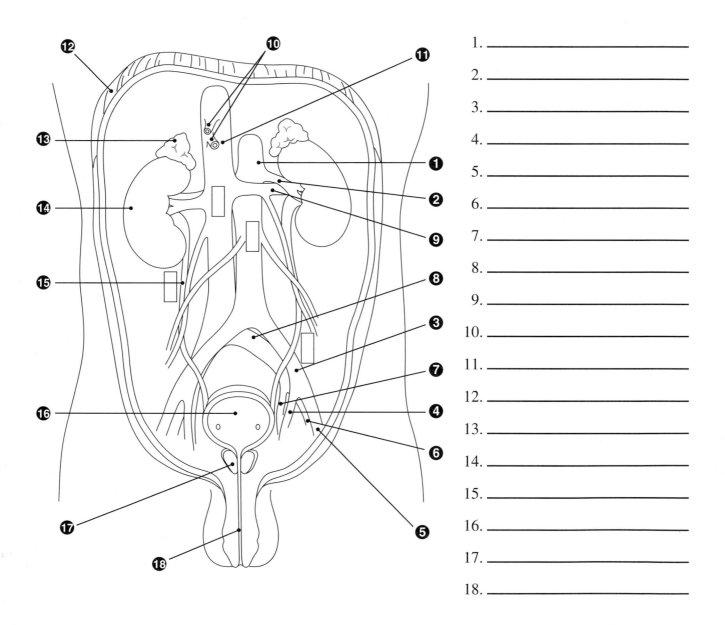

1. _____
2. _____
3. _____
4. _____
5. _____
6. _____
7. _____
8. _____
9. _____
10. _____
11. _____
12. _____
13. _____
14. _____
15. _____
16. _____
17. _____
18. _____

The Male and Female Reproductive Systems

LEARNING THE LANGUAGE: WORD ANATOMY

Word Part	Meaning	Example
1. _____	extreme end	_____
2. semin/o	_____	_____
3. _____	egg	_____
4. metr/o	_____	_____
5. fer	_____	_____
6. test/o	_____	_____
7. _____	around	_____
8. ovar, ovari/o	_____	_____

II. Labeling and Coloring Atlas

Exercise 7-29: Male Reproductive System (text Fig. 7-52)

Instructions

1. Write the names of the structures that are not part of the reproductive system on the appropriate lines 1 to 6 in different colors. Use the same color for structures 1 and 2 and for structures 4 and 5. Color the structures on the diagram.
2. Write the names of the parts of the male reproductive system on the appropriate lines 7 to 20 in different colors. Use the same color for structures 10 and 11. Color the structures on the diagram.

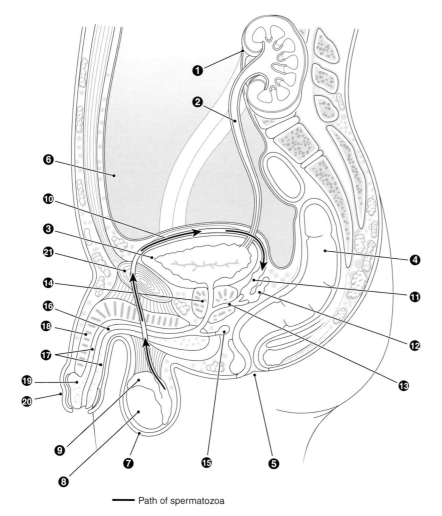

—— Path of spermatozoa

1. _____

2. _____

3. _____

4. _____

5. _____

6. _____

7. _____

8. _____

9. _____

10. _____

11. _____

12. _____

13. _____

14. _____

15. _____

16. _____

17. _____

18. _____

19. _____

20. _____

Exercise 7-30: Structure of the Testis (text Fig. 7-53)

Label the indicated parts. (Hint: the vein is more branched than the artery).

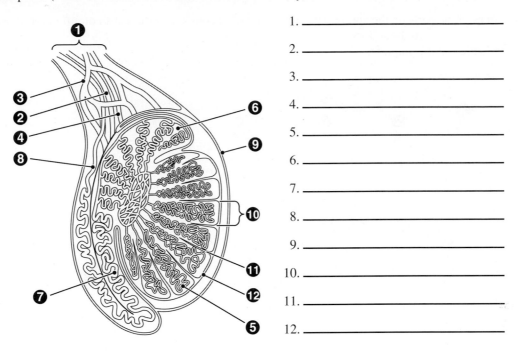

1. _____

2. _____

3. _____

4. _____

5. _____

6. _____

7. _____

8. _____

9. _____

10. _____

11. _____

12. _____

Exercise 7-31: Female Reproductive System (text Fig. 7-54)

Instructions

1. Write the names of the parts on the appropriate lines in different colors. Use the same color for parts 8 and 9, for parts 10, 11, and 13, and for parts 14 and 15.
2. Color the structures on the diagram.

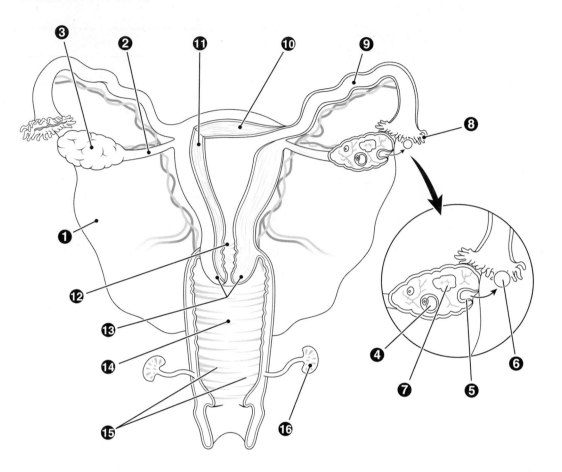

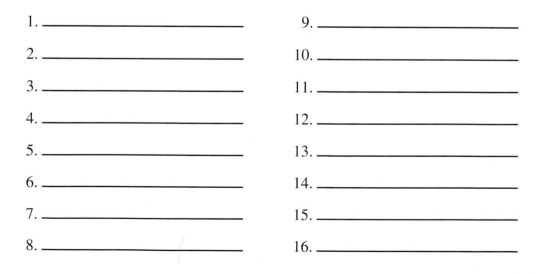

1. _____   9. _____

2. _____   10. _____

3. _____   11. _____

4. _____   12. _____

5. _____   13. _____

6. _____   14. _____

7. _____   15. _____

8. _____   16. _____

Exercise 7-32: Female Reproductive System (Sagittal Section) (text Fig. 7-56)

Instructions

1. Write the names of the structures that are not part of the reproductive system on the appropriate lines 1 to 8 in different colors. Use the same color for structures 1 and 2, for structures 3 and 4, and for structures 5 and 6. Color the structures on the diagram.
2. Write the names of the parts of the female reproductive system and supporting ligaments on the appropriate lines 9 to 19 in different colors. Use the same color for structures 15 and 16. Color the structures on the diagram.

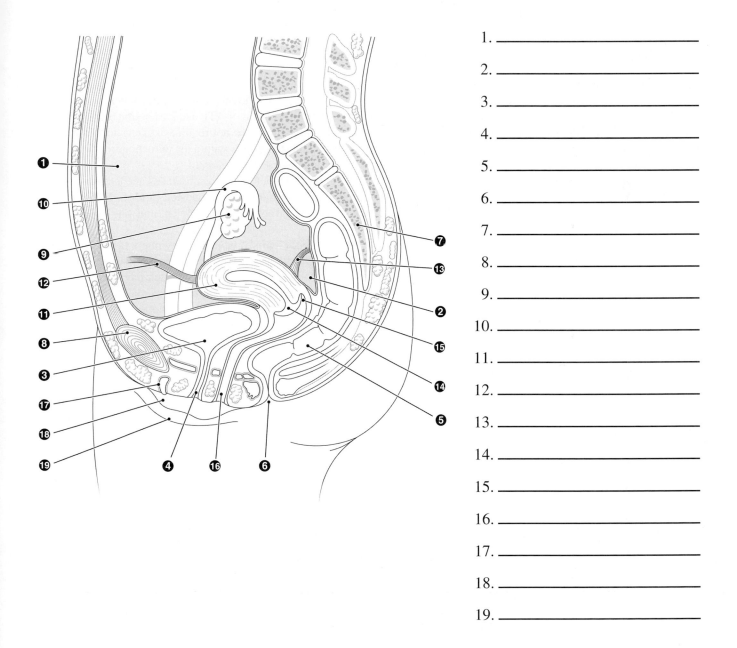

1. _____

2. _____

3. _____

4. _____

5. _____

6. _____

7. _____

8. _____

9. _____

10. _____

11. _____

12. _____

13. _____

14. _____

15. _____

16. _____

17. _____

18. _____

19. _____

8

Metabolism, Nutrition, and Body Temperature

OVERVIEW

The nutrients that reach the cells after digestion and absorption are used to maintain life. All the physical and chemical reactions that occur within the cells make up **metabolism**, which has two phases: a breakdown phase, or **catabolism**, and a building phase, or **anabolism**. Nutrients are oxidized to yield energy for the cells in the form of ATP using catabolic reactions. This process, termed **cellular respiration**, occurs in two steps: the first is **anaerobic** (does not require oxygen) and produces a small amount of energy; the second is **aerobic** (requires oxygen). This second step occurs within the mitochondria of the cells. It yields a large amount of the energy contained in the nutrient plus carbon dioxide and water.

By the various pathways of metabolism, the breakdown products of food can be built into substances needed by the body. The **essential** amino acids and fatty acids cannot be manufactured internally and must be ingested in food. **Minerals** and **vitamins** are also needed in the diet for health. A balanced diet includes carbohydrates, proteins, and fats consumed in amounts relative to individual activity levels.

The rate at which energy is released from nutrients is termed the **metabolic rate**. It is affected by many factors including age, size, sex, activity, and hormones. Some of the energy in nutrients is released in the form of heat. Heat production is greatly increased during periods of increased muscular or glandular activity. Most heat is lost through through the skin, but heat is also dissipated through exhaled air and eliminated waste products (urine and feces). The **hypothalamus** maintains body temperature at approximately 37°C (98.6°F) by altering blood flow through the surface blood vessels and the activity of sweat glands and muscles.

LEARNING THE LANGUAGE: WORD ANATOMY

Word Part	Meaning	Example
1. -lysis	_____	_____
2. _____	sugar, sweet	_____

ADDRESSING THE LEARNING OUTCOMES

I. Writing Exercise

The learning outcomes for Chapter 8 are listed below. These learning outcomes provide an overview of the major topics covered in this chapter. On a separate piece of paper, try to write out an answer to each learning outcome. All of the answers can be found in the pages of the textbook.

1. Differentiate between catabolism and anabolism.
2. Differentiate between the anaerobic and aerobic phases of cellular respiration and give the end products and the relative amount of energy released by each.
3. Define metabolic rate and name several factors that affect the metabolic rate.
4. Explain the roles of glucose and glycogen in metabolism.
5. Compare the energy contents of fats, proteins, and carbohydrates.
6. Define essential amino acid.
7. Explain the roles of minerals and vitamins in nutrition and give examples of each.
8. List the recommended percentages of carbohydrate, fat, and protein in the diet.
9. Distinguish between simple and complex carbohydrates, giving examples of each.
10. Compare saturated and unsaturated fats.
11. List some adverse effects of alcohol consumption.
12. Explain how heat is produced and lost in the body.
13. Describe the role of the hypothalamus in regulating body temperature.
14. Show how word parts are used to build words related to metabolism, nutrition, and body temperature.

MAKING THE CONNECTIONS

The following concept map deals with nutrition and metabolism. Each pair of terms is linked together by a connecting phrase into a sentence. The sentence should be read in the direction of the arrow. Complete the concept map by filling in the appropriate term or phrase. There is one right answer for each term (1–3, and 8). However, there are many correct answers for the connecting phrases. Write your phrases beside the appropriate number (if space permits) or on a separate piece of paper.

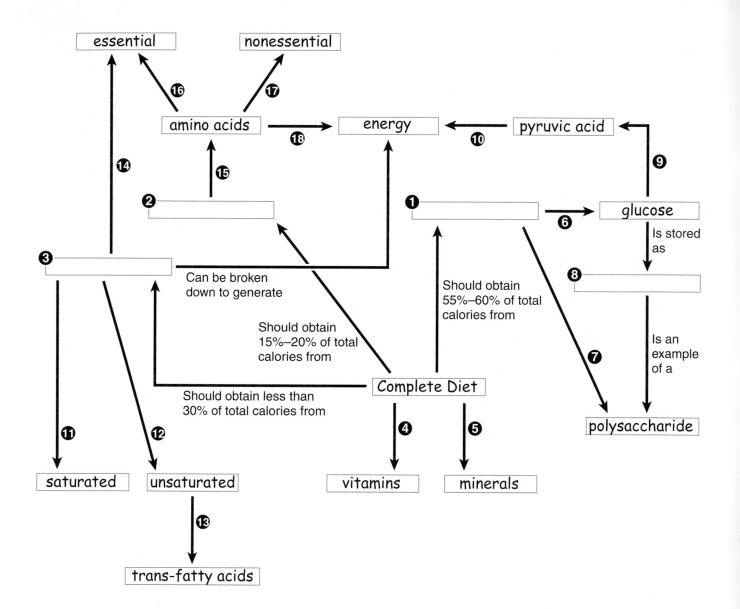

Optional Exercise: Make your own concept map based on the regulation of body temperature. Choose your own terms to incorporate into your map, or use the following list: body temperature, hypothalamus, sweating, shivering, dilation, constriction, skin, respiratory system, radiation, convection, conduction, evaporation.

9

Development and Birth

OVERVIEW

Pregnancy begins with fertilization of an ovum by a spermatozoon to form a **zygote**. Over the next 38 weeks of **gestation**, the offspring develops first as an **embryo** and then as a **fetus**. During this period, it is nourished and maintained by the **placenta,** formed from tissues of both the mother and the embryo. The placenta secretes a number of hormones, including progesterone, estrogen, human chorionic gonadotropin, human placental lactogen, and relaxin. These hormones induce changes in the uterus and breasts to support the pregnancy and prepare for parturition and lactation.

Childbirth or **parturition** occurs in four stages, beginning with contractions of the uterus and dilation of the cervix. Subsequent stages include delivery of the infant, delivery of the afterbirth, and control of bleeding. Milk production, or **lactation**, is stimulated by the hormones prolactin and oxytocin. Removal of milk from the breasts is the stimulus for continued production.

The scientific study of heredity has advanced with amazing speed in the past 50 years. Nevertheless, many mysteries remain. Gregor Mendel was the first person known to have performed formal experiments in genetics. He identified independent units of heredity, which he called factors and which we now call **genes**.

The chromosomes in the nucleus of each cell are composed of a complex molecule, **DNA**. This material makes up the many thousands of genes that determine a person's traits and are passed on to offspring at the time of fertilization. Genes direct the formation of **enzymes**, which, in turn, make possible all the chemical reactions of metabolism. Defective genes, produced by **mutation**, may disrupt normal enzyme activity and result in hereditary disorders. Some human traits are determined by a single pair of genes (one gene from each parent), but most are controlled by multiple pairs of genes acting together.

Genes may be classified as **dominant** or **recessive**. If one parent contributes a dominant gene, then any offspring who receives that gene will show the trait (e.g., Huntington disease). Traits carried by recessive genes may remain hidden for generations and be revealed only if they are contributed by both parents (e.g., albinism, cystic fibrosis, PKU, and sickle cell anemia).

LEARNING THE LANGUAGE: WORD ANATOMY

Word Part	Meaning	Example
1. _____	color	_____
2. zyg/o	_____	_____
3. _____	labor	_____
4. ox/y	_____	_____
5. chori/o	_____	_____
6. _____	body	_____
7. phen/o	_____	_____

8. _____   self   _____

9. _____   other, different   _____

10. homo-   _____   _____

ADDRESSING THE LEARNING OUTCOMES

I. Writing Exercise

The learning outcomes for Chapter 9 are listed below. These learning outcomes provide an overview of the major topics covered in this chapter. On a separate piece of paper, try to write out an answer to each learning outcome. All of the answers can be found in the pages of the textbook.

1. Describe fertilization and the early development of the fertilized egg.
2. Describe the structure and function of the placenta.
3. Briefly describe changes that occur in the fetus and the mother during pregnancy.
4. Briefly describe the four stages of labor.
5. Compare fraternal and identical twins.
6. Cite the advantages of breast-feeding.
7. Briefly describe the mechanism of gene function.
8. Explain the difference between dominant and recessive genes.
9. Compare phenotype and genotype and give examples of each.
10. Describe what is meant by a carrier of a genetic trait.
11. Define meiosis and explain its function in reproduction.
12. Explain how sex is determined in humans.
13. Describe what is meant by the term *sex-linked* and list several sex-linked traits.
14. List several factors that may influence the expression of a gene.
15. Define mutation.
16. Show how word parts are used to build words related to development and heredity.

II. Labeling and Coloring Atlas

Exercise 9-1: Fetal Circulation (text Fig. 9-2)

Instructions

1. Label the parts of the fetal circulation and placenta. Hint: you can differentiate between the uterine arterioles and uterine venules by following the path of the vessels into the umbilical arteries and vein.
2. Color the boxes in the legend using the following color scheme. Color the oxygen-rich blood box red, the oxygen-poor blood box blue, and the mixed blood box purple.
3. As much as possible, color the blood vessels on the diagram with the appropriate color, based on the oxygen content of the blood.

1. _____

2. _____

3. _____

4. _____

5. _____

6. _____

7. _____

8. _____

9. _____

10. _____

☐ Oxygen-rich blood
☐ Oxygen-poor blood
☐ Mixed blood

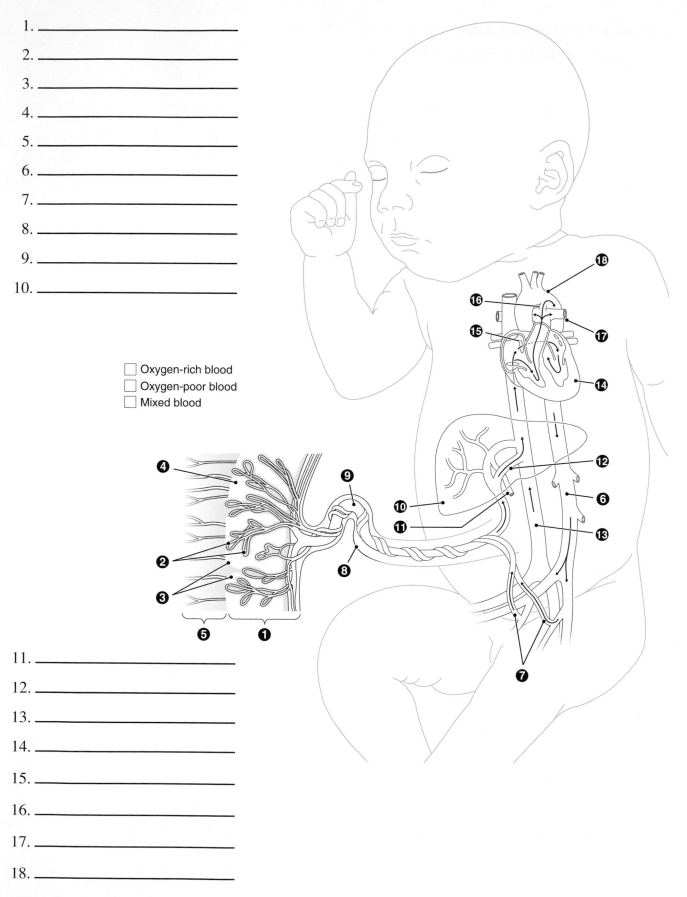

11. _____

12. _____

13. _____

14. _____

15. _____

16. _____

17. _____

18. _____

Exercise 9-2: Midsagittal Section of a Pregnant Uterus (text Fig. 9-5)

Write the name of each labeled part on the numbered lines.

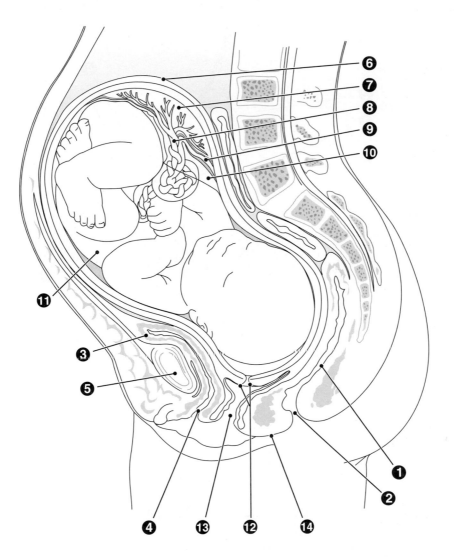

1. _____

2. _____

3. _____

4. _____

5. _____

6. _____

7. _____

8. _____

9. _____

10. _____

11. _____

12. _____

13. _____

14. _____

Exercise 9-3: Section of the Breast (text Fig. 9-7)

Write the name of each labeled part on the numbered lines.

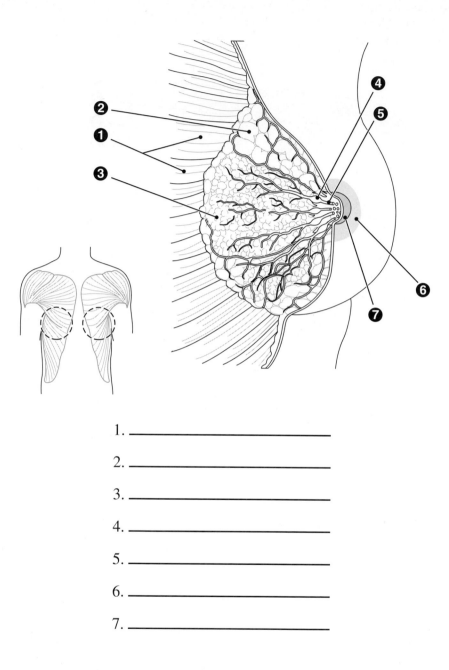

1. _____

2. _____

3. _____

4. _____

5. _____

6. _____

7. _____

MAKING THE CONNECTIONS

The following concept maps deal with different aspects of development (Map A) and heredity (Map B). Each pair of terms is linked together by a connecting phrase into a sentence. The sentence should be read in the direction of the arrow. Complete the concept map by filling in the appropriate term or phrase. There is one right answer for each term. However, there are many correct answers for the connecting phrases. Write each phrase beside the appropriate number (if space permits) or on a separate sheet of paper

MAP A

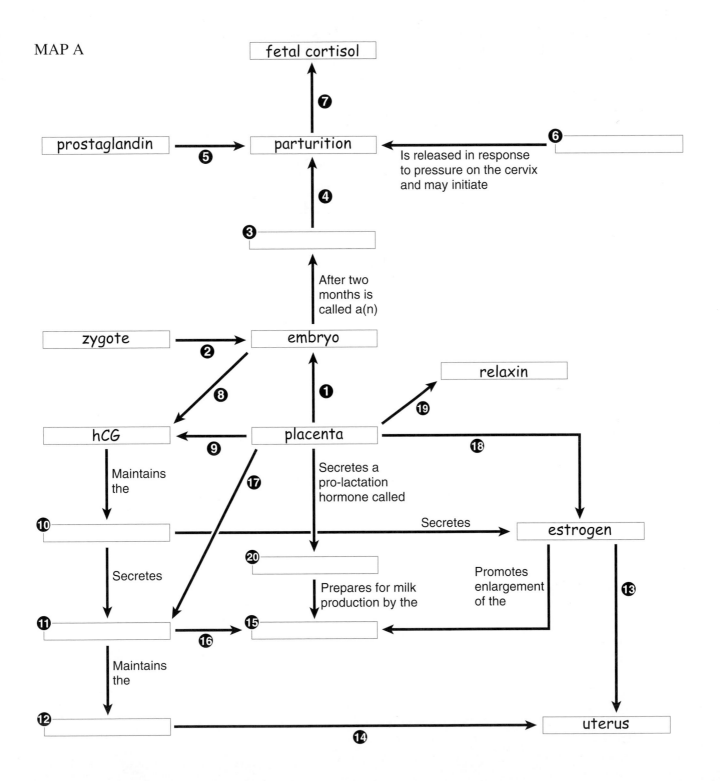

MAP B

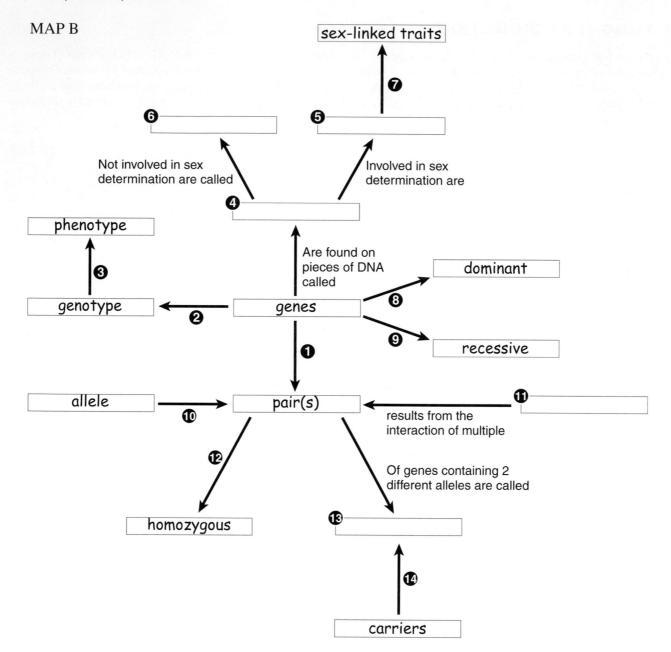

sex-linked traits

7

6 [_____]   **5** [_____]

Not involved in sex
determination are called

Involved in sex
determination are

4 [_____]

phenotype

Are found on
pieces of DNA
called

3

genotype   ←   **2**   genes   →   **8**   →   dominant

9   →   recessive

1

allele   →   **10**   →   pair(s)   ←   **11** [_____]

results from the
interaction of multiple

12

Of genes containing 2
different alleles are called

homozygous

13 [_____]

14

carriers

10

Personality and Development

Matching

Match the defense mechanism with the appropriate behavior.

a. Unhappy with her boss for his criticism, Clara turns around and takes her anger out on her husband.

b. David is unable to remember a boating accident in which his friend was killed.

c. After going to the movie the night before an exam, Molly states that she failed the exam because she did not study the right chapter.

d. An adolescent wants his mother to stay with him during a hospital stay.

e. Confined to a wheelchair, Jack becomes a computer specialist.

f. A young man who secretly desires to harm his wife appears on a television show against spousal abuse.

g. When Martha is confronted about her alcohol problem, she states she can quit anytime she chooses.

h. After taking funds out of their savings account to buy golf clubs, Hank tells his wife that the bank must have made a mistake.

1. _____ Rationalization

2. _____ Denial

3. _____ Repression

4. _____ Regression

5. _____ Projection

6. _____ Displacement

7. _____ Reaction-formation

8. _____ Sublimation

Multiple Choice

Select the best answer from the multiple-choice items.

1. A 70-year-old client states to the nurse, "My life is a shambles with nothing to show for it." The client is demonstrating what Erikson would term:

   a. Doubt
   b. Inferiority
   c. Despair
   d. Stagnation

2. A 4-year-old boy tells the nurse, "When I grow up I am going to marry Mommy." Which stage of psychosexual development is portrayed by this statement?

   a. Phallic
   b. Anal

   c. Latency
   d. Genital

3. According to Piaget, children who seek to control their world from a concentrated point of view would be in which stage of cognitive development?

   a. Sensorimotor
   b. Preoperational
   c. Concrete
   d. Formal operations

4. To avoid hurting his friend, John refrains from telling the truth to a friend whose partner is having an affair

with a co-worker. According to Kohlberg, this demonstrates which level of moral development?

a. Preconventional — stage 2

b. Conventional — stage 3

c. Postconventional — stage 5

5. Al has been arrested for physical assault. He has a history of previous aggressive offenses. Behavioral theory would explain this behavior as:

a. Feelings of repressed hostility

b. A diminished sense of self-esteem

c. An innate impulsive drive for survival

d. Reinforcement of early learning experiences

6. Surveys show that cigarette smoking and alcohol consumption are common among the adolescent population. These results reflect peer behavior and provide support for which of the following theories?

a. Social learning theory

b. Conditioning theory

c. Psychosexual theory

d. Human needs theory

7. Sue feels that her experiences have led her to a belief that she is responsible for most of the things that happen to her. According to Bowen, Sue tends to have:

a. A strong superego

b. An internal locus of control

c. A strong pseudoself

d. Strong unconscious drives

11
Grief and Loss

Matching

Match the following stages of grief with the appropriate description.

a. Deep sense of loss with withdrawal from social interaction.

b. Adjustment period in which the reality of the loss is avoided.

c. Labile moods and attempts to make deals to postpone the loss.

d. Time of peaceful letting go and allowing life to move forward.

e. Feelings of bitterness, self-blame, guilt, and hostility.

1. __b__ Denial

2. __e__ Anger

3. __c__ Bargaining

4. __a__ Depression

5. __d__ Acceptance

Multiple Choice

1. Joan is scheduled for a radical mastectomy. As the nurse enters Joan's hospital room, the client says, "It would be easier if I just didn't wake up from the surgery." The best response for the nurse to make at this time is:

   a. "You are just afraid now. Everything will look different tomorrow."

   b. "You feel it would be easier to die than to face the loss of your breast?"

   c. "Some people feel the way you do, but this does not mean the end of your life."

   d. "Why do you think it would be easier to die than to wake up after surgery?"

2. Which of the following is Joan experiencing?

   a. Resolution

   b. Conventional grief

   c. Bargaining

   d. Anticipatory grief

3. Maria has been in a comatose state for the past 8 months as a result of an automobile accident. Although doctors have told her husband, Reuben, that there is no

brain function, Reuben insists that she is showing purposeful response. Which of the following stages of grief is Reuben experiencing?

   a. Bargaining

   b. Anger

   c. Denial

   d. Depression

4. Which of the following describes how 9-year-old Jeremy would most likely respond to the death of his grandfather?

   a. Feels death happened because he went skating with a friend instead of visiting his sick grandfather.

   b. Sees the loss as interfering with his ability to determine a sense of who he is.

   c. Believes that angels took his grandfather in a chariot and went riding into the sky.

   d. Would not understand the concept of permanent loss.

12

Fundamental Communication Skills

CHAPTER COMPETENCIES

Review the information in your text that supports the following course objectives.

Learning Objectives

1. Spell and define the key terms

2. List two major forms of communication

3. Explain how various components of communication can affect the meaning of verbal messages

4. Define active listening

5. List and describe the six interviewing techniques

6. Give an example of how cultural differences may affect communication

7. Discuss how to handle communication problems caused by language barriers

8. List two methods that you can use to promote communication among hearing-, sight-, and speech-impaired patients

9. List five actions that you can take to improve communication with a child

10. Discuss how to handle an angry or distressed patient

11. Discuss your role in communicating with a grieving patient or family member

12. Discuss the key elements of interdisciplinary communication

CHAPTER OUTLINE	NOTES
Basic Communication Flow	
Forms of Communication	
Verbal Communication	
Nonverbal Communication	
Active Listening	
Interview Techniques	
Reflecting	
Paraphrasing or Restatement	
Asking for Examples or Clarification	
Asking Open-Ended Questions	
Summarizing	
Allowing Silences	

CHAPTER OUTLINE	NOTES
Factors Affecting Communication	
Cultural Differences	
Stereotyping and Biased Opinions	
Language Barriers	
Special Communication Challenges	
Hearing-Impaired Patients	
Sight-Impaired Patients	
Speech Impairments	
Mental Health Illnesses	
Angry or Distressed Patients	
Children	
Communicating With a Grieving Patient or Family Member	
Establishing Positive Patient Relationships	
Proper Form of Address	
Professional Distance	
Teaching Patients	
Professional Communication	
Communicating with Peers	
Communicating with Physicians	
Communicating with Other Facilities	

LEARNING SELF-ASSESSMENT EXERCISES

Key Terms

Define the following key terms:

anacusis _____

bias _____

clarification _____

cultures _____

demeanor _____

discrimination _____

dysphasia _____

dysphonia _____

feedback _____

grief _____

messages _____

mourning _____

nonlanguage _____

paralanguage _____

paraphrasing _____

presbyacusis _____

reflecting _____

stereotyping _____

summarizing _____

therapeutic _____

Matching

Match the definition in part 1 with the correct term in part 2.

PART 1

_____ 1. Facial expressions, gestures

_____ 2. Physical space tolerated by humans

_____ 3. Laughing, sobbing, sighing

_____ 4. Voice quality, pitch, tone

_____ 5. Verification of understanding

_____ 6. Organization of complex information

_____ 7. Restatement of exactly what patient says

PART 2

a. Paraphrasing

b. Kinesics

c. Summarization

d. Proxemics

e. Paralanguage

f. Nonlanguage

g. Reflection

Multiple Choice

1. The more accurate reflection of a person's true feelings and attitudes are demonstrated in
   a. Verbal communication
   b. Nonverbal communication
   c. Written communication
   d. All of the above

2. The limit of personal space is generally considered to be a
   a. 5-foot radius
   b. 10-foot radius
   c. 3-foot radius
   d. 1-foot radius

3. "It sounds as if . . ." is an example of which type of interviewing technique?
   a. Reflection
   b. Restatement
   c. Paraphrasing
   d. Paralanguage

4. "You were saying . . ." is an example of which type of interviewing technique?

   a. Reflection
   b. Restatement
   c. Paraphrasing
   d. Paralanguage

5. Periods of silence can
   a. Be beneficial
   b. Be natural parts of conversation
   c. Offer time for reflection
   d. All of the above

6. Factors leading to miscommunication are
   a. Language barriers
   b. Distractions
   c. Requests for feedback
   d. *a* and *b* only

7. An effective way of communicating with non–English speaking patients is
   a. Raising your voice
   b. Using commonly understood slang
   c. Speaking only to an interpreter
   d. Using simple phrases and speaking slowly

8. To communicate with patients who are hearing-impaired, you must
   a. Raise your voice pitch
   b. Raise your voice level
   c. Talk face to face
   d. None of the above

9. To facilitate communication with children, it is important to
   a. Use proper medical terms
   b. Use eye-level contact
   c. Avoid involving the parent
   d. Discourage play

Patient Education

1. Johnny is 5 years old and will be entering kindergarten in September. He is seeing Dr. Smith for his kindergarten physical. He will be receiving several immunizations. His mother tells him not to be afraid, as the shots will not hurt. She apologizes to the medical assistant when Johnny starts to cry. How can you teach Johnny's mother about his reactions?

_____

_____

_____

_____

13

Patient Education

CHAPTER COMPETENCIES

Review the information in your text that supports the following course objectives.

Learning Objectives

1. Spell and define the key terms

2. Explain the medical assistant's role in patient education

3. Define the five steps in the patient education process

4. Identify five conditions that are needed for patient education to occur

5. Explain Maslow's hierarchy of human needs

6. List five factors that may hinder patient education and at least two methods to compensate for each of these factors

7. Discuss five preventive medicine guidelines that you should teach your patients

8. Explain the kinds of information that should be included in patient teaching about medication therapy

9. Identify the components of a healthy diet and explain how to use a food guide pyramid

10. Explain the importance of teaching range-of-motion exercises to patients

11. Explain your role in teaching patients about alternative medicine therapies

12. List and explain relaxation techniques that you can teach patients to help with stress management

13. List three national organizations that can help patients with smoking cessation

14. Identify a national organization that can assist patients with treating alcoholism

15. Describe how to prepare a teaching plan

16. List potential sources of patient education materials

CHAPTER OUTLINE	NOTES
The Patient Education Process	
Assessment	
Planning	
Implementation	
Evaluation	
Documentation	
Conditions Needed for Patient Education	
Maslow's Hierarchy of Needs	
Environment	
Equipment	
Knowledge	
Resources	

CHAPTER OUTLINE	NOTES
Factors That Can Hinder Education	
Existing Illnesses	
Communication Barriers	
Age	
Educational Background	
Physical Impairments	
Other Factors	
Teaching Specific Health Care Topics	
Preventive Medicine	
Medications	
Nutrition	
The Food Guide Pyramid	
Dietary Guidelines	
Exercise	
Alternative Medicine	
Acupuncture	
Acupressure	
Hypnosis	
Yoga	
Herbal Supplements	
Stress Management	
Positive and Negative Stress	
Relaxation Techniques	
Smoking Cessation	
Substance Abuse	
Patient Teaching Plans	
Developing a Plan	
Selecting and Adapting Teaching Material	
Developing Your Own Material	

LEARNING SELF-ASSESSMENT EXERCISES

Key Terms

Define the following key terms:

alternative _____

assessment _____

carbohydrate _____

coping mechanisms _____

detoxification _____

documentation _____

evaluation _____

implementation _____

learning objectives _____

noncompliance _____

nutrition _____

placebo _____

planning _____

psychomotor _____

range-of-motion _____

stress _____

Multiple Choice

1. To educate patients effectively, a medical assistant must
   a. Involve patients
   b. Have a doctor's order
   c. Establish goals
   d. *a* and *c*

2. Teaching demonstrations can fail if they are
   a. Specific to the patient
   b. In a group setting
   c. Unrealistic
   d. None of the above

3. Evaluation of patient teaching
   a. Is not necessary
   b. Occurs only once
   c. Is an ongoing process
   d. Is done by the patient

4. A medical assistant who discovers that a patient is not compliant with goals of an educational plan should *first*
   a. Tell the physician
   b. Reevaluate the assessment

c. Check for understanding
d. Document in the chart

5. Documentation of patient teaching includes all of the following *except*
   a. Teaching aids
   b. Phone conversations
   c. Written information
   d. Laboratory values

6. The third step in patient education is
   a. Implementation
   b. Planning
   c. Evaluation
   d. Assessment

7. Which of the following must take place before learning can be achieved?
   a. Motivation of the patient
   b. Perception of need by the patient
   c. Educational plan
   d. *a* and *b*

Charting Documentation

1. With regard to the patient teaching scenario, give an example of a chart note that you might write following your patient teaching.

Date   **Time**

_____

_____

_____

_____

Matching

Match the definition in part 1 with the correct term in part 2.

PART 1

_____ 1. Most frequently abused drug

_____ 2. Impairs short-term memory

_____ 3. Reaches brain in 6 seconds

_____ 4. Stimulates central nervous system

_____ 5. Has same effect as cocaine

_____ 6. Causes physical and psychological dependence

_____ 7. LSD, PCP, mescaline, and peyote

PART 2

a. Nicotine

b. Alcohol

c. Hallucinogens

d. Cocaine and crack cocaine

e. Depressants and barbiturates

f. Marijuana and hashish

g. Stimulants and amphetamines

Skill Drills

1. Identify three factors to consider when designing a medication therapy teaching tool for a patient.

_____

_____

_____

2. List five main factors that play important roles in health.

_____

_____

_____

_____

3. Identify five components of a healthy diet.

_____

_____

_____

_____

_____

4. Identify and explain five relaxation techniques.

_____

_____

_____

_____

_____

_____

Multiple Choice

1. Nutrition is the study not only of what people eat but of
   a. How food is grown
   b. The effect of exercise on the body
   c. How the body uses food
   d. None of the above

2. In addition to identifying five food groups, the food pyramid
   a. Shows pictures of food
   b. Calculates caloric values
   c. Shows sample menus
   d. Shows maximum servings

3. Dietary guidelines are intended to improve our diet and
   a. Are government guidelines
   b. Include only items in the food pyramid
   c. Are the law
   d. None of the above

4. The role of the medical assistant with regard to physician-ordered diets is
   a. To assist in the selection of the diet
   b. To count the calories

   c. To provide patient information
   d. All of the above

5. Which factor should *not* be considered when sending patients home with a preprinted diet?
   a. Financial circumstances
   b. Religion
   c. Patient's age
   d. None of the above

6. An excellent source of information on exercise is
   a. The American Heart Association
   b. U.S. Exercise
   c. The American Red Cross Association
   d. The physician

7. Exercise can help relieve stress, maintain healthy body weight, and increase circulation and muscle tone if
   a. The heart rate exceeds 100 beats per minute
   b. It is done daily
   c. It is supervised by a physician
   d. None of the above

Critical Thinking Practice

Mrs. Greene, age 67, had a stroke 3 weeks ago and now has left hemiparesis. She is home from the hospital. Dr. Smith would like her husband to help her begin performing daily range-of-motion exercises.

1. Explain the purpose of range-of-motion exercises to Mr. Greene.

_____

_____

_____

_____

2. Describe range-of-motion exercises to Mr. and Mrs. Greene.

_____

_____

_____

_____

3. Describe the difference between positive and negative stress. Give an example of each.

_____

_____

_____

_____

4. Mr. Alexander is the president of a large manufacturing company. He is seeing Dr. Smith for frequent headaches. Dr. Smith has diagnosed the headaches as stress induced and has recommended that Mr. Alexander develop some coping mechanisms to reduce the stress in his life. As Mr. Alexander leaves the office, he questions the medical assistant about ways he can comply with Dr. Smith's recommendations. What strategies can you offer Mr. Alexander?

_____

_____

_____

_____

Patient Education

1. Mrs. Jones is taking four medications to control her hypertension and arthritis. She also takes an occasional antacid for indigestion. At a routine visit she tells the medical assistant that she is having difficulty taking all of the medication because she feels she is *always* taking pills and is not sure they are doing any good. How can you teach Mrs. Jones about her medication schedule? What critical factors should be considered before you begin a discussion with Mrs. Jones?

_____

_____

_____

_____

14
Medical Office Emergencies

CHAPTER COMPETENCIES

Review the information in your text that supports the following course objectives.

Learning Objectives

Upon successfully completing this chapter, you will be able to:

1. Spell and define the key terms.

2. Describe the role of the medical assistant in an emergency before the ambulance arrives.

3. Identify the five types of shock and the management of each.

4. Describe how burns are classified and managed.

5. Explain the management of allergic reactions.

6. Describe the management of poisoning and the role of the poison control center.

7. List the three types of hyperthermic emergencies and the treatment for each type.

8. Discuss the treatment of hypothermia.

9. Describe the role of the medical assistant in managing psychiatric emergencies.

CHAPTER OUTLINE	NOTES
Medical Office Emergency Procedures	
Emergency Action Plan	
Emergency Medical Kit	
The Emergency Medical Services System	
Patient Assessment	
Recognizing the Emergency	
The Primary Assessment	
The Secondary Assessment	
Types of Emergencies	
Shock	
Bleeding	
Burns	
Musculoskeletal Injuries	
Cardiovascular Emergencies	
Neurological Emergencies	
Allergic and Anaphylactic Reactions	
Poisoning	

CHAPTER OUTLINE	NOTES
Heat- and Cold-Related Emergencies	
Behavioral and Psychiatric Emergencies	

LEARNING SELF-ASSESSMENT EXERCISES

Key Terms

Define the following key terms:

allergen _____

anaphylactic shock _____

cardiogenic shock _____

contusion _____

ecchymosis _____

full-thickness burn _____

heat cramps _____

heat stroke _____

hematoma _____

hyperthermia _____

hypothermia _____

hypovolemic shock _____

infarction _____

ischemia _____

melena _____

neurogenic shock _____

partial-thickness burn _____

seizure _____

septic shock _____

shock _____

splint _____

superficial burn _____

Matching

Match the term in Part 1 with the correct definition in Part 2.

PART 1

_____ 1. Ischemia

_____ 2. Hypothermia

_____ 3. Shock

_____ 4. Hematoma

_____ 5. Full-thickness burn

_____ 6. Superficial burn

PART 2

a. A decrease in oxygen to tissues

b. Lack of oxygen to individual cells of the body

c. Burn that has destroyed all skin layers

d. Below-normal body temperature

e. A blood clot that forms at an injury site

f. A burn that is limited to the epidermal layer of the skin

Multiple Choice

1. Emergency medical care, when properly performed, can make a difference in several situations. Which statement is irrelevant to emergency medical attention.
   a. It can mean the difference between life and death.
   b. It can make the difference between rapid recovery and long hospitalization.
   c. It can make a difference between temporary or permanent disability.
   d. It can mean a difference between a good diagnosis and a misdiagnosis.

2. An emergency situation can occur anywhere and to anyone. What emergencies should medical personnel be prepared to handle in a medical clinic setting?
   a. Cardiac emergency, such as cardiac arrhythmia
   b. Respiratory emergency, such as anaphylaxis
   c. Hemorrhaging, such as miscarriage
   d. All of the above

3. An emergency medical kit should be kept in each medical facility. Which one of the following statements has little importance regarding emergency supplies?
   a. Contents of the kit should be checked regularly for completeness and outdates.
   b. Supplies are purchased on the basis of brand name.
   c. When supplies are used they should be promptly replaced.
   d. Supplies are based on the medical specialty of the facility.

4. Which of the following statements is not accurate?
   a. Guardians of minors must be contacted before any emergency treatment.
   b. Do not assume that the obvious injuries are the only ones present.
   c. Look for causes of the injury; they may provide clues to the extent of injury.
   d. Primary objectives are to identify and correct life-threatening problems.

5. Primary assessment of the patient includes responsiveness, airway, breathing, and circulation. What is the least likely reason for lack of responsiveness?
   a. Head trauma
   b. Electric shock
   c. Sleeping
   d. Cardiac arrest

6. An unconscious patient in a supine position may have partial or total airway obstruction. Why?
   a. Swallowed gum
   b. Air bubble swallowed while drinking water
   c. The tongue fell back into the oropharynx
   d. Small mouth and oversize tongue for the space

7. Checking circulation is an important part of patient assessment. What are some ways that circulation may be evaluated besides counting the pulse?
   a. Evaluate perfusion by checking the temperature and moisture of the skin.
   b. Observe the color of the skin and capillary filling in nail beds.
   c. Count the respirations.
   d. *a* and *b*

8. Following the primary and secondary assessment of a patient receiving emergency care, a physician does a head-to-toe physical examination. He or she will examine the arms and legs, looking for specific things. Identify the item that is least important during this examination.
   a. Moles with irregular margins
   b. Swelling
   c. Deformity
   d. Tenderness

9. The physician checks for sensation by
   a. using a safety pin or other tool to determine patient response to pain.
   b. having the patient squeeze each of the doctor's hands as hard as possible.
   c. using the tuning fork next to each of the patient's ears.
   d. having the patient push each foot against the doctor's hands as hard as possible.

10. Blunt object trauma to the body may cause injury. Some of these injuries are closed wounds. Which of the following are symptoms of closed wounds?
    a. Bleeding within a confined area or a contusion
    b. Swelling at the site
    c. A black-and-blue mark, called an ecchymosis
    d. All of the above

11. Anaphylaxis is a life-threatening allergic reaction. Which of the following is not a sign or symptom of an allergic reaction?
    a. Cough or wheeze
    b. Pale and/or moist skin
    c. Abdominal cramps
    d. Rash, hives, or wheals

12. Exposure to toxins in the home or workplace is increasing. When a parent arrives at the clinic with a child who has ingested a household chemical (i.e., chemical cleaner or medications), what steps will you take?
    a. Obtain the weight and age of the child.
    b. Ask the name of the substance and the approximate amount ingested.
    c. Obtain any previous history of chemical exposure.
    d. *a* and *b*

Matching Exercises

Matching only within each group, write the answers in the spaces provided.

➤ Group A

anatomy   tissue   organ   cell

system   physiology   chemical

1. The study of body function
   _____

2. A specialized group of cells
   _____

3. The basic unit of life
   _____

4. A combination of tissues that function together
   _____

5. The study of body structure
   _____

➤ Group B

posterior   anterior   medial

caudal   lateral   horizontal   distal

1. A term that indicates a location toward the front
   _____

2. A term that means farther from the origin of a part
   _____

3. A plane of division that also is described
   as a transverse or cross-section
   _____

4. A directional term that means away from the midline
   (toward the side)
   _____

5. A word that means nearer to the sacral (lowermost) region
   of the spinal cord
   _____

➤ Group C

hypochondriac   thoracic   sagittal   epigastric

frontal   transverse   hypogastric

1. A plane of division that is also called the coronal plane
   _____

2. A plane that divides the body into superior and inferior parts
   _____

3. Term describing the lateral regions of the abdomen
   just below the ribs
   _____

4. A term that describes the uppermost (chest) portion of the
   ventral body cavity
   _____

5. A plane that divides the body into left and right parts
   _____

6. The abdominal region below the umbilical region
   _____

➤ Group D

nervous sytem	integumentary system	cardiovascular system	urinary system
endocrine system	lymphatic system	digestive system	

1. The system that processes sensory information   _____

2. The system that delivers nutrients to body tissues   _____

3. The system that breaks down and absorbs food   _____

4. The system that includes the fingernails   _____

5. The system that includes the bladder   _____

Practical Applications

Study each discussion. Then write the appropriate word or phrase in the space provided.

➤ Group A: Directional Terms

1. The gallbladder is located just above the colon. The directional
   term that describes the position of the gallbladder with regard
   to the colon is   _____

2. The kidneys are closer to the sides of the body than is the stomach.
   The directional term that describes the kidneys with regard to the
   stomach is   _____

3. The entrance to the stomach is nearest the point of origin
   or beginning of the stomach, so this part is said to be   _____

4. The knee is located closer to the hip than is the ankle. The
   term that describes the position of the ankle with regard to the knee is   _____

5. The ears are closer to the back of the head than is the nose.
   The term that describes the position of the ears with regard
   to the nose is   _____

6. The stomach is below the esophagus; it may be described as   _____

7. The head of the pancreas is nearer the midsagittal plane than
   is its tail portion, so the head part is more   _____

➤ Group B: Body Cavities and the Metric System

Study the following cases and answer the questions based on the nine divisions of the abdomen and your knowledge of the metric system.

1. Mr. A bruised his ribs in a dirt buggy accident. He experienced
   tenderness in the upper left side of his abdomen. In which of the
   nine abdominal regions are the injured ribs located?   _____

2. Ms. D had a history of gallstones. The operation to
   remove these stones involved the upper right part of the
   abdominal cavity. Which abdominal division is this?   _____

3. After her operation, Ms. D was able to bring her stones home in
   a jar. She was told that her stones weighed 0.025 kilograms in total.
   How many milligrams do her stones weigh?   _____

4. Ms. C is 8 weeks pregnant. Her uterus is still confined to the most inferior division of the abdomen. This region is called the _____

5. Ms. C is experiencing heartburn as a result of her pregnancy. The discomfort is found just below the breastbone, in the _____

6. After the birth of her child, Ms. C opted for a tubal ligation. The doctor threaded a fiberoptic device through a small incision in her navel as part of the surgery. Ms. C will now have a very small incision in which portion of the abdomen? _____

7. Ms. C's incision was 2 millimeters in length. What is the length of her incision in centimeters? _____

➤ Group C: Body Systems

The triage nurse in the emergency room was showing a group of students how she assessed patients with disorders in different body systems. Study each situation, and answer the following questions based on your knowledge of the 11 body systems.

1. One person was describing dizziness and blurred vision. Vision is controlled by the _____

2. One person had been injured in a snowboarding accident, spraining his wrist joint. The wrist joint is part of the _____

3. A woman had attempted a particularly onerous yoga pose and felt a sharp pain in her left thigh. Now she is limping. The nurse suspected a tear to structures belonging to the _____

4. An extremely tall individual entered the clinic, reporting a headache. The nurse suspected that he had excess production of a particular hormone. The specialized glands that synthesize hormones comprise the _____

5. A middle-aged woman was brought in with loss of ability to move the right side of her body. The nurse felt that a blood clot in a blood vessel of the brain was producing the symptoms. Blood vessels are part of the _____

6. A man reporting pain in the abdomen and vomiting blood was brought in by his family. A problem was suspected in the system responsible for taking in food and converting it to usable products. This system is the _____

7. Each client was assessed for changes in the color of the outer covering of the body. The outer covering is called the skin, which is part of the _____

8. A young woman was experiencing pain in her pelvic region. The doctor suspected a problem with her ovaries. The ovaries are part of the _____

9. An older man was experiencing difficulty with urination. The production of urine is the function of the _____

Name_____   Instructor _____

Matching Exercises

Matching only within each group, write the answers in the spaces provided.

➤ Group A

tissue   **membrane**   **adipose**   **squamous**

stratified   **transitional**   **columnar**

1. A group of cells similar in structure and function   _____

2. A term that describes flat, irregular epithelial cells   _____

4. A term that means *in layers*   _____

5. Any thin sheet of tissue that separates two or more structures   _____

6. Term that describes long and narrow epithelial cells   _____

➤ Group B

bone   **myocardium**   **voluntary muscle**   **axon**

neuron   **fat**   **smooth muscle**   **neuroglia**

1. The thigh muscle is an example of   _____

2. Tissue that forms when cartilage gradually becomes
   impregnated with calcium salts   _____

3. The thick, muscular layer of the heart wall   _____

4. Visceral muscle is also known as   _____

5. A cell that carries nerve impulses is called a(n)   _____

6. Nerve impulses are carried away from the cell body by the   _____

➤ Group C

mesothelium   **serous membrane**   **cutaneous membrane**   **parietal layer**

visceral layer   **synovial membrane**   **superficial fascia**   **deep fascia**

1. The sheet of tissue that underlies the skin   _____

2. A tough membrane composed entirely of connective
   tissue that serves to anchor and support an organ or
   to cover a muscle   _____

3. The pleurae are an example of this type of membrane   _____

4. The portion of a serous membrane attached to an organ   _____

5. The connective tissue membrane that lines joint cavities

        _____

6. A tissue found in serous membranes

        _____

7. The portion of a serous membrane attached to the body wall

        _____

➤ Group D

ligament	**tendon**	**collagen**	**chondrocyte**
capsule	**fibrocartilage**	**hyaline cartilage**	**elastic cartilage**

1. A cord of connective tissue that connects a muscle to a bone

        _____

2. A tough membranous connective tissue that encloses an organ

        _____

3. The cartilage found between the bones of the spine

        _____

4. A fiber found in most connective tissues

        _____

5. A cell that synthesizes cartilage

        _____

6. A strong, gristly cartilage that makes up the trachea

        _____

➤ Group E

exocrine	**endocrine**	**periosteum**	**peritoneum**
epithelium	**mucous membrane**	**perichondrium**	

1. A term that describes glands that secrete through ducts

        _____

2. A layer of fibrous connective tissue around a bone

        _____

3. A type of tissue found in membranes and glands

        _____

4. A term that describes glands that secrete into the blood

        _____

5. The membrane that covers cartilage

        _____

6. A membrane that lines spaces open to the outside of the body

        _____

Name_____   Instructor _____

Short Essays

1. Compare and contrast connective and epithelial tissue membranes, and give an example of each. List at least one similarity and one difference in your answer.

_____

_____

_____

2. Differentiate between epithelial tissue, connective tissue, and muscle in terms of the amount and composition of the extracellular matrix.

_____

_____

_____

Completion Exercise

Write the word or phrase that correctly completes each sentence.

1. The outer layer of the epidermis, which contains flat, keratin-filled cells, is called the

   _____

2. Fingerprints are created by extensions of the dermis into the epidermis. These extensions are called

   _____

3. The main pigment of the skin is

   _____

4. The light-colored, proximal end of a nail that overlies the thicker, growing region is the

   _____

5. The muscle attached to a hair follicle that produces a "goose bump" when it contracts is the

   _____

6. The subcutaneous layer is also called the hypodermis or the

   _____

7. The ceruminous glands and the ciliary glands are modified forms of

   _____

8. Hair and nails are composed mainly of a protein named

   _____

Practical Applications

➤ Group A

Mr. B has experienced a fall in a downhill mountain biking competition. You are a first-aid volunteer at the competition and are the first person to the scene of the accident. Study each discussion. Then write the appropriate word or phrase in the space provided.

1. Mr. B has light scratches on his cheek. The scratches are not bleeding, indicating that they have only penetrated the uppermost layer of the epidermis, known as the

   _____

2. A branch tore a long jagged wound in his right arm. The wound has penetrated into the tissue underneath the dermis, known as the superficial fascia or

   _____

3. The skin of Mr B's nose is very brown. The brown color reflects the presence of a pigment called

   _____

4. Mr. B has difficulties hearing your questions. You examine his ears, and discover that they are full of ear wax. Ear wax is synthesized by modified sweat glands called

   _____

5. You note that Mr B has a rather strong body odor. Body odor reflects the secretions of glands called

   _____

6. Mr B, like many young men, suffers from acne vulgaris. This skin disease, which is characterized by pimples and blackheads, involves infection of the oil-producing glands of the skin called the

   _____

Completion Exercise

Write the word or phrase that correctly completes each sentence.

1. Normally, muscles are in a partially contracted state, even
   when not in use. This state of mild constant tension is called   _____

2. Fibers that carry impulses toward the neuron cell body are
   called   _____

3. The fatty material that covers some axons is called   _____

4. The brain and spinal cord together are referred to as the   _____

5. A nerve cell is also called a(n)   _____

6. The four chambers within the brain where cerebrospinal
   fluid is produced are the   _____

7. The three layers of membranes that surround the brain and
   spinal cord are called the   _____

8. The clear liquid that helps to support and protect the brain
   and spinal cord is   _____

9. The glands that secrete ear wax are called   _____

Practical Applications

➤ Group A

Ms. M, aged 67, experienced a serious fall at a recent bowling tournament. As a physician assistant trainee,
you are responsible for her preliminary evaluation.

1. Her right forearm is bent at a peculiar angle. You suspect a
   fracture to the radius or to the   _____

2. An x-ray reveals a broken radius as well as a number of
   fractures in the wrist bones, which are also called the   _____

3. Ms. M also reports pain in the hip region. The hip joint
   consists of the femur and a deep socket called the   _____

4. An x-ray reveals a crack in the "sitting bone" that supports
   the weight of the trunk when sitting. This bone is called the   _____

5. The large number of fractures Ms. M sustained suggests that
   she has a bone disorder called osteoporosis. The physician
   prescribes a new medication designed to increase the
   activity of cells that synthesize new bone tissue.
   These cells are called   _____

Short Essays

1. List the events that occur in an action potential.

   _____

   _____

   _____

2. Describe the structures that protect the brain and spinal cord.

   _____

   _____

   _____

3. List some functions of the structures in the diencephalon.

   _____

   _____

   _____

Matching Exercises

Matching only within each group, write the answers in the spaces provided.

➤ Group A

conjunctiva	choroid	cone	cornea
optic disk	retina	rod	sclera

1. The vascular, pigmented middle tunic of the eyeball

   _____

2. A vision receptor that is sensitive to color

   _____

3. The part of the eye that light rays pass through first as they enter the eye

   _____

4. The membrane that lines the eyelids

   _____

5. Another name for the blind spot, the region where the optic nerve connects with the eye

   _____

6. The innermost coat of the eyeball, the nervous tissue layer that includes the receptors for the sense of vision

   _____

7. A vision receptor that functions well in dim light

   _____

➤ Group B

aqueous humor	vitreous body	lens	ciliary muscle
rhodopsin	pupil	fovea centralis	iris

1. The structure that alters the shape of the lens for accommodation

   _____

2. The watery fluid that fills much of the eyeball in front of the crystalline lens

   _____

3. The jelly-like material located behind the crystalline lens that maintains the spherical shape of the eyeball

   _____

4. A pigment needed for vision

   _____

5. The depressed area in the retina that is the point of clearest
   vision   _____

6. The central opening of the iris   _____

Matching Exercises

Matching only within each group, write the answers in the spaces provided.

➤ **Group A**

anabolism	**catabolism**	**glycolysis**	**lactic acid**	**pyruvic acid**
anaerobic	**aerobic**	**glycogen**	**deamination**	

1. A term that describes any reaction that does not require oxygen   _____

2. The metabolic breakdown of complex compounds   _____

3. The storage form of glucose   _____

4. The metabolic building of simple compounds into substances needed by cells   _____

5. A modification of amino acids that occurs before they can be oxidized for energy   _____

6. An organic product of glucose catabolism that can be completely oxidized within the mitochondria   _____

7. An organic substance produced when a muscle is generating energy in the absence of oxygen   _____

8. The first anaerobic phase of cellular respiration   _____

➤ **Group B**

trans-fatty acids	**unsaturated fats**	**essential amino acids**	**nonessential amino acids**
monosaccharides	**vitamins**	**minerals**	**antioxidants**
saturated fats	**polysaccharides**		

1. Fats that are usually of animal origin and are solid at room temperature   _____

2. Fats that are artificially saturated to prevent rancidity   _____

3. Complex organic molecules that are essential for metabolism   _____

4. Protein components that must be taken in as part of the diet   _____

5. Inorganic elements needed for proper nutrition   _____

6. Protein building blocks that can be manufactured by the body   _____

7. A class of substances that stabilizes free radicals   _____

8. Carbohydrates with a low glycemic effect   _____

➤ Group C

zinc	iodine	iron	potassium	calcium
folate	calciferol	riboflavin	vitamin A	vitamin K

1. The vitamin that prevents dry, scaly skin and night blindness   _____

2. The vitamin needed to prevent anemia, digestive disorders,and neural tube defects in the embryo   _____

3. Another name for vitamin D_3, the vitamin required for normal bone formation   _____

4. The mineral component of thyroid hormones   _____

5. A mineral important in blood clotting and muscle contraction   _____

6. The characteristic element in hemoglobin, the oxygen-carrying compound in the blood   _____

7. A mineral that promotes carbon dioxide transport and energy metabolism   _____

8. A vitamin involved in the synthesis of blood clotting factors that can be synthesized by colonic bacteria   _____

➤ Group D

evaporation	conduction	epinephrine	dilation	constriction
98	37	radiation		

1. A response in the superficial blood vessels that increases heat loss   _____

2. A normal body temperature measured by the Celsius scale   _____

3. The transfer of heat to the surrounding air   _____

4. The change that occurs in blood vessels of the skin if too much heat is being lost from the body   _____

5. Heat loss resulting from the conversion of a liquid, such as perspiration, to a vapor   _____

Practical Applications

Ms. S is researching penguin behavior at a remote location in Antarctica. She will be camping on the ice for 2 months. Study each discussion. Then write the appropriate word or phrase in the space provided.

1. Ms. S is spending her first night on the ice. She is careful to wear many layers of clothing to avoid a dangerous drop in body temperature. The extra clothing will reduce the direct transfer of heat from Ms S's body to the surrounding air by the process of _____

2. She is out for a moonlight walk to greet the penguins when she surprises an elephant seal stalking a penguin. Frightened, she sprints back to her tent. Her muscles are generating ATP by an oxygen-independent pathway. Each glucose molecule is generating a small number of ATP molecules or, to be exact, _____

3. The next morning, Ms. S has soreness in her leg muscles. She attributes the soreness to the accumulation of a byproduct of anaerobic metabolism called _____

4. This byproduct must be converted into another substance before it can be completely oxidized. This substance is called _____

5. After 2 weeks on the ice, Ms. S is out of fresh fruits and vegetables, and the penguins have stolen her multivitamin supplements. She has been reading accounts of early explorers with scurvy and fears she will experience the same fate. Scurvy is caused by a deficiency of _____

6. Ms. S's diet is now reduced to luncheon meat and crackers. The crackers are still tasty because they contain significant amounts of artificially hydrogenated fats, known as _____

7. She looks forward to eating her normal diet when she returns home, which is rich in fruits, vegetables, and complex carbohydrates, also known as _____

8. Ms. S hikes to a distant penguin colony on her final day on the ice. She is dressed very warmly, and the sun is very bright. After several hours of hiking, Ms. S is sweating profusely, so she removes some clothing to cool off. Some excess heat will be lost through the evaporation of sweat. The wind will also increase heat loss by the process called _____

Completion Exercise

Write the word or phrase that correctly completes each sentence.

1. A surgical cut and repair of the perineum to prevent tearing is called a(n) _____

2. By the end of the first month of embryonic life, the beginnings of the extremities may be seen. These are four small swellings called _____

3. The mammary glands of the female provide nourishment for the newborn through the secretion of milk; this is a process called _____

4. The stage of labor during which the afterbirth is expelled from the uterus is called the _____

5. Twins that develop from the same fertilized egg are called _____

6. The normal site of fertilization is the _____

7. The clear liquid that flows from the uterus when the mother's "water breaks" is technically called _____

8. The larger sex chromosome is called the _____

9. A change in a gene or chromosome is called a(n) _____

10. The number of autosomes in the human genome is _____

11. The process of cell division that halves the chromosome number is called _____

12. An agent that induces a change in chromosome structure is called a(n) _____

Practical Applications

Study each discussion. Then write the appropriate word or phrase in the space provided.

➤ **Group A**

1. Mr. and Ms. L had been trying to conceive for 2 years. Finally, Ms. L realized her period was late and purchased a pregnancy detection kit. These kits test for the presence of a hormone produced exclusively by embryonic tissues that helps maintain the corpus luteum. This hormone is called _____

2. The pregnancy test was positive. Based on the date of her last menstrual period, Ms. L was determined to be 6 weeks pregnant. The gestational age of Ms. L's new offspring at this time would be

_____

3 During a prenatal appointment 14 weeks later, Ms. L was able to see her future offspring using a technique for visualizing soft tissues without the use of x-rays. This technique is called

_____

4 Baby L was born at 39 weeks' gestation. Ms. L immediately began to breastfeed her infant. The first secretion from her breasts was not milk, but rather

_____

➤ Group B

1. Mr. and Ms. J have consulted a genetic counselor. Ms. J is 8 weeks pregnant, and cystic fibrosis runs in both of their families. Cystic fibrosis is a disease in which an individual may carry the disease gene but not have cystic fibrosis. A term to describe this type of trait is

_____

2. Mr. and Ms. J were screened for the presence of the cystic fibrosis gene. It was determined that both Mr. and Ms. J have the gene even though they do not have cystic fibrosis. For the cystic fibrosis trait, they are both considered to be

_____

3. Ms. J wanted to know if her baby would have cystic fibrosis. Amniocentesis revealed that the fetus carried one normal allele and one cystic fibrosis allele. The fact that the alleles are different means that they can be described as

_____

4. The analysis also revealed the presence of two XX chromosomes. The gender of the baby is therefore

_____

➤ Group C

1. Mr. and Ms. B have a child with three copies of chromosome 21. This abnormality, like any change in DNA, is known as a(n)

_____

2. Chromosome 21 is one of 22 pairs of chromosomes known as

_____

Name_____   Instructor _____

3. The remainder of the child's chromosomes are normal. The total number of chromosomes in the child's cells is

_____

4. The chromosome abnormality arose during the production of gametes. The form of cell division that occurs exclusively in germ cell precursors is called

_____

FILL IN THE BLANK

Fill in the blank with the correct answer.

1. Patterns of perceiving, relating to, and thinking about ourselves and the world around us define the concept of _____.

2. _____ describes the variances in character that influence the development of personality and interpersonal relationships.

3. The process by which we bring factors together to build mental schema or connections that lead to a cognitive balance is called _____.

4. According to Piaget, _____ is the ability to incorporate new ideas and experiences into our existing mental schema.

5. Once new experiences are encountered, the ability to alter the existing schema to incorporate this new information is referred to as _____.

6. The concept that all behavior is observable or learned in response to a stimulus from the environment is the basis for the theory of _____.

7. The theory of development that states that the reasons we give to justify our choices and the behavior that results from those choices determine the level of moral development was the work of _____.

8. B. F. Skinner theorized that the human personality is formed in response to a conditioned stimulus-response of reward and punishment called _____.

9. The degree to which we define the self in terms of values and beliefs is referred to as the _____ of _____.

10. The person whose behavior is based on internal convictions and principles is defined as a _____ self.

SEEK AND FIND

Find the incorrect information in the statements below.

1. The holistic view of human beings that serves as the foundation for the nursing model of comprehensive health care delivery is based on the theory of behaviorism, which views the developing person as a total person.

2. According to Freudian theory, the division of the personality that is most closely in touch with reality is the superego.

3. The theory of psychosexual development suggests that during the latency stage, the child is discovering pleasure in genital stimulation while struggling to accept a sexual identity.

4. According to Erikson, the child begins a period of increased self-confidence and striving to become more independent in the preschool years during the stage of initiative versus guilt.

5. The person who is unable to be open and committed to a giving and sharing relationship with another is said by Erikson to be stalled in the stage of identity versus role confusion.

FILL IN THE BLANK

Fill in the blank with the correct answer.

1. _____ is defined as the emotional process of coping with a loss.

2. Those who may be expecting a major loss in the near future will usually experience _____ grief.

3. The period of time involved in the process of adapting to loss is often referred to as _____.

4. _____ describes an actual or perceived change in a relationship between a person and a valued object or other person.

5. The 5-year-old child reacts to separation from a loved person or object with _____ thinking.

6. A lack of resolution to the grief process is referred to as _____.

SCENARIO: LOST AND ALONE

The clinic nurse is assessing Art, whose wife died 6 months ago. He describes himself as "lost, forgetful, and unable to concentrate." He also states, "I seem to cry at the most inconvenient moments, so I just stay to myself."
What feelings might be responsible for Art's symptoms?

_____

_____

How should the nurse respond to Art?

_____

_____

_____

What stage of the grief process is Art most likely experiencing?

_____

_____

What referrals may be appropriate for Art?

_____

_____

_____

Skill Drills

1. Explain what it means to listen actively.

_____

_____

_____

2. Identify and explain the five stages of grief.

_____

_____

_____

_____

3. List five ways to avoid breaching confidentiality in the medical office.

_____

_____

_____

_____

_____

4. Define professional distance and explain why it is important.

_____

_____

_____

_____

Critical Thinking Practice

1. Explain how various components of communication can affect the meaning of verbal messages.

_____

_____

_____

Mrs. Smith is a 78-year-old woman with a history of gallstones. She is seeing Dr. Jones for the first time. The medical assistant approaches Mrs. Smith in a friendly manner, saying, "All right, sweetie, it's your turn," and puts her arm around her to guide her to a room. After the interview, the medical assistant leaves the room and calls to the receptionist, telling her that the gallbladder has arrived and has been roomed.

2. Explain what message or messages may have been conveyed to Mrs. Smith by the medical assistant.

_____

_____

_____

_____

3. How could the approach been improved?

_____

_____

_____

_____

Mr. Rivera's wife died a year ago. Since that time, Mr. Rivera has stopped seeing friends and participating in social activities. He visits the cemetery several times a week. Mr. Rivera has an appointment with Dr. Lee to discuss his feelings of depression and sadness. He wonders if he will ever feel any differently.

4. Are Mr. Rivera's feelings normal? Explain your answer.

_____

_____

_____

_____

5. Identify the steps in the grieving process.

_____

_____

_____

_____

Skill Drills

1. List the five major steps in patient education.

_____

_____

_____

_____

_____

2. List five factors that may hinder patient learning.

_____

_____

_____

_____

_____

Critical Thinking Practice

1. Explain the difference between a learning goal and a learning objective. Give an example of each.

_____

_____

_____

_____

2. Explain Maslow's hierarchy of needs. Give an example of each.

_____

_____

_____

_____

3. Describe how a patient who according to Maslow has reached self-actualization would approach health care.

_____

_____

_____

Name_____   Instructor _____

Patient Education

1. Mr. Applebaum is a 68-year-old diabetic who must learn to give himself insulin injections. He is nervous and afraid that the medication will not control his blood sugar. Describe four factors the medical assistant should consider that would promote learning.

_____

_____

_____

_____

_____

_____

_____

_____

Skill Drills

1. Documentation is always important. In the event of a medical emergency, name at least seven things that need to be documented about the patient.

_____

_____

_____

_____

_____

_____

_____

2. To gain an accurate impression during the secondary assessment, what four areas are assessed? Give examples from each area.

_____

_____

_____

_____

Critical Thinking Practice

1. One of the clinic patients has had a seizure. The patient's sister phones your clinic to report the incident and to ask for advice. She reports that her brother, the patient, is now "awake, but very tired." What patient history information will you need to report the episode to the doctor?

_____

_____

_____

_____

_____

2. Mrs. Clay, one of the clinic patients, phones to report that her daughter and grandson are on their way to the clinic. Her grandson is allergic to bee stings. He was stung by a yellow jacket about 5 minutes ago. She estimates that they will arrive at the clinic within the next 5–10 minutes. What would you do to prepare for their arrival?

_____

_____

_____

_____

_____

_____

_____

Name_____   Instructor _____

Patient Education

1. One of your patients is planning a backpacking trip up one of the local mountain trails. He is going with a small group and wants to be prepared for emergencies. It is late October, and the patient asks you for advice about treating hypothermia. What will you say? What additional resources might you suggest?

_____

_____

_____

_____

SKILL

PROCEDURE 12-1: Recognizing and Responding to Verbal Communications

Equipment/Supplies: Paper, writing utensil

Standards: Given the needed equipment and a place to work the student will perform this skill with _____ % accuracy in a total of _____ minutes. *(Your instructor will tell you what the percentage and time limits will be before you begin.)*

Key: 4 = Satisfactory   0 = Unsatisfactory   NA = this step is not counted

Procedure Steps

	Self	Partner	Instructor
1. Identify possible communication barriers, and obtain resources to help overcome these barriers.	☐	☐	☐
2. Begin the interview by properly greeting and addressing the patient.	☐	☐	☐
3. Begin the conversation with an open-ended question.	☐	☐	☐
4. Ask for clarification or examples as needed.	☐	☐	☐
5. Allow time for thought formation (for yourself and the patient).	☐	☐	☐
6. Paraphrase what the patient is saying to help clarify their message.	☐	☐	☐
7. Watch for and identify any paralanguage and nonverbal cues that may indicate incongruence with the verbal message.	☐	☐	☐
8. Ask closed-ended questions to get specific information.	☐	☐	☐
9. Summarize the interview for the patient and ask if there is anything else you need to discuss.	☐	☐	☐
10. Terminate the interview once you have satisfactorily discussed all of the patient's concerns.	☐	☐	☐

Calculation

Total Possible Points: _____
Total Points Earned: _____   Multiplied by 100 = _____   Divided by Total Possible Points = _____%

Pass   Fail
☐   ☐

Comments:

Student signature_____ Date_____
Partner signature_____ Date_____
Instructor's signature_____ Date_____

Name_____   Instructor _____

PROCEDURE 12-2: Recognizing and Responding to Nonverbal Communications

Equipment/Supplies: Paper, writing utensil

Standards: Given the needed equipment and a place to work the student will perform this skill with _____ % accuracy in a total of _____ minutes. *(Your instructor will tell you what the percentage and time limits will be before you begin.)*

Key: 4 = Satisfactory   0 = Unsatisfactory   NA = this step is not counted

Procedure Steps

	Self	Partner	Instructor
1. Be aware of the nonverbal cues that you are conveying to the patient. Use your body language and facial expressions to show care and concern for the patient.	☐	☐	☐
2. Identify the nonverbal communication cues that the patient is conveying.	☐	☐	☐
3. Ask appropriate questions to help verify your assumption.	☐	☐	☐
4. If the nonverbal cues do not correspond with the verbal message, convey your concern to the physician.	☐	☐	☐

Calculation

Total Possible Points: _____
Total Points Earned: _____   Multiplied by 100 = _____   Divided by Total Possible Points = _____%

Pass   Fail
☐   ☐

Comments:

Student signature_____   Date_____
Partner signature_____   Date_____
Instructor's signature_____   Date_____

PROCEDURE 13-1: Identifying Community Resources

Equipment/Supplies: Paper, writing utensil, access to local community resource book, telephone book, or internet

Standards: Given the needed equipment and a place to work the student will perform this skill with _____ % accuracy in a total of _____ minutes. *(Your instructor will tell you what the percentage and time limits will be before you begin.)*

Key: 4 = Satisfactory   0 = Unsatisfactory   NA = this step is not counted

Procedure Steps

	Self	Partner	Instructor
1. Locate a support group for patients needing help with alcohol or drug abuse and determine the contact information, services provided, hours of operation, associated fees, location and frequency of meetings, and any other pertinent information.	☐	☐	☐
2. Locate a support group for cancer patients and determine the contact information, services provided, hours of operation, associated fees, location and frequency of meetings, and any other pertinent information.	☐	☐	☐
3. Locate a food delivery program for home-bound patients and determine the contact information, services provided, hours of operation, associated fees, location and frequency of meals, and any other pertinent information.	☐	☐	☐
4. Locate area homeless shelters and determine the contact information, location, services provided, hours of operation, associated fees, and any other pertinent information.	☐	☐	☐
5. Locate financial resources for patients who do not have insurance or have financial problems affecting their ability to get appropriate medical care and determine the contact information, location, services provided, hours of operation, and any other pertinent information.	☐	☐	☐

Calculation

Total Possible Points: _____
Total Points Earned: _____   Multiplied by 100 = _____   Divided by Total Possible Points = _____%

Pass   Fail   Comments:
☐   ☐

Student signature_____ Date_____
Partner signature_____ Date_____
Instructor's signature_____ Date_____